Health Informatics

This series is directed to healthcare professionals leading the transformation of healthcare by using information and knowledge. For over 20 years, Health Informatics has offered a broad range of titles: some address specific professions such as nursing, medicine, and health administration; others cover special areas of practice such as trauma and radiology; still other books in the series focus on interdisciplinary issues, such as the computer based patient record, electronic health records, and networked healthcare systems. Editors and authors, eminent experts in their fields, offer their accounts of innovations in health informatics. Increasingly, these accounts go beyond hardware and software to address the role of information in influencing the transformation of healthcare delivery systems around the world. The series also increasingly focuses on the users of the information and systems: the organizational, behavioral, and societal changes that accompany the diffusion of information technology in health services environments.

Developments in healthcare delivery are constant; in recent years, bioinformatics has emerged as a new field in health informatics to support emerging and ongoing developments in molecular biology. At the same time, further evolution of the field of health informatics is reflected in the introduction of concepts at the macro or health systems delivery level with major national initiatives related to electronic health records (EHR), data standards, and public health informatics.

These changes will continue to shape health services in the twenty-first century. By making full and creative use of the technology to tame data and to transform information, Health Informatics will foster the development and use of new knowledge in healthcare.

More information about this series at http://www.springer.com/series/1114

Terrence Adam • Constantin Aliferis

Editors

Personalized and Precision Medicine Informatics

A Workflow-Based View

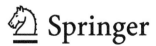 Springer

Editors
Terrence Adam
Pharmaceutical Care & Health Systems
University of Minnesota Pharmaceutical
Care & Health Systems
Minneapolis, MN
USA

Constantin Aliferis
Institute for Health Informatics
University of Minnesota
Minneapolis, MN
USA

ISSN 1431-1917   ISSN 2197-3741   (electronic)
Health Informatics
ISBN 978-3-030-18625-8   ISBN 978-3-030-18626-5   (eBook)
https://doi.org/10.1007/978-3-030-18626-5

This Springer imprint is published by the registered company Springer Nature Switzerland AG
The registered company address is: Gewerbestrasse 11, 6330 Cham, Switzerland

I dedicate this book to the memory of my sister Maria who inspired and motivated my career-long commitment to biomedical research.

Constantin Aliferis

I dedicate this book to my parents who have taught me the importance of wisdom and perseverance in approaching daily tasks and to my patients who constantly challenge me to improve our understanding and delivery of health care.

Terrence Adam

Acknowledgments

This book benefited tremendously by the extraordinary dedication, skill, and hard work of Jessica Tetzlaff. The editors are indebted to her for her contributions to the process of assembling, integrating, and copy-editing the material. We are also grateful to Jenna Lohnes for her very capable and efficient editorial administrative assistance in the last stages of the book editing and to Elizabeth Madson for excellent supervisory administrative support.

We gratefully acknowledge the following Springer-Nature staff for supporting this book: Grant Weston for being instrumental in getting the book proposal formulated and approved, and Vignesh Iyyadurai Suresh and Ganesh Ekambaram who have been critical to the execution. Our goal to create an ambitious and comprehensive text on precision medicine informatics entailed an expanded time horizon to completion, and we are grateful to the publisher for accommodating this timeline.

Last but not least, the editors are deeply grateful to all contributing authors of this volume, who generously shared in this book their remarkable knowledge across the full spectrum of personalized and precision medicine informatics.

Contents

Contributors

Terrence Adam, RPh, MD, PhD Department of Pharmaceutical Care and Health Systems, College of Pharmacy, University of Minnesota, Minneapolis, MN, USA

Institute for Health Informatics, University of Minnesota, Minneapolis, MN, USA

PhD Program in Precision Medicine Informatics, University of Minnesota, Minneapolis, MN, USA

Minneapolis Veterans Administration, Minneapolis, MN, USA

Constantin Aliferis, MD, PhD Institute for Health Informatics, Department of Medicine, School of Medicine Clinical and Translational Science Institute, Masonic Cancer Center, Program in Data Science, University of Minnesota, Minneapolis, MN, USA

Yingtao Bi, PhD Division of Health and Biomedical Informatics, Department of Preventive Medicine, Feinberg School of Medicine, Northwestern University, Evanston, IL, USA

Matthew K. Breitenstein, PhD Department of Biostatistics, Epidemiology, and Informatics, Perelman School of Medicine, University of Pennsylvania, Philadelphia, PA, USA

Donald Casey, MD, MPH, MBA IPO 4 Health, Chicago, IL, USA

Gregory F. Cooper, MD, PhD Department of Biomedical Informatics and of Intelligent Systems, University of Pittsburgh, Pittsburgh, PA, USA

Deanna Cross, PhD Department of Microbiology, Immunology, and Genetics, Health Science Center, University of North Texas, Denton, TX, USA

Erin L. Crowgey, PhD Department of Bioinformatics, Nemours Biomedical Research, Wilmington, DE, USA

Ramana V. Davuluri, PhD Division of Health and Biomedical Informatics, Department of Preventive Medicine, Feinberg School of Medicine, Northwestern University, Evanston, IL, USA

Timothy M. Herr, MS Division of Health and Biomedical Informatics, Department of Preventive Medicine, Feinberg School of Medicine, Northwestern University, Chicago, IL, USA

Pamala Jacobson, PharmD, FCCP Department of Experimental and Clinical Pharmacology, College of Pharmacy, University of Minnesota, Minneapolis, MN, USA

Division of Hematology, Oncology and Transplantation, Medical School, University of Minnesota, Minneapolis, MN, USA

Abdulrahman M. Jahhaf, MD Division of Health and Biomedical Informatics, Department of Preventive Medicine, Feinberg School of Medicine, Northwestern University, Chicago, IL, USA

Steven G. Johnson, PhD Division for Informatics Innovation Dissemination, University of Minnesota, Minneapolis, MN, USA

Institute for Health Informatics, University of Minnesota, Minneapolis, MN, USA

Michael W. Kattan, PhD The Mobasseri Endowed Chair for Innovations in Cancer Research, Department of Quantitative Health Sciences, Cleveland Clinic, Cleveland, OH, USA

Bruce Levy, MD, CPE Geisinger Commonwealth School of Medicine, Geisinger Health, Danville, PA, USA

Sisi Ma, PhD Institute for Health Informatics, Department of Medicine, School of Medicine Clinical and Translational Science Institute, Masonic Cancer Center, Program in Data Science, University of Minnesota, Minneapolis, MN, USA

Andrew J. McCarty, MS, LCGC Laboratory Services, Children's Hospital of Pittsburgh, University of Pittsburgh Medical Center, Pittsburgh, PA, USA

Catherine A. McCarty, MPH, PhD Department of Family Medicine and BioBehavioral Health, University of Minnesota Duluth, Duluth, MN, USA

Eneida Mendonca, MD, PhD Department of Biostatistics and Medical Informatics, School of Medicine and Public Health, Department of Industrial and Systems Engineering in the College of Engineering, Clinical/Health Informatics, UW Institute for Clinical and Translational Research, University of Wisconsin Madison, Madison, WI, USA

Michelle Morrow, PhD, LCGC Laboratory Services, Children's Hospital of Pittsburgh, University of Pittsburgh Medical Center, Pittsburgh, PA, USA

Christine Munro, MS, MPH, LCGC Children's Hospital of Pittsburgh, University of Pittsburgh Medical Center, Pittsburgh, PA, USA

Therese A. Nelson, AM, LSW Socio-Technical Innovation, Northwestern University Clinical and Translational Sciences, Northwestern University, Chicago, IL, USA

Eric Polley, PhD Division of Biomedical Statistics and Informatics, Department of Health Sciences Research, Mayo Clinic, Rochester, MN, USA

Luke V. Rasmussen, MS Division of Health and Biomedical Informatics, Department of Preventive Medicine, Feinberg School of Medicine, Northwestern University, Chicago, IL, USA

Jason Ross, MA OneOme, Minneapolis, MN, USA

Glenn N. Saxe, MD Department of Child and Adolescent Psychiatry, School of Medicine, New York University, New York, NY, USA

Richard Simon, DSc Computational and Systems Biology Branch, Biometric Research Program, Division of Cancer Treatment and Diagnosis, National Cancer Institute, Rockville, MD, USA

Kingshuk K. Sinha, PhD Department of Supply Chain and Operations, Carlson School of Management, University of Minnesota, Minneapolis, MN, USA

Bioinformatics and Computational Biology, University of Minnesota, Minneapolis, MN, USA

Justin B. Starren, MD, PhD Division of Health and Biomedical Informatics, Department of Preventive Medicine, Feinberg School of Medicine, Northwestern University, Chicago, IL, USA

Northwestern University Clinical and Translational Science Institute (NUCATS), Northwestern University, Chicago, IL, USA

Center for Data Science and Informatics (CDSI), Northwestern University, Chicago, IL, USA

Vigneshwar Subramanian Lerner College of Medicine, Cleveland Clinic, Cleveland, OH, USA

Umberto Tachinardi, MD, MS Department of Biostatistics and Medical Informatics, School of Medicine and Public Health, University of Wisconsin-Madison, Madison, WI, USA

UW Institute for Clinical and Translational Research, University of Wisconsin-Madison, Madison, WI, USA

UW Health, University of Wisconsin-Madison, Madison, WI, USA

Casey Overby Taylor, PhD Division of General Internal Medicine, School of Medicine, Johns Hopkins University, Baltimore, MD, USA

Division of Health Sciences Informatics, Johns Hopkins University, Baltimore, MD, USA

Shyam Visweswaran, MD, PhD Department of Biomedical Informatics and of Intelligent Systems, University of Pittsburgh, Pittsburgh, PA, USA

Jinhua Wang, MBA, PhD Institute for Health Informatics, University of Minnesota, Minneapolis, MN, USA

Cancer Bioinformatics, Masonic Cancer Center, University of Minnesota, Minneapolis, MN, USA

Marc S. Williams, MD Genomic Medicine Institute, Geisinger Health, Danville, PA, USA

Boris Winterhoff, MD, PhD Department of Obstetrics, Gynecology and Women's Health, Medical School, University of Minnesota, Minneapolis, MN, USA

Susan M. Wolf, JD Law School, University of Minnesota, Minneapolis, MN, USA

Department of Medicine, Medical School, University of Minnesota, Minneapolis, MN, USA

Consortium on Law and Values in Health, Environment and the Life Sciences, University of Minnesota, Minneapolis, MN, USA

Douglas Yee, MD Division of Hematology, Oncology and Transplantation, Medical School, University of Minnesota, Minneapolis, MN, USA

Masonic Cancer Center, University of Minnesota, Minneapolis, MN, USA

Department of Pharmacology, Medical School, University of Minnesota, Minneapolis, MN, USA

Microbiology, Immunology and Cancer Biology (MICaB) PhD Graduate Program, University of Minnesota, Minneapolis, MN, USA

Yingdong Zhao, PhD Computational and Systems Biology Branch, Biometric Research Program, Division of Cancer Treatment and Diagnosis, National Cancer Institute, Rockville, MD, USA

Computational and Systems Biology Branch, Biometric Research Program, Division of Cancer Treatment and Diagnosis, NCI, Bethesda, MD, USA

Part I
Introduction

Chapter 1
Birth of a Discipline: Personalized and Precision Medicine (PPM) Informatics

Terrence Adam and Constantin Aliferis

Introduction to PPM and Its Relationship with Informatics; Purpose of the Present Book

The terms "precision medicine", and "personalized medicine", used together in the present volume (Precision and Personalized Medicine, PPM for short) refer to the science, technology, and practice of medicine (and healthcare more broadly) such that preventative, diagnostic, and treatment decisions are tailored to the characteristics and needs of the individual [1, 2]. The delivery of the right drug to the right patient at the right time at the right dose and the right route encapsulates the widely-accepted core principles of PPM and patient safety [3, 4].

But how new is this field? The recent prominence and explosive growth of precision medicine is not a truly new conceptual development but rather reflects a

T. Adam (✉)
Department of Pharmaceutical Care and Health Systems, College of Pharmacy, University of Minnesota, Minneapolis, MN, USA

Institute for Health Informatics, University of Minnesota, Minneapolis, MN, USA

PhD Program in Precision Medicine Informatics, University of Minnesota, Minneapolis, MN, USA

Minneapolis Veterans Administration, Minneapolis, MN, USA
e-mail: adamx004@umn.edu

C. Aliferis
Institute for Health Informatics, Department of Medicine, School of Medicine Clinical and Translational Science Institute, Masonic Cancer Center, Program in Data Science, University of Minnesota, Minneapolis, MN, USA
e-mail: califeri@umn.edu

© Springer Nature Switzerland AG 2020
T. Adam, C. Aliferis (eds.), *Personalized and Precision Medicine Informatics*, Health Informatics, https://doi.org/10.1007/978-3-030-18626-5_1

recent revolution of technical approaches to prevention, medical diagnosis and treatment which have their conceptual roots to the medicine of antiquity [5, 6]. Across millennia of medical practice and health science inquiry, as researchers and scholars increased their knowledge of anatomy, physiology, biology, microbiology, biochemistry, genetics and pathophysiology they inevitably evolved systems of disease and therapeutics moving from systems with generality to systems with greater specificity.[1] Consider, as an illustrative example, the evolution of understanding of anemia. Whereas an initial distinction may focus on anemia due to reduced blood cell production (Hypoplastic or Aplastic Anemia), blood loss or increased blood cell destruction (Haemolytic Anemia) (three patient types), historical discovery of mechanisms driving each of these subtypes introduced many new subtypes (e.g., Iron deficiency anemia vs. hereditary Fanconi anemia as subtypes of aplastic/hypoplastic anemia; Sickle cell anemia vs. anemia due to systemic lupus erythematosus as subtypes of hemolytic anemias, and so on). Similar evolution from more general types of disease to more specific (i.e., with higher precision) are obvious in the evolution of understanding of jaundice/hepatitis, diabetes, cardiac failure, growth abnormalities, and most other diseases of the human body.

In addition to the *implicit* movement to PPM embedded in disease understanding and classification, some of the historical PPM forms have been *explicit*, mainly codified as *risk modeling and genetic counseling* which have existed for most of modern medicine (i.e., since the nineteenth century and onward).

However the big watershed moment that signaled the phase transition to large-scale and rapid transition to increased precision and personalization was the recent emergence of large scale genomic technologies coupled with extremely powerful computational methods. These developments introduced new and previously unimaginably powerful (and complex) forms of PPM. For example, this new PPM has had monumental influence on oncology because it has re-defined cancer on a molecular basis, has introduced targeted treatments and personalized testing and treatment modalities with great impact on outcomes. All of this has been accomplished in the span of less than 20 years.

The explosive development of modern PPM is reflected in the scientific literature which is undergoing an explosive growth in PPM publications in recent years. Indicatively, Pubmed contains 9 PPM papers that were published through 1999, 155 papers from 2000–2004, 1,353 papers from 2005–2009, 9,766 papers from 2010–2014, and 22,186 papers from 2015-May 9, 2019. [7].

---

[1] Over the years, disease categories have been refined, abolished, merged or established as underlying common mechanisms of previously thought unrelated diverse symptom clusters (syndroms). Regardless of the re-organization of the nosological taxonomies the inexorable evolutionary trend is from less refined to more refined disease subtypes and related patient groups of increasing granularity and smaller sizes.

Purpose of Present Volume

The following tenets underlie the intent of the present work:

(a) *PPM is extremely important for medicine and health.* The depth and speed of modern PPM is having great impact on the science and practice of medicine. Its potential is hard to overstate and the transition to a PPM-centric health science and healthcare of tomorrow is inevitable.

(b) *There are many different PPM formats and workflows* (for both scientific discovery and care delivery). The plurality of PPM forms often creates confusion because even PPM researchers or clinical practitioners are not typically well versed on all PPM forms. In order to remove confusion, it is essential to study and be aware of all forms of PPM and reveal their commonalities and differences.

(c) *Informatics is inextricably linked with PPM.* We define, for our purposes, informatics as the discipline that develops, validates, and applies computational methods for the capture, storage, protection and transmission of biomedical data; for the discovery of new knowledge by analysis of data and prior knowledge; and for the optimal delivery of medical knowledge for the purpose of optimal prevention, diagnosis and treatment of disease and enhancement of all aspects of health, longevity and well-being. Figure 1.1 shows a high-level view of how informatics sub-fields enable critical PPM-related areas.

(d) *A working, non-superficial understanding of PPM is by necessity interdisciplinary.* PPM requires simultaneously an understanding of, on one hand, the variety of forms of PPM and how they exist in modern health science research and healthcare; and on the other hand, an understanding of the new computational and genomics science and technology that enable PPM. Because of the relationship between informatics and PPM, professionals well-versed at the intersection will be well-positioned to advance PPM and the underlying informatics. PPM researchers or practitioners will have to be sufficiently versed in informatics that enables PPM.

(e) Informaticists are increasingly working in PPM regardless of the form of informatics they practice. PPM informatics is a meaningful interdisciplinary area of inquiry. *In the future, every informaticist will be dealing with one or more forms of PPM.*

PPM RELATED COMPONENTS → INFORMATICS ↓	Genetics, Genomics, Other Omics	Learning Health System	Evidence Based Medicine
Data capture, protection, storage and transmission			
Machine Learning, Big Data Analytics, Data Science			
Decision Support, Medical AI, EHR & Clinical Information Systems			

Fig. 1.1 Informatics enabling critical components of PPM. Green cells represent areas of very significant informatics importance

Consequently, we set out to create this edited volume with a set of concrete objectives:

Objective 1: *to review the present state of the art in PPM and the associated PPM informatics and especially to map out all major forms of PPM and systematize them for better understanding and communication.*

The focus of the present volume is on the computational part, and for reasons explained above, we need to understand PPM within the various development and delivery formats and contexts in which PPM manifests, since there are so many of them and while they do share commonalities, they also exhibit stark differences from one another. *For the lack of a better term, we chose the term "PPM workflow" to describe the type, format, context, informational architectures, and overall set of situational factors that determine the various processes via which PPM exists.* The PPM workflow builds on our traditional understanding of clinical and research workflows [8–10] and incorporates the PPM capacity.

This book will thus identify all characteristic PPM formats and workflows which address both emerging and traditional forms of PPM. Via the contributions of several highly experienced authors, who are notable researchers, practitioners and leaders in the field of PPM and PPM informatics, the book will introduce readers to how the various forms of PPM workflows and their supporting architecture function and how they are already changing both research and clinical approaches to how health sciences gather, organize and interpret information about health as well as disease. The contributing authors provide complementary perspectives on the covered topics, and occasionally use different language, but this naturally reflects the speed of development of the field and occasional lack of standards or conceptual or nomenclature consolidation across all of the PPM "tribes". We note that since PPM does not exist as a separate discipline or profession, the contributing authors were not trained in formal PPM programs; however, as the readers will find out, they have very rigorous approaches to PPM.

Objective 2: *to review trends and future developments in PPM and PPM informatics and outline concrete areas of high value research in PPM informatics.*

From the perspective of Biomedical Informatics, the core principles and best practices of the discipline of informatics remain as valid and useful a toolkit and guide to understanding and implementing PPM as anywhere else. For example, among the many necessary elements of a successful PPM effort, the value of data acquisition and storage which adheres to data representation standards; terminologies and ontologies which facilitate the development and sharing of high quality datasets (EHRs as well as omics ancillary systems) for primary (patient care) and secondary use (research and QI) is as useful as in any other form of informatics. However, the rapid growth in the types of available relevant data, such as the emerging availability of behavioral and genetic data which is being actively operationalized by innovators outside the traditional health care system, have important implications for consumer engagement to make it possible for fundamental changes in our approaches in understanding, promoting or restoring health [11–13].

An especially exciting and novel area where informatics, and data science in particular, plays an important role is in the analysis of large, multi-modal datasets with the intent to diagnose disease, re-define disease based on high-resolution instruments, predict outcomes and especially predict the effect of various actions (e.g., different prevention, care management or treatment strategies) [14]. Circa 2019, the analysis of datasets with millions of variables to elicit complex predictive patterns for example, is a routine endeavor, and a routinely successful endeavor we should add, as long as it is executed correctly.

Objective 3: to provide a consolidated and up to date PPM survey that can assist with the training of PPM researchers and practitioners (including informatics and non-informatics students and professionals). Although this book is written primarily for informaticists, because it gives a comprehensive and detailed survey of PPM, we believe that most health science researchers interested in PPM can benefit from the material here (such readers can safely ignore the most intricate informatics details).

Contents and Structure of the Book

Classical Personalized and Precision Medicine

Clinical risk assessment and prediction (Chap. 2). In earlier days of health care, providers focused on their individual clinical judgement to make decisions. However, with the availability of data for clinical risk assessment and prediction, the first elements of personalized and precision medicine began to develop informatics models of population normals, nomograms and disease staging using population science and statistical approaches to standardize and simultaneously personalize aspects of health care. Improvements in computing have facilitated the development of computational approaches to modeling disease including outcome prediction models. These risk prediction models have typically been developed with an iterative approach and incorporated new variables into the models to improve predictive capacity. The application of risk assessment and clinical decision making is explored using hypertension as a use case for disease classification and treatment in describing the *principles of guideline-driven health informatics (Chap. 3).*

Genetic counseling at the intersection of clinical genetics and informatics (Chap. 4). The traditional approaches to disease risk prediction have focused on the observation of phenotypic characteristics of patients and use of this observational data to identity subjects with genetic abnormalities and then attempt to predict the risk in subsequent generations. This type of early PPM has been challenging for non-specialist clinical providers for diagnostic and family planning purposes, resulting in the development of specialist providers to fill this clinical area. The evidentiary basis behind genetic counseling has continued to evolve alongside the understanding of genetics and this has been a key area where precision medicine is impacting health care. Traditional clinical work in newborn screening, carrier screening, diagnostics and predictive testing have been evolving with this evidence base. Results management, regulatory compliance, practice guidelines, counseling practice evolution and other legal and ethical concerns are among the issues which affect precision medicine work for the genetic counseling field in addition to the growing availability of information related to patient genetic data [15, 16].

A final area of classical personalized and precision medicine has been the *fundamentals of drug metabolism and pharmacogenomics (Chap. 5)*. The variations in response to drug therapy have been a long-standing problem requiring a series of trial and error efforts to attempt to optimize therapy for the average patient. With the observation of the variance in medication responses over time, the ability to identify individual drug responses has improved, leading to better understanding of the absorption, distribution, metabolism and excretion of medications. The understanding of individual responses to drug therapy was noted with the recognition of the p450 pathway which affects drug metabolism leading to a subsequent elucidation of a number of different p450 subtypes as well as a number of other metabolic activation and clearance pathways which affect an individual's response to drug therapy [17, 18]. Ongoing developments in pharmacogenomics will continue to influence our understanding of medication therapy with a growing number of approaches becoming available to better identify patient responses to drug treatment in a prospective fashion to predict therapeutic efficacy and avoid drug toxicity. Pharmacogenomics is a key area at the transition from traditional to emerging PPM and includes a long track record of clinically actionable information which has been made available for clinical decision making and is an essential element of a learning health system. In the efforts to create applications to use pharmacogenomics, the work at OneOme is described in *the growing medication problem: perspective from industry (Chap. 6)*. The OneOme efforts are representative of industry approaches to developing solutions to better incorporate pharmogenomics into clinical care as well as identifying some current barriers.

Newer and Emerging Forms of PPM

In recent years, developments in Machine Learning has introduced major quantitative and qualitative enhancements to the ability to use clinical data for *risk stratification and prognosis using predictive modeling and big data approaches (Chap. 7)* for patient assessment, public health and research applications. These developments have facilitated the analysis of high dimensional biomedical data with feature selection and feature extraction methods. Predictive model performance can vary among different methods and model selection is essential for optimizing productivity.

Much of the work in this space has focused on smaller data sets at individual sites, cohort studies, or with clinical consortiums. However, the growing availability of electronic health record data coupled with Machine Learning-enabled analytics allows for the creation of PPM models from patient care delivery to facilitate research and quality improvement as part of a *"Learning Healthcare System"* [19].

An additional emerging PPM area focuses on the *informatics methods for molecular profiling (Chap. 8)*. The workflows for developing and deploying molecular profiling start from feasibility assessment studies followed by clinical-grade molecular profile construction and testing. The field of molecular profiling has evolved since the late 1990s with the availability of high dimensional omics data for diagnosis and outcome prediction. Its use has been expanding since that time and currently covers a number of diseases and allows for individualized prognosis, choice of optimal treatments and the capacity to reduce healthcare costs. Molecular profiling has been established predominantly in several areas of cancer care, but is extensible to other areas as well. The primary workflows in this space support feasibility work, optimization, validation and deployment, however, this work is complex and needs to take into consideration the clinical context, data science, assays, health economics, development costs and deployment factors. A case example in ovarian cancer provides a perspective on the development of molecular profiling for patient care.

Among the organizations providing major support for cancer research discovery is the National Cancer Institute (NCI) which has provided software development resources to support biomedical scientists and statisticians by *constructing software for cancer research discovery (Chap. 9)*. The NCI workbench tools provide analytical support to address single gene queries, multi-gene correlation work, and transcription factor analysis. They can also be applied to gene expression changes over time to analyze gene pathways and other tasks of the user's interest. The availability of tools to facilitate collaboration between data analysts and biomedical scientists promotes effective team science discovery.

The ability to support *platform-independent gene-expression based classification for molecular sub-typing of cancer (Chap. 10)* is another area where informatics plays an important role in obtaining the correct diagnoses as well as optimizing treatment selection. Currently, stratification of cancer can use high-throughput platforms such as microarrays or NextGen sequencing which can reveal distinct tumor subtypes. Compared to classification of tumors using traditional histological features, the availability of molecular signatures can enhance how tumors can be classified much more effectively by incorporating large scale genomics data and providing the capacity for isoform analysis. However, the results from these high-throughput platforms have not been fully integrated into electronic health records. This critical workflow of deriving and then transferring gene-signatures at the point of care is work in progress.

Tumor sequencing (Chap. 11) has a growing role in the practice of oncology for tumor characterization and diagnosis including using next generation sequencing. Continued informatics innovations have provided support for whole genome sequencing, whole exome sequencing, and RNA transcriptome sequencing. These approaches have been applied to a number of focused cancer areas including gastric, colorectal, breast, gynecological and non-small cell lung cancers [20]. The work has identified a number of mutations and gene signatures of interest. In particular, targeted treatments for tumors may be facilitated through sequencing work to improve therapeutic responses. The cancer exome and panel sequencing work can help with finding potential new drug therapy targets and improving response rates among cancers under existing treatments. The use of next generation data also benefits from data sharing and re-use in order to understand disease prognosis and treatment optimization.

The development of *largescale distributed PPM databases (Chap. 12)* can enhance the impact on clinical care and research when data are linked across institutions to create large PPM cohorts and clinical genomics data sharing consortia. The ability to share the data across members of the consortia provides the capacity to better understand relatively rare outcomes. The large personalized and precision medicine cohorts can also enhance the understanding of common clinical conditions by providing the capacity for effective disease subtyping. The National Institutes of Health *All of Us* program is an example of national large cohort development initiative and one of several which are taking place globally [21]. Such large cohorts have substantial potential for research exploration. Large cohorts which incorporate elements from a variety of source datasets to create an individual's phenotype will require substantial data standardization and harmonization for effective use.

The use of genomics to better define disease is not confined to cancer. Genomics coupled with big data analysis has been used to re-define disease in other disease areas as well. The *Research Domain Criterion (RDoC) (Chap. 13)* initiative was launched to deal with issues around defining psychiatric disease on biological and causal terms in part by investigating pathological brain circuits incorporating genomic information [22, 23]. The RDoC includes five transdiagnostic domains that are associated with brain circuits and upstream and downstream causal processes used for diagnosis/classification. The chapter shows how this work is applied to Post-Traumatic Stress Disorder as a case study. In the realm of computational psychiatry, the initial steps of data integration are certainly not an inconsequential task and involve data integration from the patient. The data available currently promises to lead to a series of PPM modalities that will help inform decisions on the appropriate interventions to be considered for clinical care delivery. The scale of data growth has created a number of problems for providers and health systems. Applying these methods for personalized and precision medicine via machine learning approaches including the use of causal modeling is positioned to help achieve both predictive and mechanistic objectives.

PPM is helping overcome some of the limitations of traditional Clinical Trials (CTs). These studies often do not represent the broader population's variation. A newer approach is to focus on *pragmatic trials (Chap. 14)* which utilize electronic medical record data to analyze, model and understand treatment outcomes in real-life contexts across the spectrum of all patients receiving a medication. The secondary use of the EMR data is essential as are advanced informatics data analytics. The approaches can increase our capacity to improve our scientific knowledge when information can be effectively shared and exchanged across institutional boundaries. The electronic health record is, moreover, a key tool for replacing traditional phase IV trials both to explore potential new purposes for medications and also to track adverse drug events. By having shared information across sites, it is possible to identify events which may otherwise be too rare for detection at smaller individual sites. Informatics drivers for the key workflows in pragmatic trials include available pharmacovigilance reporting standards and terminologies along with natural language processing, machine learning and statistical methods to extract information for event identification.

Precision trials informatics (Chap. 15) is another modern form of PPM. Such trials can assign patients to treatment groups based on the patient's individualized molecular information and constitute a new means to maximize the effectiveness of treatments and minimize sample sizes needed for successful trials. In medication applications of precision medicine, much of the work focuses on finding the right drug to be used at the right dose at the right time. This approach is important for the day-to-day delivery of clinical care, but is also important for drug development including clinical trials. A particular focus area of great clinical interest is oncology due to the high costs of medications, the high risk of toxicity associated with the medications, and the risk to the patient of a suboptimal therapeutic response to therapy. Two key studies include the National Cancer Institute MPACT trial and the GeneMed informatics system which provide a test case and support system for precision trial management.

Informatics for a precision learning healthcare system (Chap. 16) describes a number of infrastructure elements and methods to reach consumers where they can engage the health care system to improve their health and to manage genomic data for clinical operations and research. Substantial resources must be allocated to these efforts to ensure success and they need to be accompanied with appropriate planning efforts particularly if the efforts are to align with and support a learning health care system.

Gaining an understanding of how a large integrated healthcare delivery system was able to implement and deliver precision medicine can provide important insights to other institutions considering similar efforts. Such implementation work can start by initially seeking to understand an organization's current capacity, especially areas of excellence on which PPM initiatives can be built. An understanding of the needs and interests of the patient population served is essential in helping to guide the work.

The lessons learned on how to build biobanks, link electronic health record data with whole exome data and collaborate with industry partners provide examples of how to creatively solve problems in the precision medicine space. For those intending to replicate these efforts, it is useful to understand the full development process including the consent process for patients as well as the issues with sample collection both in terms of architectural and workflow challenges. Once eligible patients are identified and consent is obtained, the specimen is collected and placed in a biorepository for sequencing and data analysis. For those with reportable results, the results are confirmed and reported to the patients and for non-reportable sequences, the exomes are saved for future work. The reporting workflows and implementation challenges are explored along with the potential for genomic decision support.

Genomic medical records and the associated OMIC ancillary systems (Chap. 17) are essential for delivery of most forms of PPM. A number of issues arise with the use of omic data including its heterogeneity related to the source of the sample, the type of data that is generated, and the clinical significance of the result interpretation. The size of omics data also creates a number of data management problems to address both in terms of data representation and its integration into the electronic health record. The omic data also has problems which are similar to typical electronic health data including knowledge management, information display, and data standards. However, omic data has more unique challenges regarding the size of data, ethical concerns and potential economic questions about its management. Ultimately, the availability of omic data follows a path to create information and knowledge and eventually generates clinical actions. This follows a similar pathway that would be pursued for the traditional translational work from the bench to the bedside, but requires management of the unique omic data characteristics for successful development and implementation efforts.

The *architecture and implementation of large-scale PPM informatics (Chaps. 18 and 19)* capabilities (e.g., at state levels or beyond) is an unavoidable stage in the evolution of PPM informatics, but one that is currently a work in progress. Architectural and workflow components include first and foremost architectures for horizontally scalable and high performance interoperable decision support but also health economics analyses, legal and technical protections of patient privacy, data security, evidence based synthesis and creation of computable guidelines, consent, integration with the EHR, portability of clinico-genomic data, feeding research and learning health system functions with the transactional care systems, and more.

An effective precision medicine workforce requires specialized PPM training for those who are currently in the workforce and for those wishing to have careers in the precision medicine space. *Personalized and precision medicine informatics education (Chap. 20)* recognizes the elements which are fundamental to the informatics world as well as those which are unique to precision medicine. This education can take various forms such as just-in-time, certificate training, specialized courses, and advanced degree training. Students may engage in PPM Informatics learning at multiple points in their professional careers.

The *landscape of PPM informatics and the future of medicine (Chap. 21)* concludes the present volume by discussing the key lessons learned about the state of the art in PPM and opportunities for implementation or new scientific discovery, across the map of PPM formats and workflows. This last chapter also provides a set of more open-ended and speculative (but testable) hypotheses about the evolution of PPM and the health sciences and healthcare around PPM.

References

1. The National Academies Collection: Reports funded by National Institutes of Health. Toward precision medicine: building a knowledge network for biomedical research and a new taxonomy of disease. Washington, DC: National Academies Press; 2011.
2. Hodson R. Precision medicine. Nature. 2016;537(7619):S49.

3. Kohn LT, Corrigan JM, Donaldson MS. To err is human: building a safer health system. Washington, DC: National Academies Press; 2000.
4. Grissinger M. The Five Rights: A Destination Without A Map. Pharmacy and Therapeutics. 2010;35(10):542
5. Dance A. Medical histories. Nature. 2016;537(7619):S52–3.
6. Egnew TR. Suffering, meaning, and healing: challenges of contemporary medicine. Ann Fam Med. 2009;7(2):170–5.
7. Health NCfBIUNLoMNIo. PubMed: National center for biotechnology information; 2019. https://www.ncbi.nlm.nih.gov/pubmed/.
8. Ramaiah M, Subrahmanian E, Sriram RD, Lide BB. Workflow and electronic health records in small medical practices. Perspect Health Inf Manag. 2012;9:1d.
9. Wetterneck TB, Lapin JA, Krueger DJ, Holman GT, Beasley JW, Karsh BT. Development of a primary care physician task list to evaluate clinic visit workflow. BMJ Qual Saf. 2012;21(1):47–53.
10. Unertl KM, Weinger MB, Johnson KB, Lorenzi NM. Describing and modeling workflow and information flow in chronic disease care. J Am Med Inform Assoc. 2009;16(6):826–36.
11. Hollister B, Bonham VL. Should electronic health record-derived social and behavioral data be used in precision medicine research? AMA J Ethics. 2018;20(9):E873–80.
12. Glasgow RE, Kwan BM, Matlock DD. Realizing the full potential of precision health: the need to include patient-reported health behavior, mental health, social determinants, and patient preferences data. J Clin Transl Sci. 2018;2(3):183–5.
13. The National Academies Collection: Reports funded by National Institutes of Health. Genomics-enabled learning health care systems: gathering and using genomic information to improve patient care and research: workshop summary. Washington, DC: National Academies Press; 2015.
14. Frey LJ, Bernstam EV, Denny JC. Precision medicine informatics. J Am Med Inform Assoc. 2016;23(4):668–70.
15. Ciarleglio LJ, Bennett RL, Williamson J, Mandell JB, Marks JH. Genetic counseling throughout the life cycle. J Clin Invest. 2003;112(9):1280–6.
16. Stoll K, Kubendran S, Cohen SA. The past, present and future of service delivery in genetic counseling: keeping up in the era of precision medicine. Am J Med Genet C Semin Med Genet. 2018;178(1):24–37.
17. Lewis DF, Watson E, Lake BG. Evolution of the cytochrome P450 superfamily: sequence alignments and pharmacogenetics. Mutat Res. 1998;410(3):245–70.
18. Tracy TS, Chaudhry AS, Prasad B, Thummel KE, Schuetz EG, Zhong XB, et al. Interindividual variability in cytochrome P450-mediated drug metabolism. Drug Metab Dispos. 2016;44(3):343–51.
19. Olsen LA, Aisner D, McGinnis JM, The National Academies Collection: Reports funded by National Institutes of Health. The Learning Healthcare System: Workshop Summary. Washington, DC: National Academies Press; 2007.
20. Beltran H, Eng K, Mosquera JM, Sigaras A, Romanel A, Rennert H, et al. Whole-exome sequencing of metastatic cancer and biomarkers of treatment response. JAMA Oncol. 2015;1(4):466–74.
21. Stark Z, Dolman L, Manolio TA, Ozenberger B, Hill SL, Caulfied MJ, et al. Integrating genomics into healthcare: a global responsibility. Am J Hum Genet. 2019;104(1):13–20.
22. Insel T, Cuthbert B, Garvey M, Heinssen R, Pine DS, Quinn K, et al. Research domain criteria (RDoC): toward a new classification framework for research on mental disorders. Am J Psychiatry. 2010;167(7):748–51.
23. Sanislow CA, Pine DS, Quinn KJ, Kozak MJ, Garvey MA, Heinssen RK, et al. Developing constructs for psychopathology research: research domain criteria. J Abnorm Psychol. 2010;119(4):631–9.

Part II
Classical PPM

Chapter 2
Clinical Risk Assessment and Prediction

Vigneshwar Subramanian and Michael W. Kattan

Overview of Early PPM Modalities

Initial attempts to apply formal PPM modalities focused on easily obtainable objective measurements, beginning with growth curves of height and weight. PPM then expanded beyond normal physiology to pathological processes. A push was made in the latter half of the twentieth century to identify factors that predisposed individuals to a disease for the purposes of screening and prevention.

Growth Curves

Growth curves have been used in a variety of fields to quantify the change in some property over time. Since the seventeenth century, biologists have used these curves to model the growth of populations of organisms, like bacteria [1]. In the sphere of personalized medicine, the concept typically refers to the practice of charting a child's height and weight to assess their growth. The first such growth chart is attributed to Count Philibert de Montbeillard in the eighteenth century, who plotted his son's height across time from birth to the age of 18 [2].

Today, the growth chart is a key screening tool in pediatric practice; a child's growth is typically plotted against a reference chart, which illustrates the distribution of growth curves from a population of healthy children [2]. This allows the

V. Subramanian (✉)
Lerner College of Medicine, Cleveland Clinic, Cleveland, OH, USA
e-mail: subramv@ccf.org

M. W. Kattan
The Mobasseri Endowed Chair for Innovations in Cancer Research, Department of Quantitative Health Sciences, Cleveland Clinic, Cleveland, OH, USA
e-mail: kattanm@ccf.org

© Springer Nature Switzerland AG 2020
T. Adam, C. Aliferis (eds.), *Personalized and Precision Medicine Informatics*, Health Informatics, https://doi.org/10.1007/978-3-030-18626-5_2

doctor to check a child's progression against a standard that reflects the diverse nature of human growth—what is healthy for a very tall child may differ from another. A person's growth can thus be expressed in the form of a percentile, where that individual is said to exhibit greater growth than that percentage of the reference population [2]. Growth curves also allow for the measurement of growth velocity; a child who is growing too quickly or too slowly may have deeper nutritional, endocrine, or behavioral issues.

Risk Factors

The term risk factor was coined in 1961 by the late Dr. William Kannel, former director of the long-running Framingham Heart study [3]. Kannel defined a risk factor as a characteristic associated with susceptibility to develop coronary heart disease [4]. Today the concept of risk factors is widely used to understand and manage essentially all diseases. Risk factors can be particular to an individual (e.g. age or BMI) or originate from an environmental exposure (e.g. pollution). Many risk factors are also biomarkers: substances or structures that can be measured as indicators of biological or disease processes [5].

Identification of new risk factors can be important for multiple reasons. For example, a new biomarker could improve our understanding of the underlying disease biology. However, new risk factors are most commonly used to improve our predictions about patients with respect to some outcome. Note that risk factors do not necessarily need to reflect disease biology, so long as their inclusion improves the accuracy of our predictions (e.g. socioeconomic status) [6].

Delivery of Classical PPM Tools at Point of Care

Risk factors for disease are an integral part of physician-patient discussions during most clinical encounters. In differential diagnosis of disease, the presence or absence of a particular risk factor can provide important clues about the underlying condition. Patient management, including treatment decisions, are also often made in the context of specific risk factors. For example, lifestyle changes are targeted at reducing BMI, cholesterol, or other such risk factors. Medication decisions can also be discussed in the same vein, e.g. the use of antihypertensives to reduce blood pressure and therefore decrease long-run risk of stroke.

Similarly, clinical prediction tools are designed to serve as decision-making aids. However, patients and physicians alike tend to have difficulty interpreting statistical risks and probabilities [7, 8]. Therefore, many classical PPM tools incorporate graphical visualizations to facilitate their use in patient counseling. Growth charts usually depict a series of curves, representing multiple percentiles of height or weight, which allows the physician to explain the trajectory of a patient's growth over multiple visits to the patient or family [2]. Similarly, nomograms enable physicians to illustrate the computation of risk in the presence of a patient by drawing out the conversion of individual risk factors to points, and demonstrating how the sum of points maps to a probability [9]. These representations enable clearer communication, improve physician and patient understanding of risks, and reduce the black box effect that often accompanies the use of these tools.

Modeling Disease Severity and Risk

When evaluating a patient, doctors must assess the severity of their disease and the risk of complications in addition to the cause. Choice of treatment, how a patient is counseled, and the disease management strategy can all change as a disease becomes more serious or an event becomes more likely. Doctors can use a patient's history and their exam findings to make judgments, but these estimates are subjective and can differ between doctors, particularly in complex cases. Objective methods of quantifying severity and risk are thus of great use in managing complicated diseases. These measures are also useful when studying outcomes, assessing quality of care, or deciding how to allocate resources.

Disease Staging

Disease staging was originally developed in the 1960s to cluster patients for quality assurance analyses [10]. Today, disease stages exist for many chronic diseases, like various cancers and neurodegenerative conditions. The goal of these systems is to classify patients into multiple groups with others who are similar with respect to prognosis (e.g. low risk, medium risk, high risk) and require similar treatments [10]. To benefit from staging, a disease must have a broad progression and heterogeneity in outcomes; otherwise there is little distinction between groups, and no real benefit to classifying patients.

Grouping of patients is done on the basis of diagnostic findings or risk factors [10]. Consider most cancers, which are usually classified into stages I–IV. The first stage usually has little to no complications, and the tumors may be relatively small. As the cancer progresses into later stages, the tumor usually grows in size and complications begin to manifest, at first locally. In stage IV, the cancer spreads to other parts of the body (i.e. metastasizes) and causes systemic damage [10]. As the stage advances, more aggressive treatments are required, and the prognosis becomes progressively poorer.

Disease staging systems have some advantages. They typically make use of commonly available tests or diagnostic criteria, and are relatively simple to implement and use [11]. However, they do not make accurate predictions about an individual's prognosis, as they group patients into relatively broad bins; the cancer staging system discussed previously makes the assumption that all patients can be grouped into four homogenous groups, whereas the condition in reality may exhibit large heterogeneity in severity and outcome [11]. Patients may also have difficulty interpreting the significance of a particular stage without the doctor's assistance. A more granular approach is needed to make personalized predictions.

Prediction Models

Clinical models are used to obtain personalized predictions based on an individual's specific risk factors. They generally require information on some combination of predictor variables, and identify each factor's relative impact on the outcome. Predictions can be made about the onset of disease (diagnosis) or the occurrence of future events during the course of a disease (prognosis). Figure 2.1 illustrates the general workflow for developing a prediction model.

Consider a patient with three risk factors, F_1, F_2, and F_3. These three factors can range from patient characteristics, like age or BMI, to their scores on clinical tests, such as a prostate-specific antigen (PSA) screening. The factors may not be equally important, and can therefore be assigned corresponding weights W_1, W_2, and W_3. If we know the weights, we can make a prediction of an outcome O [9]:

$$O = W_1F_1 + W_2F_2 + W_2F_3 \qquad (2.1)$$

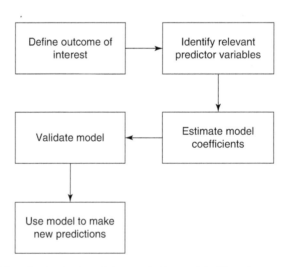

Fig. 2.1 A workflow for developing clinical prediction models. First, the outcome of interest is rigorously defined. Next, associated risk factors are identified either through literature review, preliminary analysis, or clinical judgment. The model is then derived through regression or machine learning methods. Internal and external validation are performed to assess model performance. Finally, the model can be used to aid in decision making for new patients

If we have a dataset with thousands of sets of risk factors matched with their outcomes, we can use statistical methods to estimate a set of weights. With our newly determined weights we can then predict the outcome for new patients. This approach essentially distills the characteristics of all of the individuals in our original dataset to a set of weights that best fit our particular cohort. It can be generalized to any number of risk factors, from 1 to n. The risk factors can be continuous, like age; discrete, either present or absent; or capture qualitative characteristics, like gender and ethnicity [9].

A typical family of statistical analyses used to estimate weights and generate our prediction model for an outcome is regression. We choose an appropriate regression method based on the properties of our outcome of interest. The model defined in (Eq. 2.1) is an example of a linear regression model. It is sometimes used for outcomes that vary continuously (e.g. blood levels of a pathogen).

Modeling Risk of Binary Events

More often, we are interested in predicting the probability of a binary event. In a certain period of time these events either occur or they do not. Some examples of binary events include organ transplant rejection, surgical complications, or infections. Most clinical decisions are made on the basis of preventing or treating a binary event; therefore an accurate assessment of risk can be very valuable for the purposes of stratifying patients or prescribing more aggressive treatments.

If we try to fit a linear relationship between a probability and our predictors, we run into an issue: probabilities must, by definition, take a value between 0 and 1, whereas the sum of our predictors is unbounded; i.e., $W_1F_1 + W_2F_2 + \ldots + W_nF_n$ can take any value between negative and positive infinity. To get around this, we can instead use logistic regression. We monotonically transform our probability, p, by the logit: $\log(p/1 - p)$, which is now also unbounded. We can now make the logit of our probability a linear function of our risk factors as previously:

$$\log\frac{p}{1-p} = W_1F_1 + W_2F_2 + W_2F_3 \qquad (2.2)$$

We can then solve for our probability:

$$p = \frac{1}{1 + e^{-(W1F1 + W2F2 + W3F3)}} \qquad (2.3)$$

Logistic models can predict whether an event will occur in a specified period, but give us no information about the timing of the event. Sometimes we are interested in predicting how long it will take for a specific outcome to occur (e.g. death). This is called time to event data, and we can model this outcome using Cox proportional hazards regression. Proportional hazards regression was originally proposed by Sir

David Cox in 1972 [12]; the seminal paper is one of the top 25 most cited publications in history, having been referenced over 48,000 times [13]. The hazard is defined as the instantaneous risk of failure, i.e., the probability of suffering the event of interest at a certain time, given survival to that time point. The Cox proportional hazards regression model can be written as follows:

$$h(t) = h_0(t)e^{(b1X1+b2x2...bnxn)} \qquad (2.4)$$

The outcome, h(t), is the predicted hazard at time t. The baseline hazard, $h_0(t)$, is the hazard when predictors X_1 through X_n equal zero: i.e., the effect of time. X_1 through X_n capture the effect of our risk factors or covariates.

Machine learning approaches like artificial neural networks and random forests can also be used to generate predictive models. They are generally more flexible than traditional statistical methods and do not require a linear relationship between variables [11]. However, this greater flexibility does not always result in better predictive accuracy, which is the goal of clinical modeling.

Evaluating Prediction Models

Regardless of the approach used to derive it, a prediction model's performance always heavily depends on the underlying data. If the training cohort is not representative of the broader population, or if the model fits specific characteristics of the data set too well, the results may not be generalizable. For example, a model trained on a European cohort may not be applicable to an Asian population, if the relative effects of the predictors differ between the two groups. To assess model performance, empirically derived prediction models are usually validated: external validation tests the model on an entirely new external data set (e.g., a cohort of similar patients from a different hospital), while internal validation tests the model by resampling or splitting the original data set [14].

Two common methods for internal validation are cross-validation and bootstrapping [14]. In cross-validation, the original data is partitioned into a number of equally sized training sets. The subset of the data that is not sampled in any given partition forms the validation set for that training set. A model is fit on each partition and tested on its corresponding validation set, and the individual results are combined. Conversely, in bootstrapping we generate a large number of data sets by sampling the original data set with replacement. Each bootstrapped data set is equal in size to the original data set, and will contain some observations multiple times and omit some observations entirely. A model is fit on each bootstrapped data set and tested on the original data set, and the individual results are again combined. Figure 2.2 illustrates these two methods.

Completed models are typically evaluated for discrimination, the ability to differentiate individuals with the condition from those without, and calibration, how well observed risks agree with predicted risks [14]. A model's discrimination can be

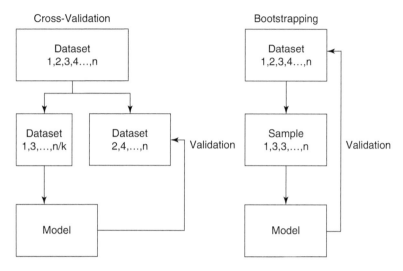

Fig. 2.2 Schematic representation of cross-validation and bootstrapping. Cross-validation involves partitioning the data into a training subset, upon which the model is fit, and a validation subset, upon which the model is tested. Bootstrapping involves generating a sample of equal size to the data set with replacement, upon which the model is fit, and validating the model on the original data Editors' note: the reader is cautioned that the Bootstrap estimator of a predictive model's error is biased, that is exhibits a systematic error that needs correction by the analyst. The cross-validation estimator by contrast is unbiased

quantified using a measure called the concordance index (also known as a c-index or c-statistic) [14]. This statistic is the probability that for any randomly selected pair of patients, the patient who experienced a worse outcome will also have a worse predicted outcome [14]. The c-index is equal to the area under the receiver operating characteristics curve, and ranges from 0.5 (chance or a coin flip) to 1 (perfect ability to rank patients) [14].

Although it is very widely used in the literature, the c-index may not be an appropriate scoring rule when predicting the risk of an event after a given number of years, as is frequently done in models of time to event outcome (such as Cox proportional-hazards) [15]. In such models, the concordance index assesses whether the predictions agree with the order of event times, instead of the order of event status, leading to the possibility to find a higher concordance index for a misspecified model than an accurate one [15].

An alternative scoring rule that does not suffer from this issue is the index of prediction accuracy (IPA) [16]. It is derived by rescaling the Brier score, a measure of predicted accuracy that is calculated as the mean squared error of the prediction [16].

IPA has several advantages relative to other measures: it is a valid scoring rule for both binary and time to event outcomes; reflects both discrimination and calibration of a model; and remains relatively straightforward to interpret (100% reflects a perfect model; values ≤ 0 reflect useless models, with negative values suggesting harm) [16].

In general, a model should be accurate while remaining relatively easy to use. If a model makes inaccurate predictions, it has no clinical value. An accurate model that is difficult to employ (e.g., requiring an uncommon lab test) is also unlikely to be used.

Selection of New Risk Factors

Identification of new risk factors is a critical step within the previously described workflow. A new marker is usually proposed on the basis of clinical suspicion or existing research. Validation of the marker requires a data set that contains information on the new marker, the outcome of interest, and existing markers that are known to be associated with the outcome. The prognostic value of the new marker—i.e., whether it improves the accuracy of predictions compared to existing models—is then investigated.

Typically, the marker is first shown to be associated with the outcome of interest [6]. If the outcome is time to event, this can be done by subsetting patients by level of the marker and using Kaplan-Meier curves (Fig. 2.3).

Although Kaplan-Meier curves demonstrate differences in time to failure for groups of patients on the basis of the new marker, established markers have not been considered [6]. This analysis does not answer the question of whether the marker provides additional predictive information that existing markers have not captured. If the new marker is perfectly correlated with an existing marker, or the survival differences demonstrated by the new marker can already be captured by some combination of existing markers, then the new marker is redundant. It offers no additional value, unless it is in some way cheaper or easier to collect than existing markers [6].

Fig. 2.3 Kaplan-Meier curves for a new marker (Reproduced from Fig. 1, Ref. [6]). The proportion of individuals for whom the event has not yet occurred (surviving individuals) is plotted as a function of time for multiple groups. Here, there are two levels: one with high expression of the new marker, and one with low expression of the new marker

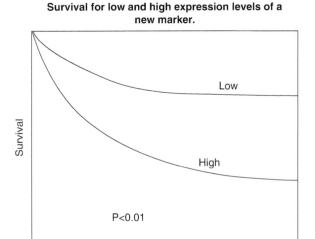

Survival for low and high expression levels of a new marker.

P<0.01

Time

Michael W. Kattan Clin Cancer Res 2004;10:822-824

Table 2.1 Multivariable analysis of new markers

(a) Conventional approach comparing effect measures. Adjusted indicates that the model incorporates some existing covariates (e.g. age, an established biomarker) in addition to the new marker.

	Adjusted hazard ratio (95% CI)	p-value
New marker 1	1.5 (1.2–1.9)	0.03
New marker 2	0.8 (0.7–0.95)	0.04

(b) Proposed approach comparing IPA as a measure of predictive accuracy.

	Increase in IPA (95% CI)	p-value
New marker 1	0.05 (0.04–0.08)	0.02
New marker 2	0.1 (0.8–0.12)	0.01

Multivariable regression analyses are usually done to test the value of new markers. A common approach is to generate a model that incorporates the existing risk factors and a new marker, for each new potential marker (Table 2.1a) [6]. The resulting measures of effect report the expected change in outcome per unit change in the marker [6]: for Cox proportional hazards regression, this is the hazards ratio; for logistic regression, the odds ratio. The p-value tests whether the measure of effect is significantly different from 1—i.e., no difference in outcome based on the level of the marker [6].

However, there are a number of issues with this approach. The numerical value of measure of effect depends to some extent on how the new and existing markers were coded (e.g. continuous vs. categorical); which other markers were included in the model; and how the variables were fit [6]. Because continuous variables tend to have smaller effect measures than categorical, this approach can encourage categorization of continuous information, which can be difficult [6]. This analysis also assumes that the modeling method used gives the most accurate predictions; an alternative approach may make better use of the existing markers and new information [6].

The purpose of including a new marker is if, given everything else already known about the patients, the new marker improves predictions by some capacity. One way to assess an improvement in predictive accuracy is to use IPA. Instead of considering an effect measure, the change in IPA can be measured when the new marker is included versus when it is omitted, in a model that also contains the existing markers (Table 2.1b) [16]. The p-value now tests whether the change in IPA is significantly different from 0 [16]. A marker that is shown to significantly improve the IPA can then be included in future models, as it improves predictive accuracy [16].

One might be tempted to ask which risk factors are most important, or make the best predictions. However, the goal is not to compare or replace existing markers, but instead to improve upon the performance of currently existing models [6]. If a new marker contributes to the ability to predict an outcome, we should consider using it, so long as it is feasible to measure and include.

Nomograms

Prediction models now exist for many diseases and outcomes of interest, but they can be difficult to use or interpret for a typical end user without a background in statistics. In the digital age, these models are commonly circulated as web forms, into which a patient's parameters can be entered to generate a prediction [9]. Although this enables widespread dissemination of prediction models, internet applications can further complicate proper interpretation by creating a black box effect: a sequence of values information is inputted into a computer and produces a mysterious output number, with no window into the underlying process [9].

Crucially, once a prediction is calculated, the doctor must be able to explain it to the patient. In order for patients to make an informed decision, they need to fully understand what the prediction means and how it was obtained. Previous research has shown both patients and doctors often have difficulty interpreting statistics and risk values [8].

Nomograms can facilitate the interpretation and explanation of prediction models by providing a visual demonstration of the computation. A nomogram is a graphical prediction tool in which points are separately determined for each of a patient's risk factors, and the sum of the points can be mapped to a predicted probability of the outcome [9]. Each risk factor occupies a separate row in the chart. The size and layout of the scale on that row corresponds to the weight for that factor from the regression model [9]. Figure 2.4 is a nomogram that predicts the prognosis of prostate cancer patients who undergo a radical prostatectomy [17].

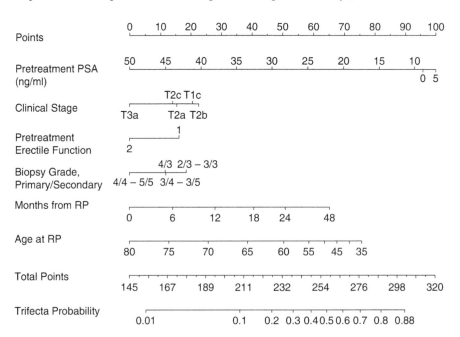

Fig. 2.4 An example nomogram (Reproduced from Fig. 4, Ref. [17])

Nomograms were invented by French engineer Maurice d'Ocagne in 1899 to facilitate graphical computation of formulas [18]. In 1928, Harvard physiologist L.J. Henderson was the first to apply the nomogram in a medical context, to describe the chemical properties of blood [18]. Medical nomograms became more common beginning in the 1950s [18], but the field truly took off with the advent of digital computing, with over 6100 related publications since 1990.

Medical nomograms offer several advantages. They simplify a mathematical model into a compact and intuitive document [9]. Unlike lookup tables, nomograms allow for the use of continuous predictors [9]. Whereas disease staging systems separate patients into homogenous groups, like low or high risk, medical nomograms produce patient-specific predictions on a continuous scale, allowing for more accurate predictions [11]. The computation can be done quickly, with sufficient precision and accuracy for clinical practice [9]. Clinicians can also use the document to demonstrate the calculation with the patient present, enabling better understanding of the prediction [9]. Nomograms are also cheap and easy to distribute, which can facilitate use of prediction models in resource-poor settings that lack reliable access to computers [9].

For each of the six factors—pretreatment PSA, clinical stage, pretreatment erectile function, biopsy grade, months from the radical prostatectomy, and age at radical prostatectomy—, the doctor traces from the patient's value on the scale up the chart to find the corresponding number of points. The doctor then traces down from the sum of points on the Total Points scale to compute the outcome, the Trifecta Probability—the probability that the patient is free of recurrence, regains continence, and regains sexual function.

Looking Forward

Early applications of PPM utilized relatively coarse, high-level information to make predictions. In recent years, the explosion of genomics, including the advent of inexpensive sequencing and functional assays, offers the potential to more finely tailor information to each individual. However, the clinical utility of such information must be further investigated. The current state of the field suggests that the individual effects of specific alleles, especially rare variants, on risk or severity of disease are likely relatively small for multifactorially determined conditions. In concert, however, multiple genes may combine to drive a significant portion of the variation in susceptibility. It is possible that most of the predictive utility of genetic information may be captured by a few genes that are most commonly altered [19].

As personalized precision medicine becomes the standard of care, nomograms will likely continue as a foundation of presenting and explaining risk modeling. From a clinician's perspective, nomograms distill a model into an inexpensive and easy-to-use document. The graphical representation of a prediction will remain a useful aid to facilitate patient counseling, and will also reduce the previously described black box effect, for clinician and patient alike. From a research perspective, nomograms remain the most effective method to display a risk model in a publication. Although a table of effect measures and p-values provide useful information about the relative impacts of each risk factor, nomograms concisely and clearly explain how a model generates predictions.

References

1. Schaechter M. A brief history of bacterial growth physiology. Front Microbiol. 2015;6:289. http://journal.frontiersin.org/article/10.3389/fmicb.2015.00289/abstract
2. Cole TJ. The development of growth references and growth charts. Ann Hum Biol. 2012;39:382–94. https://www.ncbi.nlm.nih.gov/pmc/articles/PMC3920659/
3. Langer E. Kannel, renowned medical researcher, dead at 87. Washington Post [Internet]. 2011 Aug 21; [about 2 screens]. https://www.washingtonpost.com/local/obituaries/kannel-renowned-medical-researcher-dead-at-87/2011/08/21/gIQAebbBVJ_story.html?utm_term=.c62cf783aa75
4. Kannel WB, Dawber TR, Kagan A, Revotskie N, Stokes J. Factors of risk in the development of coronary heart disease--six year follow-up experience. The Framingham Study. Ann Intern Med. 1961;55:33–50. http://www.ncbi.nlm.nih.gov/pubmed/13751193
5. Biomarkers Definitions Working Group. Biomarkers and surrogate endpoints: preferred definitions and conceptual framework. Clin Pharmacol Ther. 2001;69:89–95. http://www.ncbi.nlm.nih.gov/pubmed/11240971
6. Kattan MW. Evaluating a new marker's predictive contribution. Clin Cancer Res. 2004;10:822–4. http://clincancerres.aacrjournals.org/content/10/3/822
7. Gigerenzer G. Calculated risks: how to know when numbers deceive you. New York, NY: Simon & Schuster; 2002.
8. Gigerenzer G, Gaissmaier W, Kurz-Milcke E, Schwartz LM, Woloshin S. Helping doctors and patients make sense of health statistics. Psychol Sci Public Interest. 2007;8:53–96. http://journals.sagepub.com/doi/abs/10.1111/j.1539-6053.2008.00033.x
9. Kattan MW, Marasco J. What is a real nomogram? Semin Oncol. 2010;37:23–6. http://www.ncbi.nlm.nih.gov/pubmed/20172360
10. Gonnella JS, Louis D, Gozum M, Callahan CA, Barnes CA. Disease staging: clinical and coded criteria. Ann Arbor, MI: Thomson Medstat; 2003. https://www.hcup-us.ahrq.gov/db/nation/nis/DiseaseStagingV5_26ClinicalandCodedCriteria.pdf
11. Kattan MW. Nomograms are superior to staging and risk grouping systems for identifying high-risk patients: preoperative application in prostate cancer. Curr Opin Urol. 2003;13:111–6. http://www.ncbi.nlm.nih.gov/pubmed/12584470
12. Cox DR. Regression models and life-tables. J R Stat Soc Ser B. 1972;34:187–220. https://www.jstor.org/stable/2985181
13. Van Noorden R, Maher B, Nuzzo R. The top 100 papers. Nat News. 2014;514:550. http://www.nature.com/news/the-top-100-papers-1.16224–3.
14. Steyerberg EW, Vickers AJ, Cook NR, Gerds T, Gonen M, Obuchowski N, et al. Assessing the performance of prediction models: a framework for some traditional and novel measures. Epidemiology. 2010;21:128–38. http://www.ncbi.nlm.nih.gov/pmc/articles/PMC3575184/
15. Blanche P, Kattan MW, Gerds TA. The c-index is not proper for the evaluation of t-year predicted risks. Biostatistics. 2019;20(2):347–57. http://www.ncbi.nlm.nih.gov/pubmed/29462286

16. Kattan MW, Gerds TA. The index of prediction accuracy: an intuitive measure useful for evaluating risk prediction models. Diagnostic Progn Res. 2018;2:7. https://diagnprognres.biomed-central.com/track/pdf/10.1186/s41512-018-0029-2
17. Eastham JA, Scardino PT, Kattan MW. Predicting an optimal outcome after radical prostatectomy: the trifecta nomogram. J Urol. 2008;179:2207–11. http://www.sciencedirect.com/science/article/pii/S002253470800253X
18. Hankins TL. Blood, dirt, and nomograms: a particular history of graphs. Isis. 1999;90:50–80. https://www.jstor.org/stable/237474
19. Clayton DG. Prediction and interaction in complex disease genetics: experience in type 1 diabetes. PLoS Genet. 2009;5:e1000540. https://doi.org/10.1371/journal.pgen.1000540.

Chapter 3
Principles of Guideline-Driven PPM Informatics

Donald Casey

Guidelines Driving Precision Care

As healthcare organizations look to improve the health of the populations they serve, it is a critically important strategic priority that these entities develop and implement an effective evidence-driven standardization of care enabled by appropriate informatics infrastructure, especially for common medical conditions. In this chapter, we will highlight a use case for conceptualizing an informatics framework for electronic health records (EHRs) that can be used to effectively diagnose and manage one of the most common conditions (high blood pressure). Such EHR-delivered guidelines are important examples of established personalized and precision medicine (PPM) because they are instantiated with each specific patient's characteristics and deliver a patient-specific recommendation.

Failing to correctly diagnose and control high blood pressure can put many people at risk for cardiovascular disease, stroke, and renal failure, among other health issues. Recent analysis suggests that more than 100 million Americans currently have high blood pressure, and the 2013–14 US National Health and Nutrition Examination Survey estimated that 46% of U.S. adults had uncontrolled high blood pressure. Of that proportion, 33.1% were unaware they had the condition [1]. In addition, individuals with hypertension face on average nearly $2000 more in annual healthcare expenses compared to those without hypertension [2].

To address this critically important public health problem, the American College of Cardiology and American Heart Association (ACC/AHA) published a joint clinical practice guideline for high blood pressure diagnosis and management in 2017 [3]. This guideline includes more than 100 new recommendations for the diagnosis and treatment of high blood pressure, including:

D. Casey (✉)
IPO 4 Health, Chicago, IL, USA
e-mail: don.casey@ipo4health.com

© Springer Nature Switzerland AG 2020
T. Adam, C. Aliferis (eds.), *Personalized and Precision Medicine Informatics*,
Health Informatics, https://doi.org/10.1007/978-3-030-18626-5_3

Table 3.1 ACC/AHA blood pressure classification system

BP Classification (JNC 7 and ACC/AHA Guidelines)				
SBP		DBP	JNC7	2017 ACC/AHA
<120	and	<80	Normal BP	Normal BP
120–129	and	<80	Prehypertension	Elevated BP
130–139	or	80–89	Prehypertension	Stage 1 hypertension
140–159	or	90–99	Stage 1 hypertension	Stage 2 hypertension
≥160	or	≥100	Stage 2 hypertension	Stage 2 hypertension
• Blood Pressure should be based on an average of ≥2 careful readings on ≥2 occasions				
• Adults with SBP or DBP in two categories should be designated to the higher BP category				

- A new blood pressure classification system which categorizes blood pressure as normal, elevated blood pressure, or stage 1 or stage 2 hypertension, as highlighted in Table 3.1.
- Standardized methods for accurate measurement and documentation of blood pressure measurement.
- Appropriate treatment of high blood pressure, including recommendations pertaining to the decision to use blood pressure-lowering medications and nonpharmacological interventions through lifestyle modifications.
- Strategies for high blood pressure control including recommendations to promote lifestyle modification, implementation of comprehensive care plans by healthcare teams and accurate monitoring of patients on blood pressure medications by clinicians and in non-healthcare settings by patients.

ACC/AHA deploys a standardized approach to developing and publishing guideline recommendations. This process includes:

- A full evaluation of relevant published information by an "Evidence Review Committee"
- Grading of specific guideline recommendations based on level of evidence (LOE) (Table 3.2)
- A classification of recommendation (COR) for each recommendation
- Using a standardized lexicon for each recommendation based on specific combinations of LOE and COR where: COR = class (strength) of recommendation; EO = expert opinion; LD = limited data; LOE = level (quality) of evidence; NR = nonrandomized; R = randomized; RCT = randomized controlled trial.

With this consensus-based approach, the ACC/AHA class of recommendation and level of evidence applies to all clinical strategies, interventions, treatments, or diagnostic testing in patient care in every published guideline. The outcome or result of the intervention should be specified (an improved clinical outcome or increased diagnostic accuracy or incremental prognostic information).

COR and LOE are determined independently (any COR may be paired with any LOE). A recommendation with LOE C does not imply that the recommendation is

Table 3.2 ACC/AHA ACC/AHA strength (COR) and quality of evidence (LOE) supporting recommendations

Class (strength) of recommendation		Level (quality) of evidence	
I	Strong: Benefit >>> Risk	A	High quality evidence from >1 RCT or meta-analysis
IIa	Moderate: Benefit >> Risk	B-R	Moderate quality evidence from ≥1 RCT or meta-analysis (Randomized)
IIb	Weak: Benefit ≥ Risk	B-NR	Moderate quality evidence from ≥ 1 well designed/executed non-randomized, observational or registry studies or meta-analyses of such studies (Nonrandomized)
III: No Benefit	Moderate: Benefit = Risk	C-LD	Moderate quality evidence from randomized, observational or registry studies, meta-analyses of such studies, or physiological/mechanistic studies in humans (Limited Data)
III: Harm	Strong: Risk > Benefit	C-EO	Consensus of expert opinion (Expert Opinion)

Reproduced with permission of the American College of Cardiology and the American Heart Association

COR class (strength) of recommendation, *EO* expert opinion, *LD* limited data, *LOE* level (quality) of evidence, *NR* nonrandomized, *R* randomized, *RCT* randomized controlled trial

weak. Many important clinical questions addressed in guidelines do not lend themselves to clinical trials. Although Randomized Controlled Trials (RCTs) are often unavailable, there may be a very clear clinical consensus among experts that a particular test or therapy is useful or effective. For comparative-effectiveness recommendations (COR I and IIa; LOE A and B only), studies that support the use of comparator verbs should involve direct comparisons of the treatments or strategies being evaluated [3].

The ACC/AHA method of assessing quality of evidence continues to evolve, including the application of standardized, widely used, and preferably validated evidence grading tools and, for systematic reviews, the incorporation of an Evidence Review Committee. From an informatics standpoint, this type of approach to guideline development provides an opportunity to set priorities for automation of clinical decision support (CDS) in three dimensions as presented in the Fig. 3.1:

Hence, the COR and LOE can help to determine and prioritize the extent of automation of clinical decision support (CDS) intelligence rules based on this type of guideline recommendation classification and to help develop and determine the physical displays and nuanced syntactical/taxonomic differentiators for each classification. This process also should include the development of key parameters designed to enable rapid inclusion/exclusion decision making for guideline recommendations, especially those with lower quality of evidence and weak support.

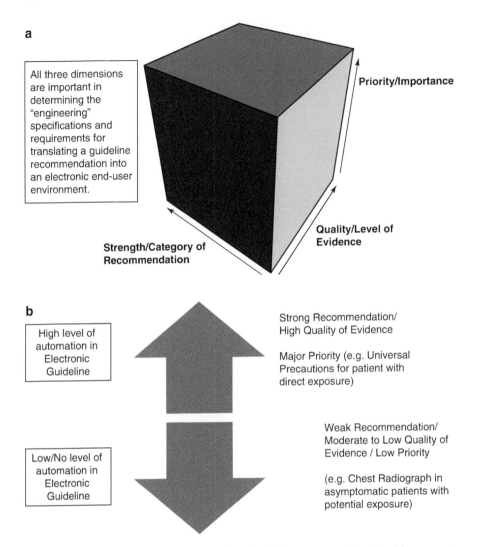

Fig. 3.1 (**a**) Dimensions for guiding translation of guidelines to computerized decision support. (**b**) High vs. low priority guideline classification for computerized decision support

Computable Guidelines and Informatics Considerations

Figure 3.2 shows an example of two critically important recommendations related to blood pressure control that have a high degree of relevance to a very large number of clinicians and patients:

An important feature of the 2017 ACC/AHA High Blood pressure guideline is that the writing committee translated related/bundled recommendations into "informatics ready" algorithmic decision trees (such as Fig. 3.3) for making decisions about specific management recommendations for each stage of High Blood Pressure:

COR	LOE	Recommendations for BP Treatment Threshold and Use of Risk Estimation* to Guide Drug Treatment of Hypertension
I	SBP: A / DBP: C-EO	Use of BP-lowering medications is recommended for secondary prevention of recurrent CVD events in patients with clinical CVD and an average SBP of 130 mm Hg or higher or an average DBP of 80 mm Hg or higher, and for primary prevention in adults with an estimated 10-year atherosclerotic cardiovascular disease (ASCVD) risk of 10% or higher and an average SBP 130 mm Hg or higher or an average DBP 80 mm Hg or higher.
I	C-LD	Use of BP-lowering medication is recommended for primary prevention of CVD in adults with no history of CVD and with an estimated 10-year ASCVD risk <10% and an SBP of 140 mm Hg or higher or a DBP of 90 mm Hg or higher.

*ACC/AHA Pooled Cohort Equations (http://tools.acc.org/ASCVD-Risk-Estimator/) to estimate 10-year risk of atherosclerotic CVD.

Fig. 3.2 Two high priority patient management recommendations from the 2017 ACC/AHA High Blood Pressure Guidelines

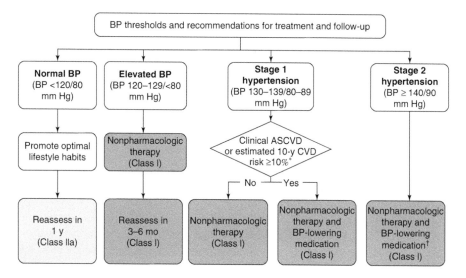

Fig. 3.3 Guidelines in decision tree format are easily computable

Informaticists also have to determine "need to know" stakeholders in terms of selection and completion of key guideline recommendations and how IT infrastructures support translation and transmission of information to end-users. This allows them to consider appropriate analytic and tracking approaches to monitoring and feedback, including alerts, gaps in care, performance dashboards, etc. The AHRQ-funded Massachusetts Clinical Decision Support Consortium [4] Knowledge Translation and Specifications (KTS) team has defined best practices for knowledge representation, data representation, and specification of knowledge content formats ranging from human readable expression of content, to expression of content for web services implementation. This foundational work included the development of a repository of CDS artifacts ranging from human-readable unstructured practice guidelines to highly structured, encoded executable knowledge. The initial clinical domains addressed for this effort included hypertension, coronary artery disease,

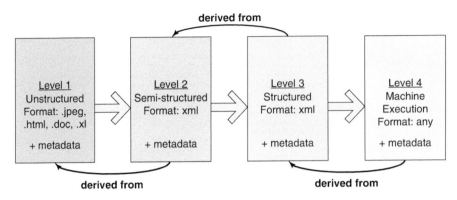

Fig. 3.4 Decision support levels of translating guideline recommendations into CDS rules [6]

and diabetes mellitus. These best practices are now being incorporated into a next generation standards framework created by HL7 through its Fast Healthcare Interoperability Resources (FHIR) [5]. The KTS team originally specified four levels of transformation and specification, which are both important to keep in mind and useful when translating guideline recommendations into CDS rules for digital health information technologies:

- Level 1—Any human readable guideline in any document format;
- Level 2—Unstructured: A guideline that has been deconstructed into rule statements and associated metadata and follows an XML schema;
- Level 3—Structured and Encoded: A Level 2 guideline that now carries with it the relevant and disambiguated encoding information to enable rendering in XML for import and interpretation by an inference engine;
- Level 4—Implementation: Either executable code, and a description, illustration, or export from an authoring-environment that details a specific implementation of a clinical decision support system (e.g., rules fully specified and encoded for a rules engine) (Fig. 3.4).

Current approaches to implementing recommendations from clinical practice guidelines (such as those published by ACC/AHA) lack standardized approaches to the translation of key parameter inputs from multiple sources of data collected at the point of patient care into Level 4 formats necessary for effective CDS interfaces.

Traditional analytic approaches to case identification have relied mainly on the use of ICD diagnosis codes from insurance claims, which has been imprecise, resulting in significant false positive and false negative diagnostic classifications of patients, thereby leading to inaccurate and incomplete assessments of an overall population such as the large one for high blood pressure. In particular, only patients with insurance claims are included in many of these analyses, which do not rely on other parameter inputs from many other common and more precise sources of patient information (such as EHRs, registries, pharmacy data, measurement and monitoring devices, self-reported patient data, etc.) See Fig. 3.5.

Fig. 3.5 Guideline-based decisions and actions may require "parameterization"

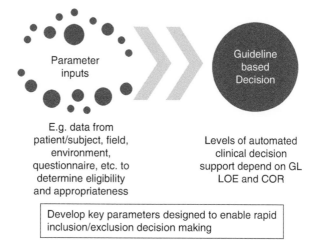

Parameter inputs

Guideline based Decision

E.g. data from patient/subject, field, environment, questionnaire, etc. to determine eligibility and appropriateness

Levels of automated clinical decision support depend on GL LOE and COR

Develop key parameters designed to enable rapid inclusion/exclusion decision making

COR	LOE	Recommendations for EHR and Patient Registries
I	B-NR	Use of the EHR and patient registries is beneficial for identification of patients with undiagnosed or undertreated hypertension.
I	B-NR	Use of the EHR and patient registries is beneficial for guiding quality improvement efforts designed to improve hypertension control.

Fig. 3.6 2017 AHA/ACC High Blood Pressure guideline recommendations for the use of EHR and Patient Registries

In the 2017 AHA/ACC guideline, there are also two new recommendations supported by moderate to high quality of evidence supporting the importance of extracting multiple key parameters related to the accurate diagnosis and proper management of patients with high blood pressure from EHRs and qualified clinical data registries (QCDRs) [7] now used in the CMS Quality Payment Program for physicians. See Fig. 3.6.

The Centers for Disease Control as of the time of this writing, is creating a standardized approach for adapting clinical guidelines for digital implementation in accordance with a number of these concepts for all of its future guideline implementation efforts for public health and disaster preparedness. The American Medical Association is also promoting its Integrated Health Model Initiative (IHMI) [8], which is a collaborative effort across healthcare and technology stakeholders that provides a continuous learning environment to create interoperable technology solutions and care models that evolve with real-world use and feedback for a common data model for organizing and exchanging information [9].

The translation of static clinical practice guideline recommendations into actionable, intelligent decision support technologies that can be embedded directly into electronic health records, qualified clinical data registries, care management data exchange platforms, and emerging patient-centered digital technologies is much closer on the horizon than ever before. This process will require the health informatics community to collaborate closely with clinical practice guideline developers, experts in evidence review and evaluation, digital technology developers, and Healthcare Information Technology regulators. Such collaboration will require each group to have fundamental understanding of the perspectives and logical reasoning of the other stakeholders to collaboratively impact the future quality and cost of patient care. Hopefully, one day in the not to distant future, all of these groups can work closely together at once in this regard.

References

1. Muntner P, Carey RM, Gidding S, Jones DW, Taler SJ, Wright JT, et al. Potential U.S. population impact of the 2017 ACC/AHA high blood pressure guideline. J Am Coll Cardiol. 2018;71:109–18. https://linkinghub.elsevier.com/retrieve/pii/S0735109717414744.
2. Kirkland EB, Heincelman M, Bishu KG, Schumann SO, Schreiner A, Axon RN, et al. Trends in healthcare expenditures among US adults with hypertension: National estimates, 2003–2014. J Am Heart Assoc. 2018;7:e008731. https://www.ahajournals.org/doi/10.1161/JAHA.118.008731.
3. Whelton PK, Carey RM, Aronow WS, Casey DE Jr, Collins KJ, Dennison Himmelfarb C, et al. 2017 ACC/AHA/AAPA/ABC/ACPM/AGS/APhA/ASH/ASPC/NMA/PCNA Guideline for the Prevention, Detection, Evaluation, and Management of High Blood Pressure in Adults: Executive Summary: A Report of the American College of Cardiology/American Heart Association Task Force on Clinical Practice Guidelines. Hypertension. 2018;71:1269–324.
4. AHRQ Agency for Healthcare Research and Quality. Clinical Decision Support Consortium (Massachusetts) | AHRQ National Resource Center; Health Information Technology: Best Practices Transforming Quality, Safety, and Efficiency [Internet]. https://healthit.ahrq.gov/ahrq-funded-projects/clinical-decision-support-consortium.
5. Health Level Seven International. Index – FHIR v3.0.1 [Internet]. [cited 2018 Oct 1]. https://www.hl7.org/fhir/.
6. Hongsermeier T, Maviglia S, Tsurikova L, Bogaty D, Rocha RA, Goldberg H, et al. A legal framework to enable sharing of clinical decision support knowledge and services across institutional boundaries. AMIA Annu Symp Proc. 2011;2011:925–33. http://www.ncbi.nlm.nih.gov/pubmed/22195151.
7. The Quality Payment Program. The quality payment Program [internet]. [cited 2018 Sep 28]. https://qpp.cms.gov/.
8. American Medical Association. AMA Integrated Health Model Initiative (IHMI) Collaboration Ecosystem|Welcome [Internet]. 2018 [cited 2018 Oct 1]. https://ama-ihmi.org/.
9. American Medical Association. Integrated health model clinical content module development methodology. Chicago, IL; 2017.

Chapter 4
Genetic Counseling at the Intersection of Clinical Genetics and Informatics

Andrew J. McCarty, Christine Munro, and Michelle Morrow

Introduction

Applied bioinformatics is the science, technology, and professional practice involving the representation, capture, collection, classification/indexing, storage, retrieval, dissemination and optimal use of biomedical knowledge. As applied to health care, clinical informatics is essentially an information-based approach to healthcare delivery. The goal of clinical informatics is to improve health outcomes through the utilization of organized information.

One pathway to this goal is through personalized or precision medicine. According to Hood et al., personalized medicine is healthcare that is "predictive, preventative, personalized, and participatory" [1]. The terms "precision medicine" and "personalized medicine" are often used interchangeably. According to definitions adopted by the National Research Council, the term "precision medicine" is preferred over the term "personalized medicine" to lessen the erroneous impression that treatments would be developed for the benefit of only one patient [2].

From a practical perspective, personalized medicine means that for each patient, information from that person's health record is incorporated into a model that creates individually tailored output. The output should be the best plan of action for that patient based on elements of his or her medical history. This approach has enormous potential to improve healthcare services, and is widely considered to be the future of medicine [3–5].

A. J. McCarty (✉) · M. Morrow
Laboratory Services, Children's Hospital of Pittsburgh, University of Pittsburgh Medical Center, Pittsburgh, PA, USA
e-mail: andrew.mccarty2@chp.edu; michelle.morrow@chp.edu

C. Munro
Children's Hospital of Pittsburgh, University of Pittsburgh Medical Center, Pittsburgh, PA, USA
e-mail: christine.munro2@chp.edu

© Springer Nature Switzerland AG 2020
T. Adam, C. Aliferis (eds.), *Personalized and Precision Medicine Informatics*, Health Informatics, https://doi.org/10.1007/978-3-030-18626-5_4

The field of clinical genetics is deeply entwined with clinical informatics and the movement toward precision medicine. The addition of more genetic and genomic information in the medical record improves our ability to create individualized management and treatment approaches. Overall, the quantity of genetic information available to providers is growing rapidly, making genetics a specialty that will gain from the application of informatics approaches. Taking another view, understanding the current models of genetic information delivery can inform the field of informatics, as it provides a springboard from which we can build and strengthen strategies for the delivery of more and increasingly varied types of healthcare information.

Genetic counseling is a clinical specialty that lies at the junction between information and clinical care. Although many of the technological advances that support informatics and precision medicine are new, the fundamental concepts underlying these innovations have been part of genetic counseling since the field's inception in the 1970s.

Genetic counselors (GC) have specialized training in genetics and counseling techniques. This combination prepares practitioners to educate patients and families about basic genetic concepts, to estimate risk for family members, to interpret genetic testing results, and to assist clients in adapting to genetic diagnoses.

This chapter will outline the ways in which the principles used in the clinical application of genetic and genomic information align with the fundamental concepts of informatics-based healthcare delivery. To better understand the current application of genetic information in clinical practice, we will first review roles of genetic counselors in the healthcare system.

Genetic Counseling: Traditional Roles and Service Delivery Models

Until recently, the majority of genetic counselors were employed as clinical providers in one of three specialties, cancer, prenatal, or pediatric genetics. Briefly, cancer genetic counselors serve individuals and families with personal or family histories suggestive of a hereditary cancer disorder. Prenatal genetic counselors serve those who are considering pregnancy and those who are currently pregnant. Prenatal counseling clients may have risk factors for having a child with a genetic condition that include family history, pregnancy history, maternal age, and/or abnormal screening tests. Pediatric genetic counselors meet with families of children with developmental and/or health concerns that raise suspicion for a genetic condition. Pediatric counselors frequently work alongside a medical geneticist to provide services in the context of a medical genetics evaluation.

In all three traditional specialties, counselors provide risk assessment based on family and medical history, provide information about the benefits and risks of genetic testing, facilitate testing, provide result interpretation with updated risk assessment, and provide resource referrals for patients and families.

In the traditional model of genetic counseling service delivery, the counselor meets with the patient and/or family in a clinic setting to determine a mutual agenda for the session, gathers data on medical and family history, and provides any combination of services including basic genetic education, risk assessment, pre-test counseling, psychosocial support in the decision-making and the post-test process. Tools to aid in this process include pedigree software, such as progeny and CDC family healthware. Additionally, informed decision-making tools are becoming more popular, such as the Genetic Support Foundations videos on prenatal screening options. Depending on the specialty, this session may or may not be done in conjunction with a physician visit. In addition to the traditional model, there are other forms of genetic counseling that have arisen to support the need.

An added consequence of an increased utilization of genetic testing is that there are currently not enough genetic counselors in the US to meet clinical demand. The genetic counseling shortage has inspired innovative changes in service delivery models. In addition to traditional clinic visits, genetic counseling services have been provided by telemedicine [6]. In some clinical settings, nurses or physicians fill genetic counseling roles including providing pre-test counseling and the delivery of negative results [7, 8]. Some institutions are making larger changes in service delivery. At UPMC Children's Hospital of Pittsburgh, a centralized genetic counseling service is now available to serve multiple divisions throughout the hospital. In non-hospital settings, several genetic testing companies offer direct to consumer (DTC) testing. These organizations employ genetic counselors who provide services as-needed via telephone or web. Experimental models are also being explored, including web-based counseling and group counseling [9, 10].

A general workflow of clinical genetic assessment is shown in Fig. 4.1.

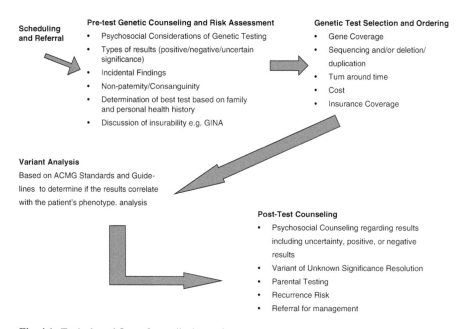

Fig. 4.1 Typical workflow of a medical genetics assessment

Genetic Testing

There are numerous forms and roles genetic testing can play in healthcare. However, to properly utilize this resource, selection of an appropriate test must occur. A genetic counselor may be a key expert in assisting with the selection of a genetic test. Regarding clinical testing criteria a genetic counselor may consider the selection of a reputable lab, reasonable turnaround time, cost, appropriate oversight, inclusion or exclusion of appropriate variants, and of course the quality of the test itself. This quality may be measured by multiple factors, but will generally include high analytic and clinical validity, high predictive value, and useful clinical utility. *Analytic validity* is the ability of a test to measure an analyte accurately. *Clinical validity* is the ability of a test to detect or predict the presence of a particular disorder or syndrome. *Predictive value*, which may be either set as positive or negative, is defined as the ability of a test to identify the presence or absence of a disease. Lastly, *clinical utility* is in reference to the ability of the test to impact clinical outcomes [11]. Examples of tools assisting with this process include genetic test selection software available at concertgenetics.com allowing comparison of multiple genetic tests in terms of cost, comprehensiveness, turn-around time, and other quality measures.

Another important factor in the selection of a clinical lab is ensuring that they are appropriately accredited by organizations for laboratory oversight. This will vary from country to country, but within the United States, there are numerous organizations available for accreditation. At minimum this will typically include Clinical Laboratory Improvement Amendments (CLIA). In addition many labs will have a minimum of two oversight organizations such as the American College of Medical Genetics, the Association of Molecular Pathologist, or the College of American Pathologists [12]. In addition to accreditation, there are varying forms of genetic testing available which may be offered at different capacities by different labs.

Genetic Testing Results

The genetic counselor plays an important role in the return of genetic testing results. The American College of Medical Genetics and Genomics has published guidelines for the interpretation of genetic testing results, which provide criteria for the classification of variants into one of five categories. In descending order of pathogenicity, these are: *pathogenic, likely pathogenic, variant of uncertain significance, likely benign, and benign* (Fig. 4.2).

Each variant is classified based on multiple lines of evidence. Considerations include whether a variant occurs at a high frequency in populations, whether computational algorithms predict that a genetic change will be harmful to a protein's structure (such as Polyphen and SIFT), whether the variant is seen in other family members with the disease, whether the variant was inherited or occurred for the first time in the patient, and whether the variant has been previously reported. Other considerations may include whether a previously reported genotype-phenotype

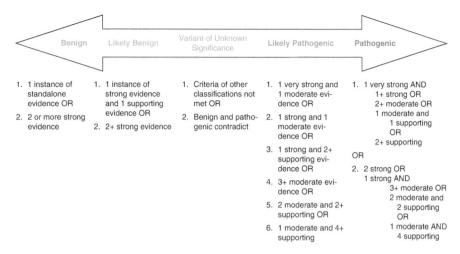

Fig. 4.2 Process to determine the pathogenicity of variants utilized by both clinicials and other genetic professionals within the laboratory. This figure is based on the Standards and Guidelines established by the American College of Medication Genetics and Genomics and the Association of Molecular Pathology

association could have an alternate explanation, or whether the patient's phenotype matches what would be expected given a defect in a particular gene [13]. ClinVar is a public database administered through the National Institutes of Health that lists variant-specific pathogenicity information from multiple laboratories, which enables a clinician to determine whether other laboratories have assessed a particular variant and how that variant was classified. Similar fee-based databases such as Mastermind and HGMD (Human Genome Mutation Database) amalgamate available pathogenicity information and link it to relevant literature. Gene and disease-specific databases also exist, such as those administered through the Leiden Open Variation Database, the dystrophinopathy-specific TREAT-UMD DMD global database, or the CFTR mutation database.

Although there are five classification criteria, generally, genetic results are explained as positive, negative, or variant of uncertain significance. In the case of a positive finding, in which a genetic variant known to be associated with a disease is identified in the patient, the counselor can provide management guidance and referrals to support resources. In the case of a negative result, the counselor can provide an appropriate interpretation, for example, distinguishing whether a negative result is informative or uninformative in the context of family history. The counselor may also offer further testing options. In the case of an equivocal result, also referred to as a variant of unknown significance, there is not enough evidence to determine whether a variant is disease-causing or benign. In this case, the counselor facilitates additional investigations as needed and provides support to assist the client in understanding and adapting to uncertainty. In both pre-test and post-test contexts, the client and the counselor work together toward the mutually agreed upon goals. A non-directive approach and shared responsibility throughout the process makes the counselor-client relationship distinct from many other healthcare settings.

When a physician and genetic counselor receive an uncertain or likely pathogenic genetic test report, they interrogate that result further to determine if it fits the patient's clinical phenotype. Examples of resources typically used include OMIM to better understand the phenotypic presentation of a particular disease and Oligo/SNP evaluation tools to investigate the genes located in a particular deletion or duplication and compare size to those previously reported. When a patient is diagnosed with a genetic condition, counselors will provide patient appropriate resources, such as Genetics Home Reference and disease specific registries and foundations.

Viewing the work of clinical genetic counselors through an information processing lens, clinical genetic counselors facilitate the input of relevant information into the lab, either through choosing an appropriate test or by providing appropriate clinical information to the lab to assist them in analysis. Upon completion of testing, the counselor receives the lab output and validates it in the context of the complete medical and family history of the patient. The counselor then completes a third stage of processing, in which he or she uses the validated lab output to determine appropriate follow up in the form of management guidelines, which are largely generated through published statements by working groups or disease-specific experts, and support resources. It would go beyond the scope of this book to discuss all types in detail but below are provided a few examples of the differing forms of genetic testing that may be performed depending on indication. The four examples below provide a rough framework of several ways genetic testing is utilized to ultimately impact the patient.

Figure 4.3 depicts the types of data used for determining benign and pathogenic variants, whereas Fig. 4.4 provides a comprehensive list of main informatics resources routinely used in the practice of clinical genetic counseling.

Pathogenic

Population Data	**MODERATE:** Not present in population databases
	STRONG: Prevalence in affected individuals increased overcontrols that is statistically significant
Computational Data	**SUPPORTING:** Computational evidence supports a pathogenic effect of the protein
	MODERATE: Missense variant at a loci where another pathogenic variant has been seen OR variant that changes protein length
	STRONG: The protein change is the same as a known pathogenic variant
	VERY STRONG: A gene where loss of function is a known cause of disease where a null variant is identified.
Functional Data	**SUPPORTING:** A missense variant in a gene with a low rate of benign missense variants and a high rate of pathogenic variants
	MODERATE: Located at mutation hotspot region or functional domain with no benign variant
	STRONG: Functional studies show a deleterious effect
Segregation Data	**SUPPORTING TO VERY STRONG:** Segregates with disease, evidence increases with increasing data
De novo Data	**MODERATE:** Variant not inherited from either parent
	STRONG: Variant not inherited from either parent (paternity/maternity confirmed)
Allelic Data	**MODERATE:** Seen in trans to a pathogenic variant
Other database	**SUPPORTING:** Other database shows a pathogenic status
Other Data	**SUPPORTING:** Phenotype or family history matches with gene phenotype

Fig. 4.3 Types of data used for determining benign and pathogenic variants

Benign

Population Data	**STRONG:** Minor allele frequency too high to be consistent with disorder
Computational Data	**SUPPORTING:** Computer models showing no impact in protein or function
	SUPPORTING: Missense variant in a gene where only truncating mutations cause disease
	SUPPORTING: Silent variant with no impact
	SUPPORTING: Inframe deletions or duplications without a
Functional Data	**STRONG:** Functional studies show no deleterious effect
Segregation Data	**STRONG:** Does not segregate with disease
Allelic Data	**SUPPORTING:** In trans phase with a dominant pathogenic variant OR in cis phase with a pathogenic recessive variant
Database	**SUPPORTING:** Unshared reliable database showing benign status
Other Data	**SUPPORTING:** Variant seen in an individual with a separate cause of disease

Fig. 4.3 (continued)

Fig. 4.4 Informatics resources commonly used in clinical genetic counseling

Population Databases
ExAC
100 Genomes Project
Exome Variant Server
dbSNP
dbVar
Disease Databases
ClinVar
OMIM
HGMD
HGVS
DECIPHER
CFTR Mutation Database
TREAT-UMD DMD
Sequence Databases
NCBI Genome
RefSeqGene
Locus Reference Genomic
MitoMap
Utilization Management
Concert Genetics
Genetic Counseling
Gene Reviews
Genetics Home Reference
Genetic Support Foundation
National Society of Genetic Counseling
American College of Medical Genetics
American Society of Human Genetics
National Comprehensive Cancer Network
Analysis Tools
SIFT
PolyPhen
GeneMatcher
Promethease
MutationTaster
GeneSplicer

Carrier Screening

Carrier screening is typically performed in several different clinical settings. The primary setting is prior to or during a pregnancy to assess the risk of an affected child for an autosomal recessive condition. In recessive conditions, if both parents are carriers they will generally not express symptoms. However, the fetus or child has a one-in-four or 25% risk for a recessive condition. Additionally, carrier testing would also be performed as follow-up testing for an individual who is identified to carry a variant of unknown significance. In such cases, carrier testing of parents may be useful to determine the risk to the patient based off of the results as well as the recurrence risk for both parents or if they themselves may be at risk [14, 15]. As an example, a genetic variant of unknown significance in an autosomal dominant gene may be identified; if this change was not inherited from a parent, the provider may be more suspicious that it is disease-causing. The genetic counselor's role in this form of testing is primarily to discuss the risks of testing as well as the resultant genetic risk determined from any additional testing. It is essential to ensure the patient or family is provided this information in an appropriately understood format.

Newborn Screening

Newborn screening, which is performed in most industrialized nations, is a form of testing that is not completely genetic in origin, but results in a significant amount of follow-up genetic testing. Newborn screening is generally performed after 48–72 h of life to determine if a child has one of a number of conditions for which interventions or treatments may improve outcome [16, 17]. The conditions include bleeding/blood disorders, congenital adrenal hyperplasia, hearing loss, immune deficiencies, and inborn errors of metabolism. Generally, the screening is not precise enough to be considered diagnostic, which leads to further functional or molecular testing. Genetic counselors hold positions in state newborn screening programs and are responsible for patient follow-up, including confirmatory testing, result disclosure, and family psychosocial support.

Diagnostic and Predictive Testing

Diagnostic genetic testing encompasses any genetic testing that may be used to rule in or rule out a genetic condition in an individual who is currently expressing symptoms. This testing has value by providing a diagnosis which may aide in the patient's treatment, redirection of care or potentially a cure. This varies from predictive testing, where an individual is not currently expressing symptoms but may have an increased risk based on family or medical history. Cancer prediction software tools are commonly used to help assess a patient's risks for carrying a hereditary cancer predisposition mutation. In cases where an individual is tested for a pathogenic variant known in the family and is found to be negative, this may be considered informative, and allow for an individual to be considered at average population risk. These individuals may not require additional surveillance or screening. Similarly, those who are pre-symptomatic but found to carry a pathogenic variant associated with a health risk, can be more informed to modify life style behaviors, obtain additional screening, and make reproductive decisions from this information. As an example, an individual may present due to a personal history of numerous polyps on colonoscopy. Pathology is suggestive of a cancer syndrome, for which their provider recommends genetic testing. In this form, the testing would be diagnostic. On return of the testing, they are found to carry a pathogenic variant in the PMS2 gene associated with Lynch Syndrome and an increased risk for colon cancer [18]. This individual has multiple siblings who would now also be at risk. If they were to have testing with no prior history of cancer to determine if they carry the same genetic change, this would be predictive testing. If they tested negative, it would be informative for their management. The genetic counselor plays a role in best test selection, result interpretation in the context of the clinical phenotype and family history, identifying appropriate family members who may carry the same diagnosis/mutation, and psychosocial counseling based on the implications and personal preferences of predictive or diagnostic testing. In addition, genetic counselors work to assess those who would obtain the most clinical utility from testing. Predictive models have been developed to better assess lifetime risk. Although beyond the scope of this chapter, some models that can be used include BRCAPRO, The Gail Model, and Claus Model which can provide information such as lifetime risk and five-year risk by integrating family history, personal history, and other important health information [11, 19].

Pharmacogenomics

An area of increasing interest in genomics is the relationship between genetic variation and the efficacy and safety of medication. A few brief examples of the use of pharmacogenomics to improve care include metabolizer status in relation to warfarin dosing and testing for thiopurine methyltransferase and metabolizer status prior to treatment with 6-mercaptopurine in childhood leukemia or autoimmune disorders both of which are considered companion diagnostics, defined as a test used to aid healthcare providers in appropriately treating by dosage, drug or intervention, including but not limited to genetic testing [20].

Genetic Counseling Practice Guidelines

As discussed, the role of a genetic counselor has continued to expand. As such the need for appropriate guidelines to encompass these broad roles has grown accordingly with this need. The practice of medical genetics and genetic counseling, has long used clinical practice guidelines due to the breadth of knowledge required to ensure appropriate clinical care for many disparate conditions [21–23].

The primary advantage to using practice guidelines is that they are formed by integrating the expertise of many expert health professionals ensuring a well-formed recommendation for use by clinicians treating a particular condition. For example, the high volume of data and information available in the field of cancer genetics has made the use of practice guidelines a necessity to ensure best patient outcome. Guidelines also serve to prevent overwhelming the healthcare system and its providers with difficult to interpret information. Prior to the use of formal informatics within this field, providers would use broad based criteria indicating the potential for an increased familial risk and utility of genetic testing. This might include the presence of bilateral primary tumors, multifocal tumors, atypical age/sex/site of tumor, rare tumor type, or a family history, to name a few. However, these criteria are non-specific and non-comprehensive. An integral tool used by providers are the National Comprehensive Cancer Network (NCCN) Diagnostic and Management Guidelines. These are employed to assist in the diagnosis, treatment, management, and surveillance of cancer. These guidelines include guidance for treatment of cancer by site; detection, prevention, and risk reduction; supportive care; and age- related recommendations as well as patient friendly material. The NCCN criteria primarily used by clinical genetic counselors are for risk assessment and assist in decision making regarding to whom genetic testing should be recommended [19, 24, 25].

Genetic Counseling Educational Standards

In addition to practice standards, genetic counseling as a profession is regulated by a number of governing bodies within the United States. Regulation is needed to establish and maintain standards, ensure competency of those entering the profession, protect the public, and centralize appropriate organization and expansion of the profession [11]. In the United States, there are three major national groups involved with the genetic counseling profession. The first is The National Society of Genetic Counselors (NSGC) whose primary roles are to promote the profession, act as a resource for professional education, and act as an advocate for policy change affecting genetic counselors as well as their patients. The second is The American Board of Genetic Counseling (ABGC), whose primary roles are to provide and update the exam that certifies genetic counselors and to study the practice of genetic counseling in order to inform practicing GCs of new developments in the field [11, 26]. This exam tests 22 core competencies organized into several core domains: genetics expertise; interpersonal, psychosocial, and counseling skills; education; and professional development and practice. These competencies are used to structure genetic counseling programs and are integral skills for competent practice and the support of complex decision making and data integration. These include the integration of the skills needed for assessment, facilitation of genetic testing options, use of a range of genetic counseling skills and models to ensure informed decision making and to promote client-centered, informed, non-coercive decision making by the patient. Additionally, many programs are incorporating bioinformatics courses into their training programs to address the information retrieval and data integration complexities of genetic testing. Accreditation and reaccreditation of programs is performed by the third organization, the Accreditation Counsel for Genetic Counseling (ACGC). This organization is charged with ensuring that the schools instructing prospective genetic counselors are providing a minimum standard to which they must achieve [11]. Of important note, currently not all states have licensure laws in place for genetic counselors. While certification in the U.S would be recognized in any state, licensure to practice as a genetic counselor is state specific and at of the time of writing, is not reciprocal [26].

Ethical and Legal Considerations

An often neglected, but meaningful, topic to discuss are the ethical and legal implications of genetic testing. Genetic testing occupies a unique space regarding testing in that it has the potential to not only impact the individual who is tested but family members as well. As such, there are several unique considerations such as bioethics, privacy concerns, the genetic information nondiscrimination act (GINA), and the duty to warn. Genetic counselors must weigh these ethical and legal considerations with every patient.

Autonomy, Beneficence, Non-maleficence, and Justice

As a provider, it is necessary to ensure the patient is receiving care in a moral and ethically appropriate manner. There are numerous ethical models for which to address these concerns; however, the most commonly cited approach is the bioethical model [27, 28]. The four primary tenants of the bioethical model are autonomy, beneficence, non-maleficence, and justice. In the setting of genetic testing, autonomy is the principle that protects an individual's freedom to make their own decisions while ensuring that the decision is made free from any false information or coercion by a third party or the provider. Beneficence describes an action performed with the goal to help others whereas non-maleficence is avoiding an action that would cause harm. In the setting of genetic testing this ensures a test is performed in the best interest of the patient. This is generally determined by weighing the benefits of an action against the risks, while ensuring that a patient's rights are maintained. Lastly the tenant of justice ensures fair distribution of limited resources and adherence to the laws where one practices.

As a clinical example of how these ethical principles may come into play, consider the following scenario:

> A 27-year-old female presents to clinic as she wishes to know her status for Huntington's disease (HD) prior to having any children. She requests this given that her paternal grandfather was diagnosed at 62 with HD. However, her father has made it clear through multiple conversations that he does not wish to know his status. If a genetic counselor saw this family they would need to consider the patient in front of them, as well as how this testing might affect others in the family, given a positive result would also diagnose the father. Considerations would include the autonomy of the father as well as the patient, ensuring that no harm, either physical or psychological comes to either, as well as ensuring a fair process to all involved. Using counseling and communication skills, a genetic counselor could attempt to facilitate a discussion for both individuals as well as the family unit to determine a decision that is mutually agreeable. However, despite counseling efforts, differences in viewpoints may remain. Such a situation would require insight by the provider and, potentially, an ethics group to come to a decision on how to proceed.

The Health Insurance Portability and Accountability Act (HIPAA)

The Health Insurance Portability and Accountability Act (HIPAA) of 1996s primary goal has been to provide legislation to ensure data privacy and security for medical information. In an era of increasingly data rich medical information which incorporates highly individualized genetic testing results, the need for patient and consumer confidence has become a priority [29]. The Act has three main sections: the privacy rule, the security rule, and the breach notification rule. The Privacy rule protects private health information (PHI) by outlining how it may be used and disclosed. PHI itself is defined as information that is individually identifiable. The Security rule is a set of standards put in place to inform how health information must be handled in order to ensure confidentiality and availability of PHI as well as the identification and anticipation of threats to PHI. Additionally, it ensures that a workforce follows these guidelines. The third rule, the Breach Notification Rule, outlines the requirements in the event of a breach of information. This is generally enforced by the US Department of Health and Human Services division, if considered a civil charge. However, if criminal charges are to be enforced, the US Department of Justice would then become involved [29, 30].

The Genetic Information Nondiscrimination Act of 2008

The primary role of the Genetic Information Nondiscrimination Act of 2008(GINA) is to prevent discrimination based on genetic information. This law applies, but is not limited, to employers, insurers, researchers, and the individual private citizens protected by the act [31].

GINA prohibits a health insurer from modifying a premium based on genetic information or forcing an individual to have a genetic test for coverage. It does allow testing in cases for coverage of certain procedures, such as risk-reducing surgeries in the presence of a genetic predisposition; however, it disallows the use of an enrollment decision based on genetic information. Similarly, the act prevents employers with more than 15 employees from discriminating for hiring, firing, or compensation based on genetic information. Employers are not allowed to collect genetic information unless required for appropriate health care. Of note, there are restrictions to GINA; it does not apply to life insurance, long-term care, and disability insurance or to those insured under the Veterans Health Administration, TRICARE, and the Indian Health Service insurance; however for these entities, separate but similar regulations are in place [11]. Genetic counselors discuss the implications of this law with patients considering genetic testing ensuring fully informed consent.

Duty to Warn

Duty to warn is the legal term stating a medical provider holds responsibility to inform or otherwise warn an individual of a particular health risk [32, 33]. This is acutely necessary if the genetic testing result may not only vastly increase a health risk for a patient but other family members as well. Numerous legal cases have been raised in regards to this issue, but at present a consensus has not been reached [32]. An area of similar discourse is the necessity of re-contacting a patient over time. Genetic testing results may often return with a variant of unknown significance. In this case, the test cannot clarify whether a genetic change impacts a health risk. Over time, these variants are eventually reclassified as benign or pathogenic, as discussed previously. Because case law is limited, there is uncertainty as to who is ultimately responsible for informing the patient of changes in the status of variants. The performing lab or provider have been suggested as responsible parties. However, given the volume of testing and resources required to re-contact, it has been difficult to reach a consensus on this issue. Arguments for re-contact might include inclusion or omission of management that could improve the patients' health outcomes or could potentially be lifesaving. Arguments against re-contact include the vast resource requirements to ensure contact and re-traumatization of a patient who, if given the choice, would elect not to discuss their genetic testing after the initial disclosure of results [32–34]. Genetic counselors have helped address these issues with patients by discussing patient responsibilities on VUS follow-up and providing patients with family letters to better help them disseminate genetic health information to extended relatives who may benefit from cascade screening. However, at the end of the day there is still lack of standardization within the industry leading to a risk to both patient and provider. The American Society of Human Genetics has published a statement attempting to address their stance stating in short that disclosure is permissive in cases where disclosure by the patient/family has been unsuccessful and where the risk for harm is high and serious and when prevention, monitoring, or treatment can vastly reduce risk. However, this discourse is ongoing, and standardization between professional groups and the law will require further assessment [32].

Expanding Roles and Service Delivery Models for Genetic Counseling

The landscape of genetic counseling has widened in recent years to include a broader range of subspecialties such as ophthalmology and neurology. In addition, so-called "nontraditional" positions within laboratories and genetic testing companies, clinical research positions, and hospital utilization management roles have increased in number [11, 12].

Genetic counselors employed in laboratory settings are fluent communicators who work collaboratively with clinicians and laboratory scientists. When a test is ordered, clinical information may or may not be sent by the ordering providers. Counselors either obtain needed information or filter the relevant clinical input and send a curated data set to the lab. On the output side, laboratory counselors offer clarification and nuanced interpretation of laboratory findings to clinical providers.

Genetic counselors in clinical research are in the challenging position of filling both a clinical and a laboratory genetic counseling role. They recruit and consent subjects for research, provide pre-test genetic counseling, and provide post-test counseling when research results are disclosed. They also work hand-in-hand with the laboratory team.

A new role for genetic counselors is utilization management. These counselors are employed in the laboratory, insurance health plan, or hospital setting to manage the ever-growing numbers of genetic testing requests and to ensure appropriate use of the resources allotted for genetic testing. Because of the newness and expense involved in genetic technologies, insurance companies have been slow to adapt, and it has been challenging for hospitals to manage costs associated with testing. These counselors utilize algorithms to ensure appropriate use of testing. They collect data and produce information that allows the hospital to justify the allocation of resources for testing. The use of population level data for genetic tests being performed may help to better understand the value of particular tests. In these roles, genetic counselors are continuing to establish cost effectiveness criteria to aide in decision making.

Genetic Counselors in Utilization Management

Healthcare costs are extremely high and constantly on the rise in the United States. With the increase in genetic test utilization, there is growing concern from a variety of healthcare stakeholders about how to balance the clinical utility and cost of genetic testing. Genetic testing costs are expected to be between $15 and $25 billion

USD by 2021 [35]. Government agencies, hospitals, healthcare insurance providers, and patients are among the major stakeholders affected by costs associated with the uptake in genetic testing. Genomic medicine will add to the cost burden of state Medical Assistance (MA) programs which may restrict availability of these services to MA members [36]. Hospitals struggle to meet the cost of genetic care when there is a lack of reimbursement from government and commercial insurance programs. Inpatient genetic testing costs are typically absorbed by the institution and outpatient institutional billing is not 100% reimbursable; however despite these difficulties, hospitals typically strive to provide state of the art care for their patients. Healthcare insurance providers strive to find a balance between best patient care practices, clinical utility of genetic testing, and costs. Patients may struggle financially with significant out of pocket costs depending on the amount of coverage their health plan may provide [36]. In order for sustained use of genetic testing, cost and benefits need to be justified and there needs to be demonstrated improvements in patient outcomes.

Pressure to reduce healthcare expenditures has highlighted the field of genetic test utilization management. Genetic counselors are playing a critical role in directing these efforts. Utilization management in genetic testing is focused on choosing the right test, for the right patient, at the right time. Limiting excessive or inappropriate testing and helping with test navigation and interpretation is leading to substantial downstream cost savings [37]. For example, studies in both commercial and academic laboratories report as high as a 30% test modification or cancellation rate, which has resulted in significant cost savings to reference laboratories, institutional laboratories, health insurance companies, and patients [35].

GCs in this role are able to identify [37]:

- Best test method

  - Single gene vs. panel
  - Reflexive testing options

- Best person to test

  - It is more informative to test a family member affected by breast cancer than testing an unaffected family member

- Best lab

  - Quality of the test reports, customer services, and turnaround times

- Best cost

  - Some commercial labs will offer volume discounts

  GCs can assist with [37]:

- Insurance prior authorization processes
- Test interpretation

  - A negative result may not rule out a diagnosis
  - Variant of uncertain significance is not a diagnosis

- Appropriate follow-up testing options
  - Parental testing may be informative if a variant of uncertain significance is identified as de novo

  GCs can detect order errors [37]:
- Duplicate test orders
  - A panel or exome test already covered the gene of interest
- Incorrect gene or test selected
  - Test indication is not matching the test ordered
- Better test strategy options
  - Sequencing is ordered for the DMD gene when copy number variations are most common

Genetic counselors are performing these tasks every day in the clinical setting, but also in specialized roles within institutional laboratories, reference laboratories, and insurance provider settings, saving costs across the genetic testing spectrum. The genetic knowledge and the communication skillset of GCs make them ideal healthcare providers for this role.

Genetic Counselors in the Public Health Setting

Public health involvement in genetic testing is nothing new, as newborn screening programs have been in existence since as early as the 1960s in many countries. However, public health involvement and policies are changing with new technologies. Public health perspectives require us to think about genetic testing in the context of communities, nations, and the world. An expansion of public health genomic programs is needed to ensure evidence-based translation of genomic information, adequate education of providers and patients, improvements in equality and access to genetic testing, and prevention of genomic discrimination [38, 39]. Genetic counselors are equipped with the knowledge and training to play a critical role in these program and policy developments, helping to find a balance between cost, information, and utility. Recently, genetic counselor programs, such as the one at the University of Pittsburgh, have started offering dual degree opportunities in genetic counseling and public health genetics.

Currently, the majority of genetic testing is offered for rare single gene disorders, however many monogenic disorders are of public health interest in the context of carrier screening (e.g., cystic fibrosis), diagnostic testing (e.g., hemochromatosis), and predictive testing (e.g., cancer predisposition genes). At this moment in time, multifactorial and monogenic diseases have very different utility in terms of predictive power and actionability in the public health framework. Testing for common multifactorial diseases such as cancer and cardiovascular disease is expected to become more prevalent as the understanding of gene-gene and gene-environment interactions improves [38].

Examining the public health utility of a genetic test involves the consideration of a number of variables in addition to examining genetic testing and its utility on an individual scale; when determining utility on a public health scale there are additional considerations [38]:

- Prevalence of the disease in the population
- Morbidity and mortality of disease
- Age of onset
- Available treatment options and their costs
- Alternative non-genetic based tests such as an enzyme assay
- Prevalence of disease-causing variants in the general population
- Penetrance of disease-causing variants in a particular gene
- Specificity and sensitivity of a genetic test
- Cost of a genetic test
- Ethical and legal issues (e.g., result disclosure and cascade testing in family members)

An example would be population-based screening of the BRCA1 and BRCA2 genes for predicting breast cancer. Breast cancer is common in the population, the penetrance of a BRCA1/2 mutation is high, and the frequency of these mutations in the general population is low. The sensitivity and specificity of the testing is high since these genes are well-characterized across different populations; therefore, the rate of variants of uncertain clinical significance may be lower than other cancer predisposition genes [40]. Costs of these tests range from the hundreds- to the thousand-dollar range. Finding a mutation in one of these genes provides women with preventative options such as increased screening, prophylactic mastectomy, and chemo preventative medications. Some experts argue that early detection would save money and improve patient outcomes. Other experts argue that increased screening can lead to unnecessary and costly biopsies and prophylactic surgeries, in turn leading to costly adverse outcomes [40]. Additionally, psychological implications and women's preferences need to be considered; some women feel empowered by the knowledge of a BRCA1/2 mutation because they can now "do something" about their risks, while other women may feel overwhelmed and anxious by the news of a mutation. Another expert concern is that the healthcare system lacks the support necessary for successful population screening. Physicians need support in order to provide individualized non-directive counseling, accurate test interpretation, and navigation of the insurance authorization process [39]. The example of BRCA1/2 population based screening highlights the complexities of assessing the public health utility of a genetic test, and it highlights the need for genetic trained experts, such as genetic counselors, to lead these conversations and initiatives.

Conclusion

Because genetic information is highly individualized, genetics professionals have long been at the forefront of the movement toward personalized medicine. Genetic counselors work at the institutional level to ensure that genetic testing is appropriately and cost-effectively managed. By doing so, they essentially curate incoming genetic information. The information can then be managed and utilized as the input for a precision medicine-based approach to patient care. GCs at the laboratory and clinical level participate in the interpretation of genetic information and the transmission of this information to medical professionals and to patients. At the clinical level, GCs also mine available expert resources to help quantify future health risks and to determine the best management strategies for patients. They use genetic information to help patients make the most appropriate choices in family planning, health management for current conditions, and engagement in preventative health practices.

In the past, testing was available for very few genes, and there were limited medical management changes for particular genotypes. Now, with the increase in accessibility of genetic testing and the push toward identifying genotype-specific treatments, genetic counselors are responsible for the accumulation and retrieval of a much wider range of genetic information. GCs interpret genetic information for both practitioners and patients and educate these groups in how to use genetic medicine to improve health outcomes.

As technology continues to advance, more genetic information will make its way into the average person's health record. A future challenge for genetic counselors and all health providers will be in assimilating large amounts of information and incorporating this information into daily practice. This challenge extends to informatics professionals, who enable efficient storage and retrieval of genetic information, and those who develop applications to assist providers in meeting this challenge. Many current electronic medical records, which are essential to an informatics-based approach to healthcare, were not designed to incorporate genetic testing information. As a result, it can be difficult for providers to find genetic information or to determine the significance of a test result. Fortunately, these challenges are now being considered and addressed [41, 42]. As the genetic testing landscape matures further, tools both on the professional and patient side will need to be developed to aide in these challenges. There are a number of online resources centered around patient driven data acquisition and analysis such as GeneMatcher and Promethease. GeneMatcher allows an individual to enter in the particular variant they have identified in an effort to be matched with other individuals with the same variant to help assist with reanalysis, whereas Promethease provides a number of available tools to further interpret data available both to scientists and the general public.

Genetic counseling service models incorporate the fundamental elements of precision medicine. Future progress in our ability to effectively utilize genetic and genomic information will depend on the ability of informatics and genetics professionals to plan and collaborate on platforms for information storage, access, retrieval, and interpretation. Together, we can make personalized health recommendations the standard of care.

References

1. Hood L, Flores M. A personal view on systems medicine and the emergence of proactive P4 medicine: predictive, preventive, personalized and participatory. New Biotechnol. 2012;29:613–24.
2. National Research Council (US) Committee on A Framework for Developing a New Taxonomy of Disease. In: The National Academies, editor. Toward precision medicine: building a knowledge network for biomedical research and a new taxonomy of disease. Washington, DC: National Academies Press; 2011.
3. Collins FS, Varmus HA. New initiative on precision medicine. N Engl J Med. 2015;372:793–5. http://www.nejm.org/doi/10.1056/NEJMp1500523.
4. Ashley EA. Towards precision medicine. Nat Rev Genet. Nature Publishing Group. 2016;17:507–22.
5. Dzau VJ, Ginsburg GS. Realizing the full potential of precision medicine in health and health care. JAMA. 2016;316:1659–60.
6. Buchanan AH, Datta SK, Skinner CS, Hollowell GP, Beresford HF, Freeland T, et al. Randomized trial of telegenetics vs. in-person cancer genetic counseling: cost, patient satisfaction and attendance. J Genet Couns. 2015;24:961–70.
7. Barr JA, Tsai LP, Welch A, Faradz SMH, Lane-Krebs K, Howie V, et al. Current practice for genetic counselling by nurses: an integrative review. Int J Nurs Pract. 2018;24:e12629.
8. Ormond KE, Hallquist MLG, Buchanan AH, Dondanville D, Cho MK, Smith M, et al. Developing a conceptual, reproducible, rubric-based approach to consent and result disclosure for genetic testing by clinicians with minimal genetics background. Genet Med. 2019;21(3):727–35.
9. Biesecker BB, Lewis KL, Umstead KL, Johnston JJ, Turbitt E, Fishler KP, et al. Web platform vs in-person genetic counselor for return of carrier results from exome sequencing. JAMA Intern Med. 2018;178:338–46.
10. Rothwell E, Kohlmann W, Jasperson K, Gammon A, Wong B, Kinney A. Patient outcomes associated with group and individual genetic counseling formats. Familial Cancer. 2012;11:97–106.
11. Uhlmann WR, Schuette JL, Yashar BM. A guide to genetic counseling. New York, NY: Wiley-Blackwell; 2009.
12. Goodenberger ML, Thomas BC, Kruisselbrink T. Practical genetic counseling for the laboratory. New York: Oxford University Press; 2017.
13. Richards S, Aziz N, Bale S, Bick D, Das S, Gastier-Foster J, et al. Standards and guidelines for the interpretation of sequence variants: a joint consensus recommendation of the American College of Medical Genetics and Genomics and the Association for Molecular Pathology. Genet Med. 2015;17:405–23. http://www.ncbi.nlm.nih.gov/pubmed/25741868.
14. Gregg AR. Expanded carrier screening. Obstet Gynecol Clin N Am. 2018;45:103–12.
15. Ong T, Marshall SG, Karczeski BA, Sternen DL, Cheng E, Cutting GR. Cystic fibrosis and congenital absence of the vas deferens. GeneReviews®. Seattle: University of Washington; 1993.
16. Howell RR. From a single child to uniform newborn screening: my lucky life in pediatric medical genetics. Annu Rev Genomics Hum Genet. 2018;19:1–14.
17. Lam MYY, Wong ECM, Law CW, Lee HHL, McPherson B. Maternal knowledge and attitudes to universal newborn hearing screening: reviewing an established program. Int J Pediatr Otorhinolaryngol. 2018;105:146–53.
18. Kohlmann W, Gruber SB. Lynch syndrome. GeneReviews®. Seattle: University of Washington; 1993.
19. Pilarski R, Buys SS, Farmer M, Khan S, Klein C, Kohlmann W, et al. NCCN Guidelines Index Table of Contents Discussion NCCN Guidelines Version 1.2018 Panel Members Genetic/Familial High-Risk Assessment: Breast and Ovarian. 2018
20. Kimmel SE, French B, Kasner SE, Johnson JA, Anderson JL, Gage BF, et al. A pharmacogenetic versus a clinical algorithm for warfarin dosing. N Engl J Med. 2013;369:2283–93.

21. Baumgartner MR, Hörster F, Dionisi-Vici C, Haliloglu G, Karall D, Chapman KA, et al. Proposed guidelines for the diagnosis and management of methylmalonic and propionic acidemia. Orphanet J Rare Dis. BioMed Central. 2014;9:130.
22. Toriello HV, Meck JM, et al. Statement on guidance for genetic counseling in advanced paternal age. Genet Med Various. 2008;10:457–60.
23. Bennett RL. The practical guide to the genetic family history. Hoboken, NJ: John Wiley & Sons, Inc.; 2010.
24. Mary Dwyer N, Ndiya Ogba M, Gupta S, Ahnen DJ, Bray T, Chung DC, et al. NCCN guidelines index table of contents discussion NCCN guidelines version 3.2017 Panel Members Genetic/Familial High-Risk Assessment: Colorectal Hereditary Colon Cancer Foundation. 2017.
25. Koh W-J, Abu-Rustum NR, Bean S, Bradley K, Campos SM, Cho KR, et al. Uterine neoplasms, version 1.2018, NCCN clinical practice guidelines in oncology. J Natl Compr Cancer Netw. 2018;16:170–99.
26. ABGC – role of genetic counselors certifications for public health.
27. Committee on Ethics. American College of Obstetricians and Gynecologists, Committee on Genetics, American College of Obstetricians and Gynecologists. ACOG Committee Opinion No. 410: Ethical Issues in Genetic Testing. Obstet Gynecol. 2008;111:1495–502.
28. AMA Code of Medical Ethics | American Medical Association.
29. HIPAA Compliance and Enforcement | HHS.gov.
30. Nass SJ, Levit LA, Gostin LO. Beyond the HIPAA privacy rule. Washington, DC: National Academies Press; 2009.
31. MH-M T. Advancing civil rights, the next generation: the Genetic Information Nondiscrimination Act of 2008 and beyond. Health Matrix Clevel. 2009;19:63–119.
32. Rothstein MA. Reconsidering the duty to warn genetically at-risk relatives. Genet Med. 2018;20:285–90.
33. Otten E, Plantinga M, Birnie E, Verkerk MA, Lucassen AM, Ranchor AV, et al. Is there a duty to recontact in light of new genetic technologies? A systematic review of the literature. Genet Med. 2015;17:668–78.
34. Fitzpatrick JL, Hahn C, Costa T, Huggins MJ. The duty to recontact: attitudes of genetics service providers. Am J Hum Genet. Cell Press. 1999;64:852–60.
35. Londre GK, Zaleski CA, Conta JH. Adding value to genetic testing through utilization management: commercial laboratory's experience. Am J Med Genet A. 2017;173:1433–5.
36. Institute of Medicine. The economics of genomic medicine. Washington, DC: National Academies Press; 2013.
37. Haidle JL, Sternen DL, Dickerson JA, Mroch A, Needham DF, Riordan CM, et al. Genetic counselors save costs across the genetic testing spectrum. Am J Manag Care. 2017;23:SP428–30.
38. Marzuillo C, De Vito C, D'Andrea E, Rosso A, Villari P. Predictive genetic testing for complex diseases: a public health perspective. QJM. 2014;107:93–7.
39. Ginsburg GS, Phillips KA. Precision medicine: from science to value. Health Aff. 2018;37:694–701.
40. Lippi G, Mattiuzzi C, Montagnana M. BRCA population screening for predicting breast cancer: for or against? Ann Transl Med. 2017;5:275.
41. Darcy DC, Lewis ET, Ormond KE, Clark DJ, Trafton JA. Practical considerations to guide development of access controls and decision support for genetic information in electronic medical records. BMC Health Serv Res. 2011;11:294.
42. Kho AN, Rasmussen LV, Connolly JJ, Peissig PL, Starren J, Hakonarson H, et al. Practical challenges in integrating genomic data into the electronic health record. Genet Med. 2013;15:772–8.

Chapter 5
Fundamentals of Drug Metabolism and Pharmacogenomics Within a Learning Healthcare System Workflow Perspective

Matthew K. Breitenstein and Erin L. Crowgey

Introduction

Advancements in pharmacologic knowledge over recent decades have included extraordinary discoveries of common, heritable genetic variants that dramatically modify human response to small molecule drug pharmacotherapies. These genetic variants—known as pharmacogenetic determinants—can profoundly modify drug absorption, distribution, metabolism or excretion, leading to reductions in therapeutic efficacy or unintended toxicity. A subset of pharmacogenetic determinants have become so clearly linked to impaired therapeutic response that they are now designated as being clinically actionable—these variants have corresponding clinical laboratory tests whose results are now readily implementable into electronic health record-based clinical workflows for precision medicine practice. To compliment these advances, our biological knowledge of pharmacogenetics has rapidly evolved to encompass a broader understanding of multiple genetic determinants (i.e. genomics) as affecting therapeutic response for any given drug. In addition to traditional drug metabolism, these genomic determinants are understood to affect series of organic reactions, branching of biochemical pathways, or as disparate determinants of physiologic response—together these genomic determinants inform our contemporary perspective of pharmacogenomics. In parallel to an ever broadening scope of

M. K. Breitenstein (✉)
Department of Biostatistics, Epidemiology, and Informatics, Perelman School of Medicine, University of Pennsylvania, Philadelphia, PA, USA
e-mail: mkbreitenstein@eihub.org

E. L. Crowgey
Department of Bioinformatics, Nemours Biomedical Research, Wilmington, DE, USA
e-mail: crowgey@nemoursresearch.org

© Springer Nature Switzerland AG 2020
T. Adam, C. Aliferis (eds.), *Personalized and Precision Medicine Informatics*,
Health Informatics, https://doi.org/10.1007/978-3-030-18626-5_5

pharmacogenomic knowledge, next-generation targeted agents (small molecule drugs, immunotherapies, and biologics) are being developed with increased sophistication so as to be therapeutically efficacious within the aberrant pathophysiology of rare disease sub-populations, as single agents or within combination regimens. While at the writing of this chapter our underlying knowledge of pharmacogenomics may not yet be amenable to informing truly personalized recommendations (i.e. for an N of 1 population), informatics within precision medicine is certainly well-poised to advance tailoring of targeted therapeutics to smaller and smaller clinic-based sub-populations within precision medicine practice.

Foundations of Pharmacogenomics for Precision Medicine Informatics

Origins of Pharmacogenetics

Throughout civilization, humans are thought to have administered biologically active organic compounds for the purpose of healing, and more generally, for the betterment of the human condition. Cuneiform clay tablets reveal that ancient Mesopotamian apothecaries, hybrid medicine-pharmacy practitioners, are amongst the earliest to connect treatments of disease symptoms to synthesis of organic compounds [1]. Fast-forwarding through the centuries, drug discovery is thought to have progressed across most civilizations, albeit in a piecemeal fashion via trial and error. Until the modern era, efficacy—or therapeutic effectiveness—of these organic compounds remained poorly understood, only recently being advanced with evidence gathered from statistical methodologies and standardized clinical trial protocols [2]. Coinciding with the maturation of chemistry in the twentieth century, advances in microbiology lead to a paradigm shift in medicine—a molecular revolution catapulting medicine into a modern clinical science with a rapidly evolving understanding of disease pathophysiology and an expanding war chest of prescriptible pharmacotherapies ('medications' or 'drugs'). In the ensuing decades, advances in pharmacotherapies led to cures for infectious diseases [3] that were previously fatal, and the human lifespan dramatically increased. However, 'diseases of age' began to appear [4]. Developed countries assumed sedentary occupations [5] while assuming elevated caloric diets loaded with sugars and processed foods [6]—chronic conditions began to permeate, and cancer incidence proliferated. Rapid development of pharmacotherapies buoyed by advancing medical knowledge helped alleviate disease symptomology and attenuate progression. However, for unknown reasons, medications deemed to be efficacious within the overall population were found to have highly variable responses by certain individuals. As we now know, heritable genetic traits—pharmacogenetic determinants—hold potential to dramatically modify therapeutic efficacy and patient response to medications [7].

The origins of pharmacogenetics as an 'observational science' trace back to 510 B.C. when Pythagoras realized that fava beans resulted in a fatal reaction, but only for certain individuals within the population [8, 9]. Our modern understanding of inheritance commenced with Mendel's establishment of the 'rules of heredity' [10, 11]. Within the famous garden pea experiments, Mendel established a model system that determined presence or absence of certain gene alleles in the parents resulted in predictable ratios of phenotypic permeation in offspring—that is, 'hidden' copies of gene alleles were present in the parent organism, but only became observable, or 'penetrant', when an offspring had two parents with 'hidden' copies of the gene allele. Of particular relevance to pharmacogenetics, Mendel established that major and minor gene allele copies dramatically modified phenotypic manifestation—and that organisms without 'observable' penetrant alleles still often carried an altered allele copy in their genome. Fast-forwarding to the mid-twentieth century, we marked the advent of pharmacogenetics [12, 13] on the heels of revolutionary breakthroughs in our understanding of deoxyribonucleic acid (DNA). Twin studies confirmed the role of heritable genome in the modification of drug metabolism and therapeutic response [14, 15]. Those early insights of the fava bean by Pythagoras became to be understood as glucose-6-phosphate dehydrogenase deficiency—now known to be one of the most common defects in human metabolism, affecting an estimated 400 million individuals worldwide [16]. Foundational understanding of polymorphisms linking to metabolic disorders and drug metabolism, included debrisoquine hydroxylase sparteine oxidase [17, 18] (later becoming known as *CYP2D6*) one of the major drug metabolizing enzymes [19] and an important human pharmacogenetic determinant [20].

Modern Pharmacogenomics

At the onset of the new millennium, pharmacogenetics began to rapidly mature into a sub-discipline of clinical pharmacology. An audacious vision was set forth for pharmacogenetics to directly inform prescribing in routine clinical practice [7, 21]. Calls for treatment personalization based on a patient's unique genome were soon to be augmented by emerging targeted therapies with increasingly refined biological specificity [22]. Advances in whole-genome sequencing [23] shifted the domain focus from single-gene pharmacogenetics, to pharmacogenomics, encompassing multiple-gene effects and pathways [7]. Pharmacogenomic inquiry placed a renewed focus on deciphering the complex molecular determinants of therapeutic response [24], drug disposition, and unintended side effects [25]. The National Institutes of Health began to support ascertainment of pharmacogenomic knowledge on a large scale through the formation of the Pharmacogenomics Research Network (PGRN) [26, 27] and the repository for pharmacogenomics knowledge 'PharmGKB' [28]. Most noteworthy for precision medicine informaticists, the PGRN enjoyed a fruitful collaboration with the eMERGE II Consortium [29], where electronic health record (EHR)-derived phenotypes where used to empower genomic medicine research [30, 31]. In pioneering work, eMERGE developed a compendium of portable EHR phenotype algorithms, that were replicated and validated across clinic-based eMERGE sites [32]. Further, the PGRN and eMERGE collaboration pioneered foundational translational informatics infrastructure and interdisciplinary scientific expertise which spurred development of large-scale linkage of EHR phenotypes to the sequenced whole-genome of consented patients for the purposes of secondary research.

Before we delve further into informatics perspectives or workflows, we felt it was important to provide the reader with a high-level overview of what pharmacogenomics encompasses as an academic discipline. Through a classical lens of pharmacology, when a patient orally ingests a medication, that compound is first absorbed, and then modified, across a series of one or many metabolic reactions. To be of intended therapeutic benefit (efficacious) to the patient, the resulting compound must be distributed from the site of primary metabolism (most often liver hepatocytes) and then succesfully uptaken into the tissue/organ site upon which the physician aims to extert a therapeutic effect. Once uptaken, the compound must be presented to the intended receptor target in an active form, or be further modified through metabolic reaction(s), to ensure robust binding affinity between the drug (ligand) and protein target. After binding between the compound and complimentary target occurs, the protein will synergistically operate so as to influence downstream enzymatic activity, exerting therapeutically efficacious perturbations upon selected downstream biological pathways. Eventually, any remaining unused or metabolized compounds will be excreted from this tissue and eliminated from the body via the renal system. How this process is synergistically modified, or unintentionally perturbed, by one or multiple heritable genetic traits is the basis for pharmacogenomics [7]. The broad physiologic mechanisms encompassing pharmacogenomics are delineated into two major classes—pharmacokinetics (PK) and pharmacodynamics (PD). In general, it is posited that a proper understanding of modification by heritable genetic traits requires considerations for multiple genes affecting drug efficacy across the PK and PD spectrum. Let us first consider pharmacokinetics/PK: While drug metabolism is a major component, PK also encompasses distinct absorption, distribution, and excretion processes occurring across various organ sites across the human body. At present, the major milestones of PK for most small molecule drugs are relatively well understood. Now we consider the much more complex, physiologic-diffuse pharmacodynamic/PD determinants: First, PD determinants are known to exert/control therapeutic efficacy through concerted regulation of downstream reaction(s) activity occuring across multiple disparate biochemical pathways. Further, while genetic variation occurring within PD determinants is thought to profoundly affect primary drug response and therapeutic efficacy, their implications towards manifestation of adverse drug reactions (ADRs) and drug-drug interactions (DDIs) are much less understood. As a general sentiment, emerging literature suggests that compositions of the human gut microbiome carry profound potential to modify drug metabolism processes (PK). Further,

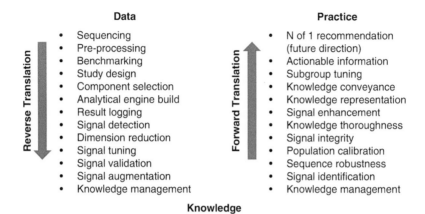

Fig. 5.1 A Translational Informatics Workflow for Pharmacogenomics as Informed by the Learning Healthcare System

advancing our understanding of PK and PD mechanisms holds potential to uncover pharmacogenomic determinants that might affect combination therapy efficacy, adverse drug reactions, and drug-drug interactions.

At present, our knowledge of single-gene pharmacogenetics has evolved to encompass over 100 clinically actionable drug-gene variant pairings. Having these clincially actionable pharmacogenomics in hand, we now stand on the cusp of another paradigm shift toward precision medicine. Particularly, where medicines are being designed with increasingly targeted specificity, and are increasingly pre-scriptible based on molecular phenotypes or sub-types of disease. The realization of pharmacogenomics at the bedside is readily achievable as a translational informatics endeavor. However, assembling pipelines from which to generate new pharmacogenomic knowledge from the Learning Healthcare System necessitates development of carefully-constructed translational informatics workflows.

Learning Healthcare System Workflow for Pharmacogenomics

Pharmacology is rooted in systematic perturbation of complex, physiologic systems for treatment of human disease. As a component of pharmacology, pharmacogenomics seeks to understand the genetic underpinnings of biochemical reactions encompassing drug metabolism and transportation, and the down-stream processes that affect drug efficacy, or the unintended manifestations of adverse drug reactions. We know that pharmacogenomics encompasses understanding biochemical reactions of multiple genes, often in sequence, that occur across the PK and PD spectrum. However, as our underlying knowledge of disease pathophysiology and availability of targeted therapeutics rapidly evolves, operationalizing pharmacogenomics considerations for a precision medicine workflow requires managing rapidly advancing knowledge and rapidly accumulating data points. This perspective operationalizes both ascertainment of additional pharmacogenomics knowledge from real-world populations and the incorporation of actionable pharmacogenetics information into clinical workflows. To guide the reader as they operationalize a translational informatics workflow for their selected precision medicine application, we have outlined key milestones below within 'A Translational Informatics Workflow for Pharmacogenomics as Informed by the Learning Healthcare System' (Fig. 5.1). We present this workflow to the reader through the lens of a learning healthcare system [33–35], where insights gleaned from translational activities inform new precision medicine knowledge [36].

Being informed by the learning healthcare systems framework, we see translational activities being most aptly delineated based on the direction of using data-driven insights to create knowledge and impact clinical practice: In reverse translation (section "Reverse Translation: Advancing Pharmacogenomics Knowledge with Real World Data"), described first, we use real-world data to create or enhance precision medicine knowledge. The informaticist synthesizes real world data in a systematic fashion so as to advance our underlying biological understanding of precision medicine. At present, such an orientation manifests primarily as research activities, but perhaps might also encompass quality improvement processes. A productive reverse translation workflow sets the stage for future treatment personalization, or tailoring therapeutic recommendations to a single patient. In the following section we describe forward translation (section "Forward Translation: Augmenting Clinical Practice with Actionable Pharmacogenomics Knowledge"). Within a forward translational workflow, the informaticist harmonizes evidence in such a way as to augment precision medicine decision making in real-world clinical practice.

Regardless of the translational workflow, the informaticist works closely with medical and pharmacology subject matter experts, sub-specialized clinical informaticists [37–39], and clinical pharmacologists to ensure the right drug is delivered to the right patient at the right dose. Informaticists are uniquely positioned to empower precision medicine utilizing quantitative skills to synthesize knowledge and help guide nuanced personalized medicine decision making. Within these sections, we outline foundational components of a precision medicine workflow for pharmacogenomics informed by the learning healthcare system.

Reverse Translation: Advancing Pharmacogenomics Knowledge with Real World Data

With the genomic revolution brought about by the Human Genome Project [40], the lightning advances in computing throughout the past three decades, and large-scale adoption of EHRs, we now have unparalleled opportunity to advance pharmacogenomics knowledge through reverse translational research.

Sequencing Technologies and Data Pre-processing

The process of sequencing DNA encompasses the precise identification and ordering of nucleotides contained within the DNA molecule. Early efforts to sequence DNA began in the 1970s when Fred Sanger and team developed a sequencing technique they termed "plus and minus system" [41]. This technique utilized polyacrylamide gel electrophoresis (known as PAGE) to amplify DNA fragments through polymerase chain reaction (PCR). With Sanger and colleagues' enhanced chain-termination or dideoxy technique [42, 43], the entirety of a single DNA molecule could be sequenced (~700 bp). Over the ensuing four decades, Sanger sequencing methodologies were further refined and high-throughput pipelines were developed. While Sanger sequencing remains a cost-effective technique for single gene or single mutation evaluation [44], it is far too costly for whole genome sequencing of large clinic-based populations, such as biobanks. Next generation sequencing (NGS) technologies have largely supplanted traditional Sanger approaches as a cost-effective, scalable sequencing technology in whole-genome discovery research.

Over the past decade, NGS technology advancements have dramatically reduced the cost and improved the speed of DNA and cDNA sequencing. In general, NGS enables the massive parallelization of DNA sequencing, or high-throughput sequencing where millions of DNA molecules can be rapidly sequenced simultaneously. NGS sequencing relies on finely-controlled 'cycle sequencing' reactions in which cycles of template denaturation, primer annealing and primer extension are performed. The types of NGS technology can be broadly categorized based on their applications for either *de novo* discovery or targeted resequencing [44]: First, in *de novo* sequencing, randomly fragmented DNA is cloned into a high-copy-number plasmid, which is then used to transform bacteria—this approach is known by the neologism 'shotgun sequencing' due to the many random fragments produced. Second, for targeted resequencing, PCR amplification is carried out with primers that flank the target. A primer is selected to contain a sequence known to flank the genetic region of interest. The output of both approaches is an amplified template, either as many 'clonal' copies or as many PCR amplicons present within a single reaction volume. Regardless of the NGS approach, bioinformatics methodologies are critical to assembling sensible data from these measurements. Overtime, NGS-based studies have broadened to encompass genome wide association studies (GWAS). NGS GWAS studies rely on known linkage disequilibrium (LD) regions to infer millions of single nucleotide polymorphisms (SNPs) (variation in base pairs) based on actual measurements of hundreds of thousands of DNA base pairs. Some of the earliest examples of GWAS applications in pharmacogenomics discovery include CYP2D6 for warfarin [45–48].

A typical workflow for an NGS assay involves: (1) the isolation of DNA, (2) the capture of DNA molecules, (3) sequencing, and (4) bioinformatics analysis of the data. Being perhaps both a humbling revelation and tremendous opportunity, NGS sequencing technologies have so rapidly matured that bioinformatics is now commonly viewed as the single biggest hurdle to applying NGS techniques in real time. The US Centers for Disease Control and Prevention (CDC) assembled a national working group, termed Next-generation sequencing: Standardization of Clinical Testing (Nex-StoCT) [49]. The goal of this initiative was to define platform-independent guidelines for using NGS in the clinical field [50–53]. These published guidelines detail key quality metrics that should be evaluated when developing and implementing a clinical NGS workflow. To ensure a robust perspective of rare and common variants, genetic epidemiologists have developed foundational quality control measurements [54]. Fine-mapping statistical approaches [55] are utilized to enhance GWAS tagging-SNP signals. In clinical trial and epidemiologic inquiry Sanger sequencing is held to be a gold standard for technical validation of GWAS signals generated using NGS technology [56]. In particular, Sanger biochemistry coupled with electrophoretic separation is the best option for continuous read-length and accuracy in DNA sequencing [44], which allows the investigator to understand the exact base pairs contained within a gene region of interest. To support NGS technical validation, commercial vendors have established NGS-to-capillary electrophoresis (CE) sequencing pipelines.

DNA sequencing techniques have revolutionized our ability to study an individual's genome in real time and enable a broader analysis approach to linking genomic alterations to specific diseases. However, next generation GWAS signals are not without limitations and caveats. Often NGS-driven GWAS studies require unsustainably sized sample cohorts to overcome Bonferroni-based corrections below the conservative $p = 0.5e^{-8}$ threshold of statistical significance [57]. Furthermore, navigating annotations of common and rare allele frequencies can be fraught with limitations based on inadequate representation of racial/ethnic minority populations within study cohorts [58]—pharmacogenomic recommendations, such as warfarin [59], often poorly represent minority populations, potentially due to under-representation in research studies. Finally, clinical significance is poorly extrapolated from many variant annotations due to limitations in underlying scientific evidence [60]. The aforementioned limitations are both a hurdle and an opportunity for informaticists to lead efforts for equitable pharmacogenomics for all populations, but particularly historically under-represented minorities.

Publicly Available Data Sources and Resources

The genomics community, spanning across government, academia, and industry, has done an excellent job of establishing data sources and resources for analyzing, interpreting, and sharing genomic data. There are numerous different types of genetic alterations, including SNPs, insertions and deletions (InDels), structural variants (SV), and various resources for these types of variants. SNPs are single-base pair substitutions, and of interest a single individual has a SNP every ~500 bp within their genome [61, 62]. There are more than 14 million SNPs that have been discovered, and they are the most studied type of polymorphism in the human genome. Of interest, the majority of these SNPs are not coded into RNA, and many have unknown biological function. There are numerous knowledge bases for depositing SNP data and extracting SNP annotations. These include, but are not limited to: The single nucleotide polymorphism database (dbSNP) [63], ClinVar [64], Exome Aggregation Consortium (ExAC) [65], the genome aggregation database (gnomAD) [66] (http://gnomad.broadinstitute.org), and the clinical pharmacogenetics Implementation Consortium (CPIC) [67].

Translational Informatics Study Design

The selection of machine learning algorithms and statistical approaches dramatically affect the ability of informaticists to detect signals within data and appropriately place results within the perspective of existing knowledge. The type of data elements required for analysis, including EHR data, biological data, and environmental factors, have signal-to-noise issues determined by the data measurement and capture techniques. Different types of data elements, for example biomarker versus EHR data, require specialized analysis approaches, so that a single modeling process capable of translating data into knowledge across all diseases and data is not realistic. Therefore, it is not surprising the full potential of pharmacogenomics can only be realized with the aid of advanced computational tools and resources, carefully selected for appropriateness in a particular application. Ensuring selection of appropriate machine learning algorithms and statistical methodologies for a particular task is a critical study design contribution of an informaticist. Very few other members of scientific or clinical teams, if any, will have training of sufficient breadth and depth to navigate these nuanced considerations spanning data science and biological measurement. It is the role of informaticists to ensure robust components within analytical engines designed for translational activities.

Technological advancements in genomics have created massive data resources, including several of the knowledgebases mentioned above, that require the support of bioinformaticists. It is essential that tools are developed that enable clinical researchers access to these data in a meaningful way, as it is not possible to manually integrate all resources. As mentioned above, data capture techniques introduce a potential noise-to-signal issue, and often important considerations for a rigorous study design are not considered. The open source notebook tool by Project Jupyter (https://jupyter.org/) can be used to ensure pipeline transparency, code interpretability, integrity of results, and potentially for publishing workflows [68]. Jupyter Notebooks deploy Python, R, and SAS code and store ascertained results within the notebook. Data science pipelines have various dependencies, package version control of these dependencies is critical to ensuring pipeline integrity and result validity. Open source package and environment management tools such as Anaconda (https://www.anaconda.com/) and Conda (https://conda.io/) ensure stable computational pipelines with precise version and dependency control. These tools run on most operating systems including macOS, Windows, and Linux, with opportunity for cloud deployments to enhance scalability.

As institutions continue to improve their meaningful use of EHR data, it is essential to develop high quality data entry, data standards, data governance and sharing plan, and security standards. Reproducibility is essential for driving better discovery of pharmacogenomic variants linked to adverse events. As the approaches for computable phenotypes and predictive modeling continue to evolve, the impact of informatics study design takes an even more prominent position in secondary research using EHR data. Even within a single institution's EHR, the specific source of EHR data fields (e.g. clinical notes vs. prescribed medications) have the potential to dramatically affect the perspective of the precision medicine phenotype ascertained [69]. Again, selection of appropriate machine learning algorithms and statistical approaches will dramatically affect detection of EHR-based signals and ascertained knowledge.

As new discoveries transition from de-identified research findings into precision medicine knowledge, and then evidence that is actionable at the clinical bedside, the law requires that clinically informative measurements be generated using clinically validated laboratory technology. This entails in practice using measurements ascertained through CLIA-certified clinical laboratory tests [70] generated within a lab CLIA-certified to run that particular test. Outside the realm of genetic and genomic tests that inform clinical decisions, for sequencing measurements used for research, informaticists bear great responsibility for generating sequencing results of the best possible quality for the research design needs at hand, by using robust analytical engines and appropriate informatics best practices.

Agnostic Signal Detection and Dimensionality Reduction

A difficult challenge in deploying supervised methods to study pharmacogenomics, or other pharmaco-'omics' big data projects, is the ability to quickly and accurately develop models that represent the inputted labeled features. While it might be empirically justifiable to deploy a single machine learning algorithm (e.g., random forests, linear discriminant analysis, or relief-based methods) when modeling a pharmacogenomics question, it is important to recognize that any single modeling approach is unlikely to capture all of the biologically-relevant variation, even within a single pharmacogenomics study. To streamline model identification and feature selection, research software has been developed to quasi-automate development of machine learning models [71, 72]. Such pipelines simultaneously i) recommend optimal machine learning models that best represent the data amongst a pre-loaded suite of algorithms, and then ii) selects features contained within the model(s) based on their relative importance to the model pipeline. Enhancing ascertained models with tandem perspectives of individual feature accuracy and rank/fit/importance hold opportunity to guide selection of biologically-relevant feature thresholds in agnostic pharmaco-'omic' profiling endeavors [73]. In supervised learning more broadly, regardless of the analytical engine, selected methods must be reasonably computationally efficient—so as to successfully complete the desired analytical tasks—, highly accurate, sensitive to complex or redundant signals [74]—so as to retain these informative features for downstream modeling—, and finally, output results that are readily human interpritable. Properly selecting machine learning, deep learning, or statistical methods to most appropriately address the scientific question and generate biologically-informative insights is paramount to robust informatics study/workflow design for pharmacogenomics inquiry.

Dimensionality reduction, the process of reducing the number of random variables and data features, is also an important approach in pharmacogenomic data modeling endeavors. In particular, there are three main types of feature-related terms and concepts that are essential for understanding dimensionality reduction in either hypothesis-testing or hypothesis-generating endeavors: (1) feature extraction, (2) feature transformation, and (3) feature selection. Often data features can be in a format that is not analysis ready, and require complex extraction, called feature extraction. Application of feature extraction methods often reduce the number of features available for analysis (i.e. feature reduction), while enhancing the meaningfulness of those extracted. Feature transformation, on the other hand, is the process of inputting raw data and transforming them into entirely new feature matrices. Finally feature selection is the process in which data features are selected based on relevance to answering the question at hand, guided by an analytical engine. It is important to note that when navigating deployment of supervised vs. unsupervised algorithms/pipelines there are varying considerations when performing feature selection and developing model predictions [75]. Research also suggests that deep learning pipelines outfitted with autoencoders might be suited for dimensionality reduction, due to their purported capability for generating human-interpretable feature matrices [76].

Signal Tuning and Validation

A powerful and important deliverable from machine learning efforts, is the ability to do predictive modeling, or rather the ability to develop a model using test and training data that is capable of then "predicting" the outcome of blinded samples [77]. Oftentimes the challenge with developing these predictive models pharmacogenomics studies/workflows is optimizing, or tuning, the machine learning algorithm due to having too few observations with labeled features. There are several issues related to algorithm tuning, including overfitting, and underfitting, when optimizing parameters. Overfitting happens when the model leared from training data matches the training data but does not provide an accurate representation of the validation data, (alternatively, the concepts learned from the training data to not apply to the validation data). On the other hand, underfitting occurs when a model cannot appropriately utilize the training and test data, and therefore cannot be applied to the validation data (but does not perform well in training data either). An important principle dictates that a validation dataset should always be used only for validating a machine learning algorithm, and should be withheld from the model (test and training data) until the model is optimized.[1]

---

[1] Editors' note: for more details on machine learning algorithm and model selection, error estimation and avoiding over- and under-fitting the reader can refer to Chap. 8.

Signal Augmentation and a Priori Knowledge

The pharmacogenomics knowledgebase, termed PharmGKB [78], is a publicly available resource that includes dosing guidelines, potentially clinically actionable gene-drug associations and genotype-phenotype information. The PharmGKB is a platform which collects, curates and disseminates knowledge about genetic variation and drug response (https://www.pharmgkb.org/about). The PharmGKB consists of (as of October 2018): 645 drugs with variant annotations, 132 pathways implicated in pharmacogenomics, 100 dosing guidelines, and 509 annotated drug labels.

The PharmGKB consists of a partnership between CPIC [67], Pharmacogenomics Research Network (PGRN) [27], PrecisionFDA [79], and that Pharmacogenomics Clinical Annotation Tool, called PharmCat [80]. PharmGKB has submitted 396 entries to ClinVar (https://www.ncbi.nlm.nih.gov/clinvar/submitters/500295/), a knowledgebase that aggregates information about genomic variation and relationship to human health. ClinVar [64] is publicly available and facilitates access to and the relationships between human variation and observed health status, along with the history of interpretation. This resource facilitates all levels of data submissions, from the simple representations of an allele and its interpretation, to detailed reports from multiple structure observational studies.

The Online Mendelian Inheritance in Man (OMIM) knowledgebase is also relevant to pharmacogenomics, as it is a comprehensive resource of genes and genetic phenotypes [81]. The OMIM resource sites 6267 phenotypes for which a molecular basis is known, and 3967 genes with phenotype-causing mutations (https://www.omim.org/statistics/geneMap).

General knowledgebase resources that might be of interest to the informaticist for annotating potentially novel variant findings, include ReactomeFIViz [82], KEGG [83], STRING [84], and UniProt [85]—these resources are focused on protein level data and connecting signaling molecules together. For example, Wilke et al. [86] have proposed a data analysis approach to large-scale pharmacogenomics studies that relies on a pathway-based step that informs subsequent downstream analytics and variation interpretation. These types of approaches are gaining momentum and have led to novel discoveries, such as Grados et al., [87] which utilized a pathway approach to identify several potential pharmacological targets for glutamate drugs. Gene ontologies (GO) [88], are also helping to drive new approaches for associating genotypes with biological implication. The Gene Ontology Consortium [89] maintains a knowledge base (http://www.geneontology.org) that defines concepts and classes descriptive of gene functions, and the relationships between these concepts. There are three different types of classifiers: molecular function, cellular component, and biological process. Ontologies can increase knowledge integration by providing structured and standardized biomedical knowledge [90]. To inform a cheminformatics perspective, DrugBank [91] combines drug data with drug target information and a Comparative Toxicogenomics Database (CTD) [92] which contains curated relations between chemicals, genes and diseases to create a chemical-gene-disease network for predicting novel relations [90].

Forward Translation: Augmenting Clinical Practice with Actionable Pharmacogenomics Knowledge

In forward translation, the informaticist harmonizes evidence in such a way as to augment precision medicine decision making in real-world clinical practice. This might encompass fine-tuning of models that help navigate potentially ambiguous or conflicting precision medicine recommendations. It also involves working closely with subject matter medical experts and providers, clinical informaticists and clinical pharmacologists, to ensure the right drug is delivered at the right dose to the right patient. Close collaborations between groups of experts will only become more critical in the precision medicine era—where informaticists are uniquely empowered to utilize quantitative skills to synthesize knowledge and nuanced personalized medicine decisions and considerations. A learning healthcare system that is capable of delivering precision medicine has to incorporate genomic data into a knowledge-generating infrastructure [93]. Ultimately, patient care has to drive and inform research, and research must drive and inform care [36]. The use of EHR systems has been essential in helping to create the foundation for these concepts and drive precision medicine knowledge.

"N of 1" and Comparable Populations

A major barrier for implementing pharmacogenomic testing at the bedside is the translation of a genomic variant into an actionable event when prescribing drugs. CPIC is focused on alleviating some of this burden by providing publicly available, peer-reviewed, evidence-based, updatable, and detailed gene and drug clinical practice guidelines (https://cpicpgx.org). Providing these types of guidelines is only one key aspect for implementing clinical use of pharmacogenomics data, however.

Signal Robustness and Sequencing Technology Considerations

As technologies continue to fuel data-driven discovery approaches, it is difficult to translate these types of tests into something actionable [94, 95]. Often clinicians and researchers struggle to decide whether a variant is clinically actionable, as is evident in ClinVar and other resources where institutions deposit genomic findings. Traditionally, pharmacogenomics studies rely on assays that focus on known gene candidates and common SNPs. Sanger single molecule sequencing, is ideal for technical validation for these types of variants. For example, SNP variants in thiopurine S-methylatransferease (TPMT), a cytosolic metabolizing enzyme, can cause severe hematopoietic toxicities. Several common SNPs are known in this enzyme and are often screened for in cancer subjects receiving thiopurine drugs. Fortunately, the methodologies and analysis approaches for univariate single candidate gene and SNPs-phenotype association are simple and easy to interpret allowing for a controlled probability of type I error rate (i.e., false positives), small sample size and low costs (when appropriate). However, these approaches have suboptimal ability to discover more genetically complex traits, since they are based on a monogenic trait paradigm.

Knowledge Management and Representation

Present day management of genomics data in a meaningful way within a clinic-based EHR represents a major challenge. Often pharmacogenomic results are returned to providers via scanned PDFs and lack granular data entry. The results are viewed as static and in non-computational readable formats, preventing scalability. Furthermore, the lack of clinical decision support tools within an EHR system can dramatically influence the use of these data at the bedside. It is essential that clinical providers have appropriate training on how best to prioritize and utilize pharmacogenomic results, and that computerized decision support provides timely evidence-driven guidance (and education-on-demand) at the point of need. Collectively, an effective implementation approach that involves a multi-disciplinary team of informaticist methodologists, clinical informaticists, medical subject experts, clinical geneticists, and clinical pharmacologists are suggested to create a high-quality and sustainable solution capable of realizing the impact of pharmacogenomic results.

Software tools such as ANNOVAR [96] allow for functional annotation of genetic variants. However, it is important to note our understanding of a specific genomic variant can change with time, commonly from technical changes in human genome reference builds intended to enhance reference accuracy and coverage of protein-coding genes [97, 98] or less frequently due to changes in our scientific understanding of a gene coding capabilities [99, 100].

Frequently, high-throughput genomic projects generate numerous variants of unknown significance (VUS); however, these variants can be described as benign or pathogenetic with additional research, and highlight the importance of an effective pharmacogenomic data management system needing a robust re-analysis technique. There is no hard rule about how often and how to run these types of re-analysis and how to best represent the data. There are several commercial platforms for this type of work, including ActX (https://www.actx.com/info/about), but a single interoperable system is not yet available.

Computational Tools to Navigate Signals

Implementation science, the movement of evidence-based practice into routine clinical usage, is becoming a key focus for pharmacogenomics [101]. There is often a major gap between incorporating translational research findings into clinical care.

Clinical decision support (CDS) tools need to increase clinical workflow efficiencies, avoiding alert fatigue, and preventing liabilities. They have the potential to enhance efficiency by influencing (1) when a pharmacogenomics test is ordered, (2) how the results are interpreted and used, and (3) the use of the genomics data across the lifespan of a patient. It is essential that providers receive appropriate educational resources for pharmacogenomics as this cannot be assumed to be part of the traditional training background of clinicians. It is also essential that patients are provided with educational materials and have access to appropriate clinical resources, such as genetic counselors, who are responsible for interacting with patients to help them understand their genetic findings and impact.

The NHGRI and NCI-sponsored Implementing GeNomics In Practice (IGNITE) Network [102] was established in 2013 for development, investigation, and dissemination of genomic medicine practice models that integrate genomic data into EHRs. The complimentary Clinical Sequencing Evidence-Generating Research (CSER) Consortium [103], also supported by NHGRI and NCI, was recently launched with similar goals, albeit focused on serving historically underrepresented or underserved populations. Both of these initiatives study a spectrum of disease phenotypes within a variety of healthcare settings. Beyond developing foundational methods for integrate genomic data, or implementing CPIC recommendations into clinical practice, these initiatives aim to identify real-world barriers to integrating genomic within a healthcare system to populate a knowledgebase with utility to inform precision medicine clinical decision recommendations [93].

Appropriate Conveyance of Knowledge

It is important to note, incorporation of pharmacogenomic-guided decision making into instutional EHRs workflows have been deliberately metered, with only a few premiere healthcare organizations, including Mayo Clinic, having implemented point-of-care programs. This metered uptake has been partially attributed to gaps in outcomes research that might inform needed best practice standards [104]. However, numerous other challenges exist, including development of secure cloud resources-connected to the local EHR, optimization of clinical workflows, standardization of processing and use of data procedures, education for providers, and evidence-based studies that support the clinical and financial benefit of altering care based on genomics [105]. Although CPIC provides suggestions for altered clinical dosing recommendations based on genotypes (e.g. attenuated dosing of compound based on a genomic variant), a consensus for implementing these practices at the bedside across institutions remains to be developed. In addition "alert fatigue" is a well-documented issue for providers [106] which likely affects delivery of pharmacogenomics via clinical alerts within the EHR. Further, it is also important to recognize the "evolving" nature of data, and often times a variant may not be actionable at the one time, but perhaps it might be deemed to be clinically actionable a few years later. The rhetorical question quickly becomes, 'how does a precision medicine workflow adapt to changes in foundational knowledge?' Finally, successful implementation of pharmacogenomics at the bedside is absolutely dependent on disseminating pharmacogenomics lab results in a meaningful way, particularly in a format that is readily interpretable by the provider [105].

Future Directions

At the writing of this chapter, the U.S. Food and Drug Administration's Center for Drug Evaluation & Research and Center for Biologics Evaluation & Research Office have launched an audacious challenge to generate informative knowledge from 'real world data'. Within this 'Real World Knowledge' [107] program, data from the 'real world' (e.g. insitutional EHRs, patient wearbles, and other emerging data modalities) will be used to streamline drug approvals and inform future therapeutic respositioning endeavors. This grand challenge places translational informaticians at the foci of drug development, including ascertainment of pharmacogenomic knowledge for traditional small molecule drugs and within the emerging class of biologic modalities—Biologics and designer therapies hold potential to disrupt the current understanding of pharmacogenomics. Within this framework the role of informatics in pharmacogenomics is simultaneously generating real world evidence from existing clinical practice data, and computationally overcoming knowledge gaps to generate real world knowledge.

Overcoming gaps in our knowledge of pharmacogenomics and computationally investigating counterfactual situations is a critical endeavor, and uniquely places informatics to advance precision medicine. Implementation of pharmacogenomics rules is amongst the lowest-hanging fruit in approaching precision medicine in the clinic. Spanning our existing pharmacogenomics knowledge to tailor it for special populations and predict potential drug-drug interactions in therapeutic combinations that have never been truly evaluated in the clinic are important areas for inquiry with the potential to enhance medication safety.

Summary and Conclusion

Prescribing the right drug to the right patient by tailoring clinical treatment decisions informed by an individual patient genome within the context of current knowledge is a primary goal of pharmacogenomics. In broadening our perspective of pharmacogenomics to encompass precision medicine, pharmacogenomics also seeks to maximize opportunity for drug efficacy and minimizes risk of potential ADRs or DDIs, all based on a patient's unique molecular composition.

To foster the proliferation of precision medicine, we as informaticists must press to expand upon pharmacogenomics' foundational focus on heritable traits, towards encompassing the complexity of a patient's unique molecular make-up. We must develop rigorous quantitative engines inclusive of modifiable molecular processes that affect therapeutic availability, delivery, and physiologic control. Further, informaticists hold important professional responsibilities, within broad scientific and caregiving institutional endeavors, to ensure both accuracy and equitability in accruing additional pharmacogenomics knowledge and actionability within the clinical setting. Informaticists must recognize that we hold special scientific roles with potential to profoundly affect the quality and scope of newly discovered pharmacogenomic knowledge. Most pronounced, informaticists have significant opportunities to lead, or significantly contribute to, broader efforts that ensure health equity surrounding pharmacogenomics knowledge. Finally, informaticists must ensure that pharmacogenomics be utilized to reduce opportunity for health and healthcare disparities, particularly amongst traditionally underserved populations of color. This might be accomplished by both ensuring that these minority populations are appropriately sampled (with sufficient statistical power) within local pharmacogenomic knowledgebases, and remaining vigilant to safeguard against potentially endangering these same patients from inappropriate EHR-based recommendations that either lack appropriate specificity or where the underlying pharmacogenomic knowledge was obtained from non-representative training data.

References

1. Borchardt JK. The beginnings of drug therapy: ancient mesopotamian medicine. Drug News Perspect. 2002;15(3):187–92.
2. Chalmers I, Clarke M. Commentary: the 1944 patulin trial: the first properly controlled multicentre trial conducted under the aegis of the British Medical Research Council. Int J Epidemiol. 2004;33(2):253–60.
3. Fleming A. On the antibacterial action of cultures of a Penicillium, with special reference to their use in the isolation of B. influenzæ. Br J Exp Pathol. 1929;10(3):226–36.
4. Finch CE. Evolution of the human lifespan and diseases of aging: roles of infection, inflammation, and nutrition. PNAS. 2010;107(Suppl 1):1718–24.
5. Booth FW, Roberts CK, Laye MJ. Lack of exercise is a major cause of chronic diseases. Compr Physiol. 2012 Apr;2(2):1143–211.
6. Popkin BM. Global nutrition dynamics: the world is shifting rapidly toward a diet linked with noncommunicable diseases. Am J Clin Nutr. 2006;84(2):289–98.
7. Weinshilboum R, Wang L. Pharmacogenomics: bench to bedside. Nat Rev Drug Discov. 2004;3(9):739–48.
8. Nebert DW. Pharmacogenetics and pharmacogenomics: why is this relevant to the clinical geneticist? Clin Genet. 1999;56(4):247–58.
9. Pirmohamed M. Pharmacogenetics and pharmacogenomics. Br J Clin Pharmacol. 2001;52(4):345–7.
10. Abbott S, Fairbanks DJ. Experiments on plant hybrids by Gregor Mendel. Genetics. 2016;204(2):407–22.
11. Mendel G. Experiments on plant hybrids. Verhandlungen des naturforschenden Vereines in Brunn. 1866;4:3–44.
12. Motulsky AG. Drug reactions, enzymes, and biochemical genetics. JAMA. 1957;165(7):835–7.
13. Vogel F. Moderne Probleme der Humangenetik. In: Heilmeyer L, Schoen R, de Rudder B, editors. Ergebnisse der Inneren Medizin und Kinderheilkunde. Berlin, Heidelberg: Springer; 1959. p. 52–125.

14. Vesell ES, Page JG. Genetic control of drug levels in man: phenylbutazone. Science. 1968;159(3822):1479–80.
15. Vesell ES, Page JG. Genetic control of drug levels in man: antipyrine. Science. 1968;161(3836):72–3.
16. Cappellini M, Fiorelli G. Glucose-6-phosphate dehydrogenase deficiency. Lancet. 2008;371(9606):64–74.
17. Eichelbaum M, Spannbrucker N, Steincke B, Dengler HJ. Defective N-oxidation of sparteine in man: a new pharmacogenetic defect. Eur J Clin Pharmacol. 1979;16(3):183–7.
18. Mahgoub A, Dring LG, Idle JR, Lancaster R, Smith RL. Polymorphic hydroxylation of debrisoquine in man. Lancet. 1977;310(8038):584–6.
19. Gonzalez FJ, Vilbois F, Hardwick JP, McBride OW, Nebert DW, Gelboin HV, et al. Human debrisoquine 4-hydroxylase (P450IID1): cDNA and deduced amino acid sequence and assignment of the CYP2D locus to chromosome 22. Genomics. 1988;2(2):174–9.
20. Kimura S, Umeno M, Skoda RC, Meyer UA, Gonzalez FJ. The human debrisoquine 4-hydroxylase (CYP2D) locus: sequence and identification of the polymorphic CYP2D6 gene, a related gene, and a pseudogene. Am J Hum Genet. 1989;45(6):889–904.
21. Goldstein DB. Pharmacogenetics in the laboratory and the clinic. N Engl J Med. 2003;348(6):553–6.
22. Evans WE, Relling MV. Moving towards individualized medicine with pharmacogenomics. Nature. 2004;429:464–8.
23. Zhang J, Chiodini R, Badr A, Zhang G. The impact of next-generation sequencing on genomics. J Genet Genomics. 2011;38(3):95–109.
24. Weinshilboum RM. Inheritance and drug response. N Engl J Med. 2003;348:529–37.
25. Evans WE, McLeod HL. Pharmacogenomics – drug disposition, drug targets, and side effects. N Engl J Med. 2003;348(6):538–49.
26. Davis A, Long R. Pharmacogenetics research network and Knowledge Base: 1st Annual Scientific Meeting. Pharmacogenomics. 2001;2(3):285–9.
27. Giacomini KM, Brett CM, Altman RB, Benowitz NL, Dolan ME, Flockhart DA, et al. The pharmacogenetics research network: from SNP discovery to clinical drug response. Clin Pharmacol Ther. 2007;81(3):328–45.
28. Klein TE, Chang JT, Cho MK, Easton KL, Fergerson R, Hewett M, et al. Integrating genotype and phenotype information: an overview of the PharmGKB project. Pharmacogenomics J. 2001;1(3):167–70.
29. Gottesman O, Kuivaniemi H, Tromp G, Faucett WA, Li R, Manolio TA, et al. The electronic medical records and genomics (eMERGE) network: past, present, and future. Genet Med. 2013;15(10):761–71.
30. Manolio TA, Chisholm RL, Ozenberger B, Roden DM, Williams MS, Wilson R, et al. Implementing genomic medicine in the clinic: the future is here. Genet Med. 2013;15(4):258–67.
31. Rasmussen-Torvik LJ, Stallings SC, Gordon AS, Almoguera B, Basford MA, Bielinski SJ, et al. Design and anticipated outcomes of the eMERGE-PGx project: a multicenter pilot for preemptive pharmacogenomics in electronic health record systems. Clin Pharmacol Ther. 2014;96(4):482–9.
32. Kirby JC, Speltz P, Rasmussen LV, Basford M, Gottesman O, Peissig PL, et al. PheKB: a catalog and workflow for creating electronic phenotype algorithms for transportability. J Am Med Inform Assoc. 2016;23(6):1046–52.
33. Etheredge LM. A rapid-learning health system. Health Aff. 2007;26(2):w107–18.
34. Mandl KD, Kohane IS, McFadden D, Weber GM, Natter M, Mandel J, et al. Scalable collaborative infrastructure for a learning healthcare system (SCILHS): architecture. J Am Med Inform Assoc. 2014;21(4):615–20.
35. McGinnis JM, Aisner D, Olsen L. The learning healthcare system: workshop summary. Washington, DC: National Academies Press; 2007.
36. Tenenbaum JD, Avillach P, Benham-Hutchins M, Breitenstein MK, Crowgey EL, Hoffman MA, et al. An informatics research agenda to support precision medicine: seven key areas. J Am Med Inform Assoc. 2016;23(4):791–5.

37. Gardner RM, Overhage JM, Steen EB, Munger BS, Holmes JH, Williamson JJ, et al. Core content for the subspecialty of clinical informatics. J Am Med Inform Assoc. 2009;16(2):153–7.
38. Safran C, Shabot MM, Munger BS, Holmes JH, Steen EB, Lumpkin JR, et al. Program requirements for fellowship education in the subspecialty of clinical informatics. J Am Med Inform Assoc. 2009;16(2):158–66.
39. Shortliffe EH. President's column: subspecialty certification in clinical informatics. J Am Med Inform Assoc. 2011;18(6):890–1.
40. Lander ES, Linton LM, Birren B, Nusbaum C, Zody MC, Baldwin J, et al. Initial sequencing and analysis of the human genome. Nature. 2001;409(6822):860–921.
41. Sanger F, Coulson AR. A rapid method for determining sequences in DNA by primed synthesis with DNA polymerase. J Mol Biol. 1975;94(3):441–8.
42. Sanger F, Nicklen S, Coulson AR. DNA sequencing with chain-terminating inhibitors. PNAS. 1977;74(12):5463–7.
43. Sanger F, Air GM, Barrell BG, Brown NL, Coulson AR, Fiddes JC, et al. Nucleotide sequence of bacteriophage φX174 DNA. Nature. 1977;265(5596):687–95.
44. Shendure J, Ji H. Next-generation DNA sequencing. Nat Biotechnol. 2008;26(10):1135–45.
45. Cooper GM, Johnson JA, Langaee TY, Feng H, Stanaway IB, Schwarz UI, et al. A genome-wide scan for common genetic variants with a large influence on warfarin maintenance dose. Blood. 2008;112(4):1022–7.
46. Limdi NA, Veenstra DL. Warfarin pharmacogenetics. Pharmacotherapy. 2008;28(9):1084–97.
47. Limdi NA, Veenstra DL. Expectations, validity, and reality in pharmacogenetics. J Clin Epidemiol. 2010;63(9):960–9.
48. Motsinger-Reif AA, Jorgenson E, Relling MV, Kroetz DL, Weinshilboum R, Cox NJ, et al. Genome-wide association studies in pharmacogenomics: successes and lessons. Pharmacogenet Genomics. 2013;23(8):383–94.
49. Gargis AS, Kalman L, Berry MW, Bick DP, Dimmock DP, Hambuch T, et al. Assuring the quality of next-generation sequencing in clinical laboratory practice. Nat Biotechnol. 2012;30(11):1033–6.
50. Gargis AS, Kalman L, Bick DP, da Silva C, Dimmock DP, Funke BH, et al. Good laboratory practice for clinical next-generation sequencing informatics pipelines. Nat Biotechnol. 2015;33(7):689–93.
51. Lih C-J, Takebe N. Considerations of developing an NGS assay for clinical applications in precision oncology: the NCI-MATCH NGS assay experience. Curr Probl Cancer. 2017;41(3):201–11.
52. Lubin IM, Kalman L, Gargis AS. Guidelines and approaches to compliance with regulatory and clinical standards: quality control procedures and quality assurance. In: Wong L-JC, editor. Next generation sequencing: translation to clinical diagnostics. New York, NY: Springer New York; 2013. p. 255–73. https://doi.org/10.1007/978-1-4614-7001-4_14.
53. Strom SP. Current practices and guidelines for clinical next-generation sequencing oncology testing. Cancer Biol Med. 2016;13(1):3–11.
54. Panoutsopoulou K, Walter K. Quality control of common and rare variants. In: Evangelou E, editor. Genetic epidemiology: methods and protocols. New York, NY: Springer New York; 2018. p. 25–36. https://doi.org/10.1007/978-1-4939-7868-7_3.
55. Schaid DJ, Chen W, Larson NB. From genome-wide associations to candidate causal variants by statistical fine-mapping. Nat Rev Genet. 2018;19(8):491–504.
56. Gudbjartsson DF, Helgason H, Gudjonsson SA, Zink F, Oddson A, Gylfason A, et al. Large-scale whole-genome sequencing of the Icelandic population. Nat Genet. 2015;47(5):435–44.
57. Johnson RC, Nelson GW, Troyer JL, Lautenberger JA, Kessing BD, Winkler CA, et al. Accounting for multiple comparisons in a genome-wide association study (GWAS). BMC Genomics. 2010;11(1):724.
58. Popejoy AB, Fullerton SM. Genomics is failing on diversity. Nat News. 2016;538(7624):161–4.
59. Martin A, Downing J, Maden M, Fleeman N, Alfirevic A, Haycox A, et al. An assessment of the impact of pharmacogenomics on health disparities: a systematic literature review. Pharmacogenomics. 2017;18(16):1541–50.

60. Ackerman MJ. Genetic purgatory and the cardiac channelopathies: exposing the variants of uncertain/unknown significance issue. Heart Rhythm. 2015;12(11):2325–31.
61. Kwok PY. Methods for genotyping single nucleotide polymorphisms. Annu Rev Genomics Hum Genet. 2001;2:235–58.
62. Roses AD. Pharmacogenetics and the practice of medicine. Nature. 2000;405:857–65.
63. Kitts A, Sherry S. The single nucleotide polymorphism database (dbSNP) of nucleotide sequence variation. Bethesda, MD: National Center for Biotechnology Information (US); 2011. https://www.ncbi.nlm.nih.gov/books/NBK21088/
64. Landrum MJ, Lee JM, Benson M, Brown G, Chao C, Chitipiralla S, et al. ClinVar: public archive of interpretations of clinically relevant variants. Nucleic Acids Res. 2016;44(D1):D862–8.
65. Lek M, Karczewski KJ, Minikel EV, Samocha KE, Banks E, Fennell T, et al. Analysis of protein-coding genetic variation in 60,706 humans. Nature. 2016;536(7616):285–91.
66. Karczewski K. The genome Aggregation Database (gnomAD). MacArthur Lab. 2017. https://macarthurlab.org/2017/02/27/the-genome-aggregation-database-gnomad/
67. Relling MV, Klein TE. CPIC: clinical pharmacogenetics implementation consortium of the pharmacogenomics research network. Clin Pharmacol Ther. 2011;89(3):464–7.
68. Kluyver T, Ragan-Kelley B, Pérez F, Granger BE, Bussonnier M, Frederic J, et al. Jupyter notebooks-a publishing format for reproducible computational workflows. In: ELPUB. 2016. p. 87–90.
69. Breitenstein MK, Liu H, Maxwell KN, Pathak J, Zhang R. Electronic health record phenotypes for precision medicine: perspectives and caveats from treatment of breast cancer at a single institution. Clin Transl Sci. 2018;11(1):85–92.
70. Government Printing Office. Clinical Laboratory Improvement Amendments (42 USC 263a) [Internet]. 42. Sect. § 263a. Certification of laboratories; 1988. p. 371–8. https://www.govinfo.gov/content/pkg/USCODE-2011-title42/pdf/USCODE-2011-title42-chap6A-subchapII-partF-subpart2-sec263a.pdf.
71. Olson RS, Bartley N, Urbanowicz RJ, Moore JH. Evaluation of a tree-based pipeline optimization tool for automating data science. In: Proceedings of the genetic and evolutionary computation conference 2016. New York, NY: ACM; 2016. p. 485–92. (GECCO'16). https://doi.org/10.1145/2908812.2908918.
72. Olson RS, Urbanowicz RJ, Andrews PC, Lavender NA, Kidd LC, Moore JH. Automating biomedical data science through tree-based pipeline optimization. In: Squillero G, Burelli P, editors. Applications of evolutionary computation. Switzerland: Springer International Publishing; 2016. p. 123–37.
73. Orlenko A, Moore JH, Orzechowski P, Olson RS, Cairns J, Caraballo PJ, et al. Considerations for automated machine learning in clinical metabolic profiling: altered homocysteine plasma concentration associated with metformin exposure. Pac Symp Biocomput. 2018;23:460–71.
74. Urbanowicz RJ, Meeker M, La Cava W, Olson RS, Moore JH. Relief-based feature selection: introduction and review. J Biomed Inform. 2018;85:189–203.
75. Ali M, Aittokallio T. Machine learning and feature selection for drug response prediction in precision oncology applications. Biophys Rev. 2019;11(1):31–9.
76. Breitenstein, Matthew K, Hu, Vincent, Bhatnagar, R, Ratnagiri, M. Approaching neural net feature interpretation using stacked autoencoders: gene expression profiling of systemic lupus erythematosus patients. In: Proceedings of the AMIA 2019 Informatics Summit. San Francisco, CA; 2019. p. 8.
77. Crowgey EL, Marsh AG, Robinson KG, Yeager SK, Akins RE. Epigenetic machine learning: utilizing DNA methylation patterns to predict spastic cerebral palsy. BMC Bioinformatics. 2018;19(1):225.
78. Whirl-Carrillo M, McDonagh EM, Hebert JM, Gong L, Sangkuhl K, Thorn CF, et al. Pharmacogenomics knowledge for personalized medicine. Clin Pharmacol Ther. 2012;92(4):414–7.
79. Kass-Hout TA, Litwack D. Advancing precision medicine by enabling a collaborative informatics community. FDA Voice. 2015. https://web.archive.

org/web/20151222181400/http://blogs.fda.gov/fdavoice/index.php/2015/08/advancing-precision-medicine-by-enabling-a-collaborative-informatics-community/

80. Klein TE, Ritchie MD. PharmCAT: a pharmacogenomics clinical annotation tool. Clin Pharmacol Ther. 2018;104(1):19–22.

81. Amberger JS, Hamosh A. Searching Online Mendelian Inheritance in Man (OMIM): a knowledgebase of human genes and genetic phenotypes. Curr Protoc Bioinformatics. 2017;27(58):1.2.1–1.2.12.

82. Wu G, Dawson E, Duong A, Haw R, Stein L. ReactomeFIViz: a Cytoscape app for pathway and network-based data analysis. F1000Res. 2014;3:146.

83. Kanehisa M, Sato Y, Kawashima M, Furumichi M, Tanabe M. KEGG as a reference resource for gene and protein annotation. Nucleic Acids Res. 2016;44(D1):D457–62.

84. Szklarczyk D, Morris JH, Cook H, Kuhn M, Wyder S, Simonovic M, et al. The STRING database in 2017: quality-controlled protein–protein association networks, made broadly accessible. Nucleic Acids Res. 2017;45(D1):D362–8.

85. The UniProt Consortium. UniProt: the universal protein knowledgebase. Nucleic Acids Res. 2017;45(D1):D158–69.

86. Wilke RA, Mareedu RK, Moore JH. The pathway less traveled: moving from candidate genes to candidate pathways in the analysis of genome-wide data from large scale Pharmacogenetic association studies. Curr Pharmacogenomics Person Med. 2008;6(3):150–9.

87. Grados MA, Specht MW, Sung H-M, Fortune D. Glutamate drugs and pharmacogenetics of OCD: a pathway-based exploratory approach. Expert Opin Drug Discov. 2013;8(12):1515–27.

88. Ashburner M, Ball CA, Blake JA, Botstein D, Butler H, Cherry JM, Davis AP, Dolinski K, Dwight SS, Eppig JT, Harris MA. Gene ontology: tool for the unification of biology. Nat Genet. 2000;25(1):25.

89. Gene Ontology Consortium. Expansion of the gene ontology knowledgebase and resources. Nucleic Acids Res. 2017;45(D1):D331–8.

90. Hoehndorf R, Dumontier M, Gkoutos GV. Identifying aberrant pathways through integrated analysis of knowledge in pharmacogenomics. Bioinformatics. 2012;28(16):2169–75.

91. Wishart DS, Feunang YD, Guo AC, Lo EJ, Marcu A, Grant JR, et al. DrugBank 5.0: a major update to the DrugBank database for 2018. Nucleic Acids Res. 2017;46(D1):D1074–82.

92. Davis AP, Grondin CJ, Johnson RJ, Sciaky D, King BL, McMorran R, et al. The comparative toxicogenomics database: update 2017. Nucleic Acids Res. 2016;45(D1):D972–8.

93. Ginsburg GS, Phillips KA. Precision medicine: from science to value. Health Aff. 2018;37(5):694–701.

94. Becquemont L. Pharmacogenomics of adverse drug reactions: practical applications and perspectives. Pharmacogenomics. 2009;10(6):961–9.

95. Innocenti F. Genomics and pharmacogenomics in anticancer drug development and clinical response. Berlin: Springer Science & Business Media; 2008. p. 379.

96. Wang K, Li M, Hakonarson H. ANNOVAR: functional annotation of genetic variants from high-throughput sequencing data. Nucleic Acids Res. 2010;38(16):e164.

97. Guo Y, Dai Y, Yu H, Zhao S, Samuels DC, Shyr Y. Improvements and impacts of GRCh38 human reference on high throughput sequencing data analysis. Genomics. 2017;109(2):83–90.

98. Schneider VA, Graves-Lindsay T, Howe K, Bouk N, Chen H-C, Kitts PA, et al. Evaluation of GRCh38 and de novo haploid genome assemblies demonstrates the enduring quality of the reference assembly. Genome Res. 2017;27(5):849–64.

99. Ezkurdia I, Juan D, Rodriguez JM, Frankish A, Diekhans M, Harrow J, et al. Multiple evidence strands suggest that there may be as few as 19 000 human protein-coding genes. Hum Mol Genet. 2014;23(22):5866–78.

100. Uhlén M, Fagerberg L, Hallström BM, Lindskog C, Oksvold P, Mardinoglu A, et al. Tissue-based map of the human proteome. Science. 2015;347(6220):1260419.

101. Bauer MS, Damschroder L, Hagedorn H, Smith J, Kilbourne AM. An introduction to implementation science for the non-specialist. BMC Psychol. 2015;3:32.

102. Weitzel KW, Alexander M, Bernhardt BA, Calman N, Carey DJ, Cavallari LH, et al. The IGNITE network: a model for genomic medicine implementation and research. BMC Med Genet. 2016;9:1.

103. Amendola LM, Berg JS, Horowitz CR, Angelo F, Bensen JT, Biesecker BB, et al. The clinical sequencing evidence-generating research consortium: integrating genomic sequencing in diverse and medically underserved populations. Am J Hum Genet. 2018;103(3):319–27.
104. Nishimura AA, Tarczy-Hornoch P, Shirts BH. Pragmatic and ethical challenges of incorporating the genome into the electronic medical record. Curr Genet Med Rep. 2014;2(4):201–11.
105. Caraballo PJ, Bielinski SJ, St Sauver JL, Weinshilboum RM. Electronic medical record-integrated pharmacogenomics and related clinical decision support concepts. Clin Pharmacol Ther. 2017;102(2):254–64.
106. American Medical Association. The hidden dangers of EHR pop-up fatigue | American Medical Association. 2015. https://www.ama-assn.org/practice-management/digital/hidden-dangers-ehr-pop-fatigue
107. U.S. Food & Drug Administration. Framework for FDA's Real-World Evidence Program. 2018. https://www.fda.gov/downloads/ScienceResearch/SpecialTopics/RealWorldEvidence/UCM627769.pdf

Chapter 6
The Growing Medication Problem: Perspective from Industry

Jason Ross

Introduction

According to the IMS Institute for Healthcare Informatics, over four billion pre-scriptions are filled each year [1]. While many people experience effective therapy, not all drugs are effective for all people. In fact, response rates for many drugs are only 50–75% [2]. In addition, adverse drug reactions produce more than 3.5 million physician office visits [3] and approximately 1 million emergency department visits [4] annually, as well as contributing an estimated $3.5 billion to U.S. healthcare costs [5]. These issues are largely thought to be related to a few paradigms in drug delivery and development. First, today's standard of care for prescribing medica-tions is still largely dependent on a "trial and error" approach. Second, pharmaceuti-cal companies utilize observed population averages to establish medication guidelines, including dosages, disease effectiveness and side effects. Third, our genetics play a significant role in the effectiveness of many medications, however, very few providers have access to, understand, or use this information effectively when making prescription decisions.

In 2014, following the discovery that advances in genomic testing and interpreta-tion can help to mitigate issues with today's prescribing practices, leading pharma-cogenomic experts from Mayo Clinic co-founded OneOme. Their vision was to give healthcare providers access to high quality pharmacogenomic solutions to help

J. Ross (✉)
OneOme, Minneapolis, MN, USA
e-mail: jasonross@oneome.com

© Springer Nature Switzerland AG 2020
T. Adam, C. Aliferis (eds.), *Personalized and Precision Medicine Informatics*,
Health Informatics, https://doi.org/10.1007/978-3-030-18626-5_6

them make more informed prescription decisions based on an individual's specific genetic makeup, and to make those solutions available to everyone.

RightMed® Comprehensive Solution

Since 2014, OneOme has been focused on creating and providing the most credible, comprehensive pharmacogenomic solution in the world. OneOme identified the most relevant medications influenced by genetics for common medical conditions. This process led OneOme to develop complex pharmacological and genetic models that have the ability to predict drug response for over 250 medications. These models are the foundation of the RightMed® comprehensive solution, which samples an individual's DNA (obtained by cheek swab), performs genetic testing for 27 different genes, and predicts how variants in your genome may impact the medication response for all 250 medications, spanning over 30 medical conditions.

Precision Medicine Information Challenge

One of the largest challenges within precision medicine is making complex scientific information understandable and actionable for healthcare providers. Even in the age of precision medicine, many providers have limited genetic training and require solutions that aid them in interpretation and clinical action. For pharmacogenomics, this involves providing genetic results, explaining how these results affect an individual's response to medication(s), and providing relevant clinical action (when possible). OneOme has addressed this challenge in the RightMed comprehensive report, through the use of icons, colors, graphics and concise information to help providers to quickly identify potential medication issues for a patient. In addition to the comprehensive report, OneOme offers additional reports and interactive applications that enables providers to tailor the level and amount of information presented based on the providers' medical specialty and patient needs.

Another challenge is that commercial electronic health record (EHR) systems dictate most providers' workflows and access to clinical information. These systems are wonderful at offering standardized information and functionality for common, well established diagnostic testing; however they often are unable to manage and utilize a patient's genomic information. To overcome this challenge, OneOme has developed solutions to integrate with the providers' EHR. Integration capabilities include direct test ordering in the EHR and real-time alerts at the point of prescribing. This solution creates further value by providing only relevant information about the patient, as needed.

OneOme Future Plans

Pharmacogenomics is at the forefront of bringing precision medicine into routine care and has the potential to impact each and every person utilizing medication therapies. Yet, barriers still remain to adoption, including lack of provider understanding, limited clinical evidence, and problems with workflow integration. To address these barriers we need to develop innovative solutions and awareness through provider education. At OneOme, we continue focusing on all of these barriers through the following approaches: (1) Creation of educational events and programs that allow providers to experience testing and benefits for themselves; (2) Completion of clinical trials to demonstrate clinical utility; (3) Provision of educational materials to patients about the issues and benefits of pharmacogenomics; (4) Development of technology solutions that provide real-time medication insight to providers within existing EHR systems; (5) Building tools to help identify patients who are at higher risk of adverse events or poor therapeutic response.

The promise of precision medicine is real and can fundamentally change the practice of healthcare in the near future. We need to be ready to understand and leverage these rapid advancements so that potential patient benefits become reality.

References

1. QuintilesIMS Institute. Medicines Use and Spending in the U.S.: A Review of 2016 and Outlook to 2021 [Internet]. Parsippany, NJ; 2017. https://structurecms-staging-psyclone.netdna-ssl.com/client_assets/dwonk/media/attachments/590c/6aa0/6970/2d2d/4182/0000/590c6aa069702d2d41820000.pdf?1493985952.
2. Spear BB, Heath-Chiozzi M, Huff J. Clinical application of pharmacogenetics. Trends Mol Med. 2001;7:201–4. http://www.ncbi.nlm.nih.gov/pubmed/11325631.
3. Bourgeois FT, Shannon MW, Valim C, Mandl KD. Adverse drug events in the outpatient setting: an 11-year national analysis. Pharmacoepidemiol Drug Saf. 2010;19(9):901–10.
4. Budnitz DS, Pollock DA, Weidenbach KN, Mendelsohn AB, Schroeder TJ, Annest JL. National surveillance of emergency department visits for outpatient adverse drug events. JAMA. 2006;296(15):1858.
5. Institute of Medicine Committee on Identifying and Preventing Medication Errors. Preventing medication errors: quality chasm series. Washington, DC: The National Academies Press; 2006.

Part III
Emerging PPM

Chapter 7
Risk Stratification and Prognosis Using Predictive Modelling and Big Data Approaches

Shyam Visweswaran and Gregory F. Cooper

Introduction to Predictive Models in Medicine

Prediction is critical to many activities in clinical medicine, such as assessing risk of developing disease in the future (risk assessment and stratification), determining the presence or absence of disease at the current time (diagnosis), forecasting the likely course of disease (prognosis), and predicting treatment response (therapeutics) [1]. In addition to clinical medicine, prediction plays a critical role in public health and in biomedical research. Predictive models that are derived from data can improve predictions and help guide decision-making in clinical medicine and in public health. Often predictive models are probabilistic models that compute the prediction as a probability, and such models are typically estimated from data using statistical and, more recently, machine-learning methods.

The better the predictive models, the better the decisions and the ensuing outcomes are likely to be for the individual and for the public at large. Even small improvements in predictive performance can have meaningful impact on individual and public health outcomes and costs. The burgeoning field of precision and personalized medicine aims to tailor risk assessment, diagnosis, prognosis and therapeutics to the characteristics of individuals that go beyond those measured during routine clinical care. The goal is to deliver the right treatment at the right time to the right patient based on complex patient characteristics that may be obtained from a range of molecular, clinical, and environmental measurements.

Traditionally, predictive models in medicine have been developed from data such as clinical findings, laboratory test results, and findings from clinical imag-

S. Visweswaran (✉) · G. F. Cooper
Department of Biomedical Informatics and of Intelligent Systems, University of Pittsburgh, Pittsburgh, PA, USA
e-mail: shv3@pitt.edu; gfc@cbmi.pitt.edu

© Springer Nature Switzerland AG 2020
T. Adam, C. Aliferis (eds.), *Personalized and Precision Medicine Informatics*, Health Informatics, https://doi.org/10.1007/978-3-030-18626-5_7

ing studies. Recent advances in two areas are making available big biomedical data at an unprecedented scale for use in clinical medicine, public health, and research. Electronic health records (EHRs) are widespread and are capturing ever more clinical data. EHR data coupled with administrative claims data are increasingly used for characterization of disease progression and outcomes, comparative effectiveness of treatments, and predictive and prognostic modeling. Such observational healthcare data sets contain data on millions to tens of millions of patients and hold the promise of enabling research into less frequent diseases and outcomes. Another advance is the burgeoning use of low cost omics technologies, which is producing a rich base of high-throughput molecular data, such as genomic variant, gene expression, proteomic, and metabolomic data. Omics data in conjunction with EHR data hold the promise of better prediction of diseases before their occurrence, increased accuracy of diagnosis of complex diseases, and more precisely targeted therapies.

Examples of Applications

Predictive models have applications in the domains of clinical practice, in public health, and in biomedical research. Table 7.1 gives illustrative examples of the application of predictive models for risk assessment across all three domains.

In *clinical medicine*, both predictive models and clinical decision rules are useful in assisting clinicians with decision making. Predictive models generate probabilities but do not recommend actions and the interpretation of the probabilities is left to the clinician. Clinical decision rules, in addition, suggest actions based on probabilities generated by a predictive model. Risk assessment models are useful in evaluating risk for developing disease that informs the initiation of preventive measures. An example of a risk assessment model is the Framingham Risk Score that predicts the 10-year risk of developing coronary heart disease from age, total and HDL cholesterol, blood pressure, diabetes, and smoking status [2]. This score is used clinically to identify those at high risk and initiate life style changes and cholesterol lowering pharmacotherapy.

Table 7.1 Illustrative examples of prediction that guide decision-making

Domain	Prediction task	Decision to make
Clinical medicine	Will an individual have a heart attack in the coming year?	Prescribe aspirin or not
Public health	How many residents of a county will have a heart attack in a year?	Determine the number of paramedics to be trained to perform electrocardiograms in ambulances
Biomedical research	How many heart attacks are likely to occur in the control arm of a clinical trial?	Enroll fewer or more participants

Predictive models are also useful for deciding whether or not to perform diagnostic testing. When the probability of the presence of disease is relatively high, diagnostic testing is indicated to confirm or rule out disease, while if the probability is low, no immediate testing is indicated. For example, sepsis is a relatively rare but a life-threatening cause of infection, and the definitive diagnostic test is a blood culture to detect bacteremia (presence of viable bacteria in circulating blood). A clinical decision rule has been described to selectively perform blood cultures in Emergency Department patients who are predicted to be at high risk of bacteremia. Features of the history, co-existing illnesses, physical examination, and laboratory testing were used to create a clinical decision rule that consists of major and minor criteria, and blood culture is indicated if at least one major criterion or two minor criteria are present [3, 4].

Furthermore, predictive models are useful for selecting treatment such that the anticipated benefit exceeds the risk of harm. For example, in patients with atrial fibrillation, antithrombotic agents are effective in reducing the risk of stroke while concurrently increasing the risk of serious bleeding. Predictive models that estimate a patient's stroke risk and bleeding risk are useful in identifying the appropriate antithrombotic agent for which the reduction in the risk of stroke most strongly outweighs the increased risk of bleeding [5].

In *public health*, predictive models are useful in surveillance and forecasting of epidemics like influenza. Traditional surveillance that is provided, for example, by the Centers for Disease Control and Prevention (CDC) relies on clinical findings, virology laboratory results, hospital admissions, and mortality data. Newer digital surveillance employs sources such as over-the-counter retail sales of medications, social network activity, and internet search engine queries [6]. Such surveillance produces forecasts that assist health officials to inform public health actions and allocate resources.

In *biomedical research*, predictive models may be useful in selection and stratification of participants in terms of baseline as well as predicted characteristics for a study such as a clinical trial. This allows enrollment of more refined subgroups and improves statistical analyses. For example, a trial in traumatic brain injury may exclude patients with high likelihood of a poor outcome. A prognostic model that predicts 6-month mortality in traumatic brain injury can be used to select patients who have a small probability of mortality [7].

Prognostic Versus Predictive Factors

Some authors in the biomedical literature differentiate between prognostic and predictive factors or biomarkers. A prognostic factor is defined as a clinical or biological characteristic that is associated with a clinical outcome such as development or progression of disease, irrespective of the treatment. A predictive factor is defined as a characteristic that is associated specifically with response or lack of response to a particular therapy [8, 9]. For example, a prognostic factor for primary breast cancer is any measurement available at the time of diagnosis or surgery that is associated with disease-free or overall survival in the absence of systemic adjuvant therapy, while a predictive factor is one that is associated with response or lack of response to systemic adjuvant therapy [8]. In this framework, a prognostic factor is predictive of a clinical outcome and a predictive factor is predictive of differences in response to a therapy. However, in this chapter, the terms prognostic and predictive are considered to be synonymous and denote the ability of a factor to predict outcomes.

Workflow of Development and Validation of Predictive Models

The development of predictive models in medicine consists of two phases, namely, derivation (or training) and validation (or external validation) [10, 11]. The workflow in the two phases is shown in Fig. 7.1. The derivation phase consists of collection of training or derivation data, preprocessing of the data that includes handling missing values and feature selection, building a multivariable model, and performing internal validation to assess the model's predictive performance for discrimination and calibration. Internal validation is performed by splitting the data into training and test, by cross-fold validation or by leave-one-out validation. To perform cross-fold validation, data is partitioned into several equal parts; all parts except one are combined and the model is derived from it and evaluated on the left out part; this process is performed once for each part.

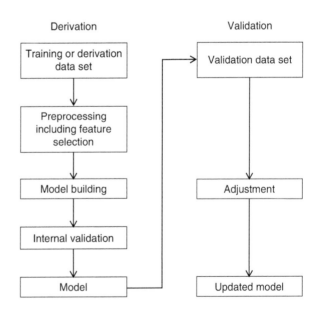

Fig. 7.1 Workflow of development of clinical predictive models. The two phases are derivation followed by validation. (Adapted from Fig. 1 in Ref. [10])

In the external validation phase, the predictive performance of the model is evaluated on data that is obtained independently of the derivation data. External validation is needed to assess generalizability of the model, such as temporal generalizability across data from different time periods, geographical generalizability across data obtained from different physical locations, and spectrum generalizability across data that possess differing disease severity or varying prevalence of the outcome. When external validation suggests that model performance needs to be improved, the model may have to be rebuilt or updated using the validation data. If the model is updated, the new model should be assessed for external validity on data that is obtained independently of the derivation and validation data before it is considered for deployment.

Emerging Informatics Methods

Challenges abound in the development of predictive models. This chapter focusses on four challenges and new approaches to surmount them. A critical challenge in the developing predictive models from big data is dimensionality reduction, which is the process of reducing the number of features in the data. Another challenge is the development of models that can not only adequately discriminate between individuals who will have an outcome and those who will not but also possess adequate calibration to predict accurately the actual risk of outcome [12]. For example, the European System for Cardiac Operative Risk Evaluation Score (EuroSCORE), a model to predict mortality from cardiac surgery, showed excellent discrimination but had poor calibration because it overestimated the risk of mortality in elderly patients (e.g., the model predicted mortality risk of 15% when the actual risk of dying after surgery was 8.8%) [13]. An updated version of the score called EuroSCORE II was developed to improve calibration [14]. A third challenge is developing models that perform well not only on the population as a whole but also perform well in the individual. Personalized modeling approaches can produce high performing and simpler models that are tailored to the individual. Finally, explanations for predictions produced by predictive models are necessary for real-world deployment.

Dimensionality Reduction

Two main approaches to dimensionality reduction are feature selection and feature extraction. Feature selection is the process of selecting a subset of the original set of features, to obtain a smaller subset, and feature extraction is the process of creating a new, smaller set of features from the original set of features. Thus, feature selection preserves a subset of the original features while feature extraction creates new ones.

In biomedical data sets where the number of features is in the tens of thousands or more, many of the potential predictor features are either redundant or irrelevant for predicting the target outcome. Predictive modeling techniques, including regression and classification methods, often perform poorly when all features are included, due to irrelevant features introducing noise. One approach is to preprocess the data set by selecting a reduced subset of features, and use that subset for predictive modeling. In addition to improving the predictive model's performance, feature selection reduces the computational cost and may provide better interpretability of the underlying processes that generated the data [15].

A good feature selection method identifies the smallest number of features that deliver maximal predictive performance. Feature selection methods can be broadly categorized into wrapper and filter methods. Wrapper methods evaluate feature subsets using the predictive model and select the best performing subset. Filter methods do not use the predictive model but instead apply statistical criteria to select the features and then construct the model with the selected features.

A filter-type feature selection approach that has been investigated extensively is based on identifying the Markov blanket of the outcome or target [16]. The Markov blanket of a target is defined as a minimal set conditioned on which all other measured features become independent of the target. A variety of Markov blanket discovery algorithms have been developed and evaluated on biomedical data [17].

Markov Blanket Algorithms

A Bayesian network (BN) model is a graphical model that represents probabilistic relationships among a set of features X. A BN contains a graphical model structure that is a directed acyclic graph (DAG) that contains a node for every feature X_i and an arc between every pair of nodes if the corresponding features are directly probabilistically dependent. Conversely, the absence of an arc between a pair of nodes denotes probabilistic independence (often conditional) between the corresponding features. In addition, a BN contains a set of parameters θ that encode the probability distributions. In a BN, the immediate predecessors of a node X_i are called the parents of X_i, the immediate successors are called the children of X_i, and the remote successors are called the descendants of X_i. The joint probability distribution over X, represented by the parameters θ can be factored into a product of probability distributions defined on each node in the network.

The Markov blanket (MB) of a target X_i, is a set of features such that conditioned on the MB, X_i is conditionally independent of all other features. The MB consists of the parents, the children, and the parents of the children of X_i (see Fig. 7.2). The MB of a node X_i is noteworthy because it identifies a minimal set of features that are maximally predictive of X_i. A comprehensive review of the methods for the discovery of MBs from data is provided in [17, 18].

One of the earliest algorithms that discover MBs from data is the Grow-Shrink (GS) algorithm that works in two stages [19]. In the growing phase, it identifies

Fig. 7.2 An example MB. The MB of the node X_6 (shown stippled) consists of parents, X_2 and X_3, children, X_8 and X_9, and parents of the children, X_5 and X_7. Nodes X_1, X_4, X_{10} and X_{11} are not part of the MB of X_6

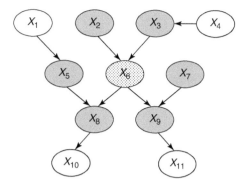

features that are strongly associated with the target and in the shrinking phase, it reduces the estimated MB from the growing phase using conditional independence tests. The shrinking phase of the GS algorithm is not sound; this phase is improved in the Incremental Association Markov Blanket (IAMB) algorithm [20]. The growing phase of IAMB identifies all features that have a strong association with the target using a conditional mutual information test that conditions on the features in the MB so far. Falsely included features are removed in the shrinking phase that uses a conditional independence test between each feature in the MB and the target given the remaining features in the MB. The IAMB was shown to select MB features that when used in predictive models out performed classification algorithms when applied directly to the data without filtering. Moreover, though the MB itself can be used directly as a predictive model, it was out performed by other classification algorithms that used the features selected by IAMB [20]. Furthermore, IAMB and its variants were the first of the MB algorithms that were shown to scale to high-dimensional data sets.

More efficient and scalable algorithms that were introduced after IAMB include HITON and Max-Min Markov Blanket (MMMB) [21, 22]. These algorithms were shown to find MBs in a scalable and efficient manner. When HITON was evaluated in clinical, text, genomic, structural and proteomic data it was shown to have excellent performance in terms of parsimony and classification performance. Progress in developing scalable MB algorithms continues including the development of better conditional independence tests such as the kernel-based tests [23].

Biologically Motivated Feature Extraction

A commonly used technique of feature extraction is Principal Component Analysis that constructs a small set of discriminative features from the original features. Another technique is to use available knowledge to extract features. For example, features in gene expression data that contain measurements of individual genes are combined to create pathway features based on current knowledge of known genes that are members of signaling and metabolic pathways. The pathway features are used to develop predictive models such as outcomes in cancer. This approach can also be viewed as automated, biologically inspired dimensionality reduction where the features are extracted automatically inspired by the types of pathways that are likely driving outcomes.

Model Averaging

When predictive models are estimated from data, multiple models often fit the data more or less equally well. It is usual, then, to select one of the models according to some criteria like model fit to the data or predictive performance of the model. The selection of one model over others that are almost as good can lead to overconfident predictions since it ignores the uncertainty in choosing one model to the exclusion of all others. Hence, it is desirable to model this source of uncertainty by appropriate selection and combination of multiple models. One coherent approach to dealing with the uncertainty in model selection is Bayesian model averaging (BMA) that is an extension of standard Bayesian inference. Typical Bayesian inference models parameter uncertainty through prior distributions, and BMA extends this approach to model uncertainty by estimating posterior distributions for both model parameters and the model structure [24].

BMA estimates the outcome as a weighted average of the outcome predictions of a set of models, with more probable models influencing the prediction more than less probable ones. In practical situations, the number of models to be considered may be enormous, and averaging the predictions over all of them by enumerating each model is infeasible. In selected model families, a closed form solution is available. The next section describes one such example where prediction using the naïve Bayes model can be performed efficiently by averaging over all naïve Bayes models. In most situations, a closed form solution will not be available. A pragmatic approach, then, is to average over a few good models, termed selective Bayesian model averaging, which serves to approximate the prediction obtained from averaging over all models.

Madigan and Raftery show that BMA is expected to have better predictive performance than any single model [25]. Empirically, the superior performance of BMA is supported by a range of case studies. Yeung et al. applied BMA to select genes from DNA microarray data to predict prognosis in breast cancer and showed that BMA identified smaller numbers of relevant genes that had comparable prediction accuracy to other methods that identified larger numbers of genes [26]. Wei et al. applied BMA to high-dimensional single nucleotide polymorphism (SNP) data and showed that it has better predictive performance than model selection [27]. A good overview of BMA is provided in [24] and a comprehensive review of the applications of BMA is described in [28].

Model Averaged Naïve Bayes

Bayesian model averaging of naïve Bayes (NB) models can improve predictions over a single NB model. The single NB model is widely used because of good discriminative performance and computational efficiency. However, on high-dimensional data sets, such as genome-wide single nucleotide polymorphisms (with features in the hundreds of thousands to millions), the predictions of NB tend to be poorly calibrated so that the predictions are too extreme with probabilities that are too close to 0 and 1. The model-averaged naïve Bayes (MANB) algorithm produces predictions by performing BMA over all possible NB models produced by feature selection on a given set of available predictors [29]. MANB averages over the predictions of these models, weighted by the posterior probability of each model. Compared to NB, MANB addresses the challenges of feature selection and tends to have better calibration than NB. MANB has almost the same computationally efficiency as NB. When evaluated on a genome-wide association dataset to predict late-onset Alzheimer's disease, MANB performed significantly better than NB, in terms of both discrimination and calibration [27].

Personalized Modeling

Much of predictive modeling in biomedicine has been based on the expected outcome of an average patient. Data from a population of patients with the same disease are pooled together for statistical analysis, and models derived from the analysis inform the management of future patients. In other words, the typical approach for modeling clinical outcomes is to derive a single predictive model from a dataset of individuals for whom the outcomes are known, and then to apply the model to predict outcomes for future individuals. Such a model is called a *population-wide model* since it is intended to be applied to an entire population of future individuals and is optimized to have good predictive performance on average on all members of that population. This approach has often been quite successful; however, it ignores important individual differences during model *construction*, such as differences in treatment response. Precision medicine aims to tailor clinical therapy to individual patients, with the goal of delivering the right treatments at the right time to the right patient [30]. An approach for better capturing individual differences during modeling is called *patient-specific modeling*, and it focuses on learning models that are tailored to the characteristics of the individual at hand for whom we wish to make a prediction. The basic notion is that patient-specific models that are optimized to perform well for a specific individual are likely to have better predictive performance for that patient than a population-wide model that is optimized to have good predictive performance on average on all future individuals [31, 32].

Personalized Decision Trees

An example of a patient-specific modeling method is the personalized decision tree model that takes advantage of the particular features of an individual [33]. The authors introduce several methods that derive personalized decision trees (a decision path, in fact). When compared to the Classification And Regression Tree (CART) population-wide decision-tree model, the personalized methods performed better in both discrimination and calibration.

Personalized Bayesian Model Averaging

Another example that combines personalized modeling with BMA is a patient-specific algorithm that uses MB models, carries out Bayesian averaging over a set of models to predict the outcome for an individual, and employs a patient-specific heuristic to locate a set of suitable models to average over [31, 34]. When compared to a range of population-wide models, the MB patient-specific models had better performance in both discrimination and calibration.

Explanations

With the increasing complexity of predictive models, a critical bottleneck in their widespread use is the availability of explanations that describe the basis of individual predictions [35]. For example, the insight that an explanation provides about why a particular patient is predicted with high probability to develop a disease, may lead a clinician receiving it to gain trust in that prediction. Such explanations may assist clinicians in making clinical decisions. Explanations differ from model interpretability that refers to understandability or intelligibility of the model in terms of structure and parameters. Some predictive models, such as logistic regression and decision trees, are easier to interpret. Most machine learning models are more opaque. Predictive explanation provides reasoning for the prediction that is made by a model for an individual. Good explanations are parsimonious so that they are readily and rapidly understood by the clinician user and use concepts that are understandable to the user, such as clinical features that are not modified or transformed [36]. Predictive explanations are potentially more useful than interpretable models in the context of clinical decision making, although they are complementary.

Predictive explanations may be based on the structure and parameters of the predictive model that yielded the prediction or may be based on an independent method that is applied after the predictive model has produced its prediction. The latter types of methods can be used with any type of predictive model and have wider applicability. A recently developed method is the Local Interpretable Model-Agnostic Explanations (LIME) that provides an explanation for a prediction by learning an interpretable model locally around the patient for whom we wish to make a prediction [37]. Figure 7.3 provides an example of the application of LIME to explain a clinical outcome prediction.

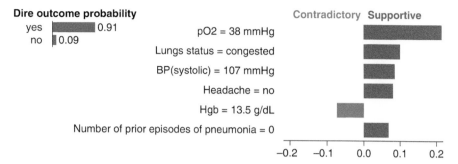

Fig. 7.3 An example explanation obtained from LIME for a patient with pneumonia who was predicted to have a very high probability of a dire outcome (i.e., death or severe complication). The plot at the top left shows the predicted probability distribution for dire outcome. The plot on the right shows the explanation for the prediction. The explanation is limited to six top ranked features by magnitude. The magnitude on the horizontal axis represents the weight of a feature. Green bars represent the magnitude of predictors that support the predicted outcome, while red bars represent the magnitude of contradictory features

Emerging Informatics Standards and Technologies

While many clinical predictive models are developed, few are validated externally, and even fewer are adopted in clinical practice. A key obstacle to the more widespread use of predictive models is the paucity of reporting standards, computable standards, and technologies. Moreover, while the workflow for development and validation of predictive models from research study data is well developed (see section "Workflow of Development and Validation of Predictive Models"), similar workflow for development of models from observational healthcare data is not yet mature.

Transparent Reporting of Predictive Models

One issue has been the poor quality and nonstandard reporting in published articles of descriptions of predictive models in medicine. The lack of a comprehensive, standard way of reporting the key details of studies that develop and validate models makes it difficult for the scientific and healthcare community to judge the validity and applicability of multivariable predictive models. To address this obstacle, a guideline for the Transparent Reporting of a multivariable predictive model for Individual Prognosis Or Diagnosis (TRIPOD) was introduced [38]. It provides a 22-item checklist that focuses on reporting how a predictive model study was designed, conducted, analyzed, and interpreted. This checklist provides guidance on reporting of items such as title, abstract, descriptions of predictors, outcomes and blinding, descriptions of development and validation data, model specification, development, performance and updating for both model development and external validation (see Table 7.2). A recent study showed that more than half of the items on the checklist were either absent or inadequately reported. Critical information for

Table 7.2 TRIPOD checklist for predictive model development and validation

Section/topic	Item		Checklist item
Title and abstract			
Title	1	D;V	Identify the study as developing and/or validating a multivariable predictive model, the target population, and the outcome to be predicted.
Abstract	2	D;V	Provide a summary of objectives, study design, setting, participants, sample size, predictors, outcome, statistical analysis, results, and conclusions.
Introduction			
Background and objectives	3a	D;V	Explain the medical context (including whether diagnostic or prognostic) and rationale for developing or validating the multivariable predictive model, including references to existing models.
	3b	D;V	Specify the objectives, including whether the study describes the development or validation of the model or both.
Methods			
Source of data	4a	D;V	Describe the study design or source of data (e.g., randomized trial, cohort, or registry data), separately for the development and validation data sets, if applicable.
	4b	D;V	Specify the key study dates, including start of accrual; end of accrual; and, if applicable, end of follow-up.
Participants	5a	D;V	Specify key elements of the study setting (e.g., primary care, secondary care, general population) including number and location of centers.
	5b	D;V	Describe eligibility criteria for participants.
	5c	D;V	Give details of treatments received, if relevant.
Outcome	6a	D;V	Clearly define the outcome that is predicted by the predictive model, including how and when assessed.
	6b	D;V	Report any actions to blind assessment of the outcome to be predicted.
Predictors	7a	D;V	Clearly define all predictors used in developing or validating the multivariable predictive model, including how and when they were measured.
	7b	D;V	Report any actions to blind assessment of predictors for the outcome and other predictors.
Sample size	8	D;V	Explain how the study size was arrived at.
Missing data	9	D;V	Describe how missing data were handled (e.g., complete-case analysis, single imputation, multiple imputation) with details of any imputation method.
Statistical analysis methods	10a	D	Describe how predictors were handled in the analyses.
	10b	D	Specify type of model, all model-building procedures (including any predictor selection), and method for internal validation.
	10c	V	For validation, describe how the predictions were calculated.
	10d	D;V	Specify all measures used to assess model performance and, if relevant, to compare multiple models.
	10e	V	Describe any model updating (e.g., recalibration) arising from the validation, if done.
Risk groups	11	D;V	Provide details on how risk groups were created, if done.

Table 7.2 (continued)

Section/topic	Item		Checklist item
Development vs. validation	12	V	For validation, identify any differences from the development data in setting, eligibility criteria, outcome, and predictors.
Results			
Participants	13a	D;V	Describe the flow of participants through the study, including the number of participants with and without the outcome and, if applicable, a summary of the follow-up time. A diagram may be helpful.
	13b	D;V	Describe the characteristics of the participants (basic demographics, clinical features, available predictors), including the number of participants with missing data for predictors and outcome.
	13c	V	For validation, show a comparison with the development data of the distribution of important features (demographics, predictors and outcome).
Model development	14a	D	Specify the number of participants and outcome events in each analysis.
	14b	D	If done, report the unadjusted association between each candidate predictor and outcome.
Model specification	15a	D	Present the full prediction model to allow predictions for individuals (i.e., all regression coefficients, and model intercept or baseline survival at a given time point).
	15b	D	Explain how to the use the predictive model.
Model performance	16	D;V	Report performance measures (with CIs) for the predictive model.
Model-updating	17	V	If done, report the results from any model updating (i.e., model specification, model performance).
Discussion			
Limitations	18	D;V	Discuss any limitations of the study (such as nonrepresentative sample, few events per predictor, missing data).
Interpretation	19a	V	For validation, discuss the results with reference to performance in the development data, and any other validation data.
	19b	D;V	Give an overall interpretation of the results, considering objectives, limitations, results from similar studies, and other relevant evidence.
Implications	20	D;V	Discuss the potential clinical use of the model and implications for future research.
Other information			
Supplementary information	21	D;V	Provide information about the availability of supplementary resources, such as study protocol, web calculator, and data sets.
Funding	22	D;V	Give the source of funding and the role of the funders for the present study.

Adapted from Table 1 in Ref. [38]

Items relevant only to the development of a predictive model are denoted by D, items relating solely to a validation of a predictive model are denoted by V, and items relating to both are denoted D;V

using the model, including model specification and performance, was inadequately reported for more than 80% of the models [39]. Increased adherence and further refinement of the TRIPOD checklist will enhance more transparent reporting of clinical predictive models.

Computable and Portable Predictive Models

Widespread use of predictive models in clinical medicine requires deployment of models in computable formats so that they can be applied to EHRs to automatically provide predictions and recommend actions in the context of a patient. Currently, well-described human-readable predictive models require manual translation to computable formats that is slow and resource -intensive. Rapid deployment of computable models will require development of new standards and technologies. These include the creation of standards for a computable representation of predictive models, development of tools to enable standards-based authoring of models, construction of infrastructure for execution of models in a variety of EHR systems, and digital libraries for collecting, storing, and sharing models.

In the domain of data, the FAIR Data Principles are a set of guiding principles that have been put forth to make data findable, accessible, interoperable, and reusable [40]. These principles facilitate the ability of computers to automatically find and use data and enable its reuse. A similar set of principles are needed for making computable predictive models findable, accessible, interoperable, and reusable. As an example, a computable phenotype is defined as a set of clinical features that can be determined from the data in EHRs, and efforts are ongoing to develop a set of standards for developing a computable phenotype representation that is easily authored, portable and executable. The recently described Knowledge Object Reference Ontology provides a framework to help make computable biomedical knowledge that includes computable phenotypes and predictive models findable, accessible, interoperable, and reusable [41].

Modeling Using Large Scale Observational Data

Observational healthcare data, that includes EHRs and administrative claims data, are increasingly available for secondary use and research through federated data networks. The PCORnet, funded by the PCORI, is a U.S.-wide federated network of EHR, claims, and patient reported outcome data on over 100 million patients [42]. The Accrual to Clinical Trials (ACT) network, funded by the NIH, is another U.S. federated network of EHR and claims data on over 40 million patients [43]. The Observational Health Data Sciences and Informatics (OHDSI) collaboration is a network of loosely collaborating sites with EHR and claims data on hundreds of millions of patients [44]. These networks have adopted similar data models that specify standardized structure and content for observational data. In contrast to research study data that consist of specified measurements that are expressly measured for the study, observational healthcare data consists of clinical measurements across a range of domains (such as diagnoses, procedures, medications, and laboratory test values) that are captured during the process of care. Compared to study data, observational healthcare data are typically much larger with tens of thousands of measurements on tens of millions of individuals. For research use, healthcare data are standardized to common terminologies, such as ICD-9 and ICD-10 codes for diagnoses and procedures, RxNorm and National Drug Codes (NDC) for medications, and Logical Observation Identifiers Names and Codes (LOINC) for laboratory test results. Standardization of the data requires considerable time and resources to map the source data to standard terminologies and transform it in accordance to the data model specifications.

The use of healthcare data for predictive modeling is still in its infancy. It holds the promise of revolutionizing clinical predictive modeling on very large scales and across several different diagnoses, outcomes, and treatments simultaneously. The OHDSI community has introduced a framework for developing and validating predictive models using observational healthcare data. Moreover, open-source software is available that implements this framework for data that has been transformed to the Observational Medical Outcomes Partnership (OMOP) data model. This framework was applied to develop predictive models using several machine learning methods for 21 different outcomes in a population of pharmaceutically-treated depression patients across four observational data sets that contained a total of over 230 million patients. For some outcomes, high performing models were obtained while for other outcomes the models performed poorly, suggesting that observational data sets are likely to be useful for some outcomes but not for all, and that, healthcare data complement research study data [45].

Policy, Ethical, and Legal Challenges

The increasing availability of big biomedical data and the growing application of new statistical and machine learning methods for developing complex models from big data provide an opportunity for widespread development of clinical predictive models. When such models are deployed to provide targeted care, to improve outcomes, and to lower healthcare costs, several policy, ethical, and legal challenges arise. A comprehensive consideration of such issues is presented in a recent publication [46], and a few key issues are summarized in the next paragraph.

A primary consideration is that data used in model derivation and validation is representative of the whole population. Historically, members of certain racial and ethnic groups, people with disabilities, individuals in prison, and members of other vulnerable groups have been underrepresented in research studies. Such inequitable representation can lead to models that are not valid for parts of the population. In addition to extensive validation, models need to be evaluated in real-world settings before deployment. A second consideration is that the models are developed both in human-readable and machine-readable forms using standards that are transparent and replicable. A third consideration is liability. Makers as well as users of predictive models may face liability if there are errors in the model or the model malfunctions. A fourth consideration is that population-wide models that are designed to improve outcomes in a population may produce a sub-optimal prediction for a specific patient. As a simple illustrative example, a population-wide model that predicts future morbidity may not include human immunodeficiency virus (HIV) status as a predictor because the proportion of HIV positive patients in the data is very small. Such a model will produce sub-optimal predictions for patients with positive HIV status, and a patient-specific model that includes HIV status as a predictor will provide better predictions. Ethical obligations of clinicians to act in the best interests of a patient may lead to increased use of patient-specific models over population-wide ones.

Conclusions

With increasing availability of big biomedical data, valid and high-performing predictive modeling methods are needed to leverage the data for clinical medicine, public health, and biomedical research. Several current trends indicate that biomedical data will become more readily available and that will accelerate the development of predictive models in medicine. For example, the National Institutes of Health's strategic plan for data science provides a roadmap for storing, managing, standardizing and publishing the vast amounts of data produced by biomedical research [47]. The Director of the National Library of Medicine at the National Institutes of Health anticipates an important role for a library of models that will identify, collect and archive biomedical models [48]. In addition to the expertise in academia, companies with expertise in artificial intelligence like Microsoft, Google, Baidu, and Apple are developing predictive models for healthcare [49]. The General Data Protection Regulation (GDPR) that was recently adopted by the European Union includes a "right to explanation" with regard to predictive models that seeks to enforce the availability of explanations for predictions made by models [50]. Thus, the coming decade will likely see increasing development and validation of predictive models from big biomedical data and will include advances in feature selection, high performance, personalization of models, and explanations of predictions.

References

1. Moons KGM, Altman DG, Vergouwe Y, Royston P. Prognosis and prognostic research: application and impact of prognostic models in clinical practice. Br Med J. 2009;338:b606.
2. Wilson PWF, D'Agostino RB, Levy D, Belanger AM, Silbershatz H, Kannel WB. Prediction of coronary heart disease using risk factor categories. Circulation. 1998;97:1837–47.

3. Jessen MK, Mackenhauer J, Hvass AMSW, Ellermann-Eriksen S, Skibsted S, Kirkegaard H, et al. Prediction of bacteremia in the emergency department: an external validation of a clinical decision rule. Eur J Emerg Med. 2016;23:44–9.
4. Shapiro NI, Wolfe RE, Wright SB, Moore R, Bates DW. Who needs a blood culture? A prospectively derived and validated prediction rule. J Emerg Med. 2008;35:255–64.
5. LaHaye SA, Gibbens SL, Ball DGA, Day AG, Olesen JB, Skanes AC. A clinical decision aid for the selection of antithrombotic therapy for the prevention of stroke due to atrial fibrillation. Eur Heart J. 2012;33:2163–71.
6. Brownstein JS, Freifeld CC, Chan EH, Keller M, Sonricker AL, Mekaru SR, et al. Information technology and global surveillance of cases of 2009 H1N1 influenza. N Engl J Med. 2010;362:1731–5.
7. Steyerberg EW. Clinical prediction models: a practical approach to development, validation, and updating. New York: Springer; 2008.
8. Clark GM, Zborowski DM, Culbertson JL, Whitehead M, Savoie M, Seymour L, et al. Clinical utility of epidermal growth factor receptor expression for selecting patients with advanced non-small cell lung cancer for treatment with erlotinib. J Thorac Oncol. 2006;1:837–46.
9. Sechidis K, Papangelou K, Metcalfe PD, Svensson D, Weatherall J, Brown G. Distinguishing prognostic and predictive biomarkers: an information theoretic approach. Bioinformatics. 2018;1:12.
10. Labarère J, Bertrand R, Fine MJ. How to derive and validate clinical prediction models for use in intensive care medicine. Intensive Care Med. 2014;40:513–27.
11. Hendriksen JMT, Geersing GJ, Moons KGM, De Groot JAH. Diagnostic and prognostic prediction models. J Thromb Haemost. 2013;11:129–41.
12. Alba AC, Agoritsas T, Walsh M, Hanna S, Iorio A, Devereaux PJ, et al. Discrimination and calibration of clinical prediction models: users' guides to the medical literature. J Am Med Assoc. 2017;318:1377–84.
13. Collart F, Feier H, Kerbaul F, Mouly-Bandini A, Riberi A, Mesana TG, et al. Valvular surgery in octogenarians: operative risks factors, evaluation of Euroscore and long term results. Eur J Cardio Thoracic Surg. 2005;27:276–80.
14. Nashef SAM, Roques F, Sharples LD, Nilsson J, Smith C, Goldstone AR, et al. Euroscore II. Eur J Cardio Thoracic Surg. 2012;41:734–45.
15. Guyon I, Elisseeff A. An introduction to variable and feature selection. J Mach Learn Res. 2003;3:1157–82.
16. Zeng Y, Luo J, Lin S. Classification using Markov blanket for feature selection. IEEE International Conference on Granular Computing. 2009. p. 743–7.
17. Aliferis CF, Statnikov A, Tsamardinos I, Mani S, Koutsoukos XD. Local causal and Markov blanket induction for causal discovery and feature selection for classification part I: algorithms and empirical evaluation. J Mach Learn Res. 2010;11:171–234.
18. Aliferis CF, Statnikov A, Tsamardinos I, Mani S, Koutsoukos XD. Local causal and Markov blanket induction for causal discovery and feature selection for classification part II: analysis and extensions. J Mach Learn Res. 2010;11:235–84.
19. Margaritis D, Thrun S. Bayesian network induction via local neighborhoods. Proc Adv Neural Inf Process Syst. 2000:505–11.
20. Tsamardinos I, Aliferis CF, Statnikov AR, Statnikov E. Algorithms for large scale Markov blanket discovery. Proc Florida Artif Intell Res Soc. 2003:376–80.
21. Aliferis CF, Tsamardinos I, Statnikov A. HITON: a novel Markov blanket algorithm for optimal variable selection. AMIA Annu Symp Proc. 2003;2003:21–5.
22. Tsamardinos I, Brown LE, Aliferis CF. The max-min hill-climbing Bayesian network structure learning algorithm. Mach Learn. 2006;65:31–78.
23. Strobl EV, Visweswaran S. Markov blanket ranking using kernel-based conditional dependence measures. arXiv Prepr arXiv14020108. 2014.
24. Hoeting JA, Madigan D, Raftery AE, Volinsky CT. Bayesian model averaging: a tutorial. Stat Sci. 1999;14:382–401.

25. Madigan D, Raftery AE. Model selection and accounting for model uncertainty in graphical models using Occam's window. J Am Stat Assoc. 1994;89:1535–46.
26. Yeung KY, Bumgarner RE, Raftery AE. Bayesian model averaging: development of an improved multi-class, gene selection and classification tool for microarray data. Bioinformatics. 2005;21:2394–402.
27. Wei W, Visweswaran S, Cooper GF. The application of naive Bayes model averaging to predict Alzheimer's disease from genome-wide data. J Am Med Inform Assoc. 2011;18:370–5.
28. Fragoso TM, Bertoli W, Louzada F. Bayesian model averaging: a systematic review and conceptual classification. Int Stat Rev. 2018;86:1–28.
29. Dash D, Cooper GF. Exact model averaging with naive Bayesian classifiers. Proc Int Conf Int Conf Mach Learn. 2002:91–8.
30. Collins FS, Varmus H. A new initiative on precision medicine. N Engl J Med. 2015;372:793–5. https://doi.org/10.1056/NEJMp1500523.
31. Visweswaran S, Angus DC, Hsieh M, Weissfeld L, Yealy D, Cooper GF. Learning patient-specific predictive models from clinical data. J Biomed Inform. 2010;43:669–85.
32. Visweswaran S, Cooper GF. Learning instance-specific predictive models. J Mach Learn Res. 2010;11:3333–69.
33. Visweswaran S, Ferreira A, Ribeiro GA, Oliveira AC, Cooper GF. Personalized modeling for prediction with decision-path models. PLoS One. 2015;10:e0131022.
34. Visweswaran S, Cooper GF. Patient-specific models for predicting the outcomes of patients with community acquired pneumonia. AMIA Annu Symp Proc. 2005;2005:759–63.
35. Suermondt HJ, Cooper GF. An evaluation of explanations of probabilistic inference. Comput Biomed Res. 1993;26:242–54.
36. Caruana R, Lou Y, Gehrke J, Koch P, Sturm M, Elhadad N. Intelligible models for healthcare: predicting pneumonia risk and hospital 30-day readmission. Proceedings of the 21th ACM SIGKDD International Conference on Knowledge Discovery and Data Mining, ACM; 2015. p. 1721–30.
37. Ribeiro MT, Singh S, Guestrin C. Why should I trust you?: explaining the predictions of any classifier. Proceedings of the ACM SIGKDD International Conference on Knowledge Discovery and Data Mining 2016. p. 1135–44.
38. Moons KGM, Altman DG, Reitsma JB, Ioannidis JPA, Macaskill P, Steyerberg EW, et al. Transparent reporting of a multivariable prediction model for individual prognosis or diagnosis (TRIPOD): explanation and elaboration. Ann Intern Med. 2015;162:W1–73.
39. Heus P, Damen JAAG, Pajouheshnia R, Scholten RJPM, Reitsma JB, Collins GS, et al. Poor reporting of multivariable prediction model studies: towards a targeted implementation strategy of the TRIPOD statement. BMC Med. 2018;16:120.
40. Wilkinson MD, Dumontier M, Aalbersberg IJ, Appleton G, Axton M, Baak A, et al. The FAIR guiding principles for scientific data management and stewardship. Sci Data. 2016;3:160018.
41. Flynn AJ, Friedman CP, Boisvert P, Landis-Lewis Z, Lagoze C. The knowledge object reference ontology (KORO): a formalism to support management and sharing of computable biomedical knowledge for learning health systems. Learn Heal Syst. 2018;2:e10054.
42. Collins FS, Hudson KL, Briggs JP, Lauer MS. PCORnet: turning a dream into reality. J Am Med Inform Assoc. 2014;21:576–7.
43. Visweswaran S, Becich MJ, D'Itri VS, Sendro ER, MacFadden D, Anderson NR, et al. Accrual to clinical trials (ACT): a clinical and translational science award consortium network. JAMIA Open. 2018;1:147–52. https://doi.org/10.1093/jamiaopen/ooy033.
44. Hripcsak G, Duke JD, Shah NH, Reich CG, Huser V, Schuemie MJ, et al. Observational health data sciences and informatics (OHDSI): opportunities for observational researchers. Stud Health Technol Inform. 2015;216:574.
45. Reps JM, Schuemie MJ, Suchard MA, Ryan PB, Rijnbeek PR. Design and implementation of a standardized framework to generate and evaluate patient-level prediction models using observational healthcare data. J Am Med Inform Assoc. 2018;25:969–75.

46. Cohen IG, Amarasingham R, Shah A, Xie B, Lo B. The legal and ethical concerns that arise from using complex predictive analytics in health care. Health Aff. 2014;33:1139–47.

47. National Institutes of Health. NIH strategic plan for data science [Internet]. [cited 2018 Oct 21]. p. 1–26. https://grants.nih.gov/grants/rfi/NIH-Strategic-Plan-for-Data-Science.pdf.

48. Brennan PF. Models: the third leg in data-driven discovery – NLM musings from the mezzanine [internet]. 2017 [cited 2018 Oct 21]. https://nlmdirector.nlm.nih.gov/2017/12/12/models-the-third-leg-in-data-driven-discovery/.

49. Ravi D, Wong C, Deligianni F, Berthelot M, Andreu-Perez J, Lo B, et al. Deep learning for health informatics. IEEE J Biomed Heal Informat. 2017;21:4–21. http://ieeexplore.ieee.org/document/7801947/.

50. Voigt P, von dem Bussche A. The EU General Data Protection Regulation (GDPR): a practical guide. Cham: Springer; 2017.

Chapter 8
Informatics Methods
for Molecular Profiling

Constantin Aliferis, Sisi Ma, and Boris Winterhoff

Introduction

A molecular profile is a computational model that accepts as inputs omics assay results, plus other contextual data such as clinical and demographic variables, and outputs a number of predictions.

The predictions can be one or more of the following: (1) an estimate of the patient's expected outcomes of interest (typically: survival, recurrence, metastasis) if untreated; (2) an estimate of the patient's outcomes of interest if given specific treatments. (3) Sometimes (but less often) a molecular profile is used for more accurate diagnosis or early diagnosis of difficult to diagnose (or differentially diagnose) conditions.

The assay is typically a multivariate gene expression assay although other types of omics assays can and have been used such as proteomics, metabolomics, microbiomics, miRNAs, copy number variation, methylation, etc. The assay can be executed on DNA or RNA extracts from targeted or circulating somatic or tumor or microbial tissue or cells (or combinations thereof).

This chapter is a revised version of Winterhoff, Boris, et al. "Developing a Clinico-Molecular Test for Individualized Treatment of Ovarian Cancer: The interplay of Precision Medicine Informatics with Clinical and Health Economics Dimensions." AMIA Annual Symposium Proceedings. Vol. 2018. American Medical Informatics Association, 2018, used with permission.

C. Aliferis (✉) · S. Ma
Institute for Health Informatics, Department of Medicine, School of Medicine Clinical and Translational Science Institute, Masonic Cancer Center, Program in Data Science, University of Minnesota, Minneapolis, MN, USA
e-mail: califeri@umn.edu; sisima@umn.edu

B. Winterhoff
Department of Obstetrics, Gynecology and Women's Health, Medical School, University of Minnesota, Minneapolis, MN, USA
e-mail: winterh@umn.edu

© Springer Nature Switzerland AG 2020
T. Adam, C. Aliferis (eds.), *Personalized and Precision Medicine Informatics*,
Health Informatics, https://doi.org/10.1007/978-3-030-18626-5_8

Molecular profiling using high dimensional omics data emerged in the late 1990s with the first FDA-approved test (Mammaprint), approved in 2007. This form of PPM currently used across several diseases, allows for individualized prognosis, choice of optimal treatment for reducing toxicities or other adverse events and for enhancing effectiveness, as well as for reducing healthcare system costs. The majority of modern molecular profiling tests address various forms of cancer and use gene expression profiles, although the science and technology of molecular profiling can be used for virtually any disease and a large variety of clinico-molecular assays.

General Workflow for Molecular Profile-Based PPM

The overall framework for developing, validating and deploying precision tests based on molecular profiling are depicted in Fig. 8.1. As can be seen, informatics plays a central role in the research design, modeling, model optimization and clinical deployment phases.

A critical observation is that while informatics methods and implementation is an essential component of discovery and clinical deployment of molecular profiles, all informatics work exists within a complex context of socio-technical and healthcare considerations that includes the following dimensions: (a) defining clear and compelling clinical objectives, (b) ability to construct robust models that accurately

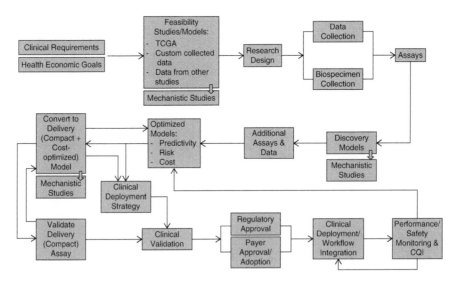

Fig. 8.1 Process for development and clinical validation of clinico-molecular profiling precision medicine tests. Used with permission from Winterhoff, Boris, et al. "Developing a Clinico-Molecular Test for Individualized Treatment of Ovarian Cancer: The interplay of Precision Medicine Informatics with Clinical and Health Economics Dimensions." AMIA Annual Symposium Proceedings. Vol. 2018. American Medical Informatics Association, 2018, figure 1

predict outcomes under a variety of conditions, (c) choosing assays to maximize value of information while satisfying economic and technical feasibility constraints, (d) economic affordability for the healthcare system (established via health economics analysis), (e) development costs optimization (measured in time and financial costs), (f) deployment cost optimization, (g) seamless deployment at the point of care.

The present chapter provides an introduction to the above topics, starting from general principles for informatics data modeling essential for molecular profiling development and then in the context of a real-life case study of developing a precision test for bevacizumab for treating patients with ovarian cancer.

The two most important informatics dimensions in developing molecular profiling based PPM tests are: (a) data analysis and modeling and (b) delivery at the point of care (Fig. 8.2).

The successful analysis of clinico-molecular data involves a first stage of "upstream" *analysis* and a second stage of "downstream" *analysis*. The upstream analysis involves operation of (typically "omic") assay instruments and mapping of biochemical and physical signals to measurements of absolute or relative concentration or abundance (depending on what is measured). Typical upstream analysis is tied to instruments such as deep sequencers [1–3], microarray instruments [4, 5] spectrometry [6–9], or multiplexed PCR [10]. Such instruments are capable of measuring gene copy number variation, gene expression levels, genetic mutations in germline (hereditary mutations) or somatic cells (acquired mutations), genetic polymorphisms, protein and peptide abundance, metabolites, sequences of microbiota and their genetic alterations, micro RNAs, epigenetic (e.g., methylation) markers, etc. [2, 5, 9, 11, 12]. The assays may be targeted (1 or a few dozen measured variables), or genome wide (from hundreds of thousands to, potentially, billions of variables).

Common themes include normalization of measurements against reference values [5], removal of so-called "batch effects" (when assays are conducted in batches across time/labs and with different operators or operating protocols [13–15]),

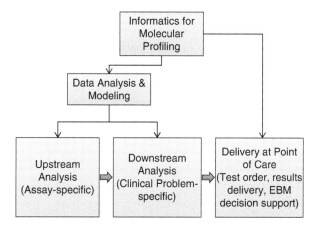

Fig. 8.2 Informatics for molecular profiling

assembly of information (e.g., assembly of whole genomes from shorter genetic sequences [12]), contrasting measured variables against reference values (e.g., identification of patients' mutations relative to a reference genome [1, 16]), mapping of measured variables to reference entities (e.g. mapping of microbial sequences to microbial species [17–19], or mapping of RNA sequences to genes [12, 17]).

The specific informatics methods and tools employed for upstream analysis are closely tied to the type and generation of the assay technology used and furthermore as new technologies enter and older ones are leaving the translational and clinical research realm, there is a constant cycle of innovation and introduction of new upstream informatics methods. For details about upstream analysis we will refer the interested reader to the references provided above since this informatics component is removed from the purview of the clinicians, and it is highly specialized (often conducted in the genome or proteomic assay facility before handed over to informatics specialists tasked to downstream analysis). Chapter 9 of the present volume also provides an introduction to next generation sequencing upstream informatics.

Similarly *ordering and delivery of send out lab tests* from within the EHR is a commodity feature of modern EHRs, whereas *delivery of clinical decision support related to MP* does not differ from any other form of PPM DS (see for example Chap. 16 on how to do so in a highly scalable manner within and across health systems).

By contrast, downstream data analysis involves a large array of important scientific challenges and methodologies that we will discuss in more focused detail. Many of these methodologies and principles are very robust and thus interoperable across different molecular profiling projects.

After establishing the general principles, we will provide a description of a case study where these different components are brought together in a coherent design and applied in context. Chapters 7 and 8 discuss related issues such as informatics tools for biomarker discovery and cross-platform molecular profiling discovery.

Main Principles of Downstream Bioinformatics Data Analysis for Molecular Profiling

Model Seletction, Model Fitting, and Error Estimation

In general, downstream analysis for MP involves three interrelated and essential activities: (a) model selection, (b) model fitting, and (c) error estimation. Model selection is the process of systematic consideration of different classes of models and their instantiation to the data at hand. Model fitting is the process of fitting parameters of a model family in order to obtain an instantiated model to the data at hand. Error estimation is the process of estimating how well the fitted models will perform in future patient data samples from the same population and assayed with same protocols.

Perhaps the most prominent modern form of model selection for MP develop-ment is the "grid design" combined with cross-validation [20–23] where a number of modeling method families are evaluated across a number of high-level (data inde-pendent) parameters called "hyper-parameters" [21]. Each method family is instan-tiated according to the hyper parameter values on a *training* portion of the data and then evaluated using cross validation in another independent *validation* portion (the coupling between a discovery—training- dataset and a validation one is the essen-tial principle of cross validation for model fitting). Then the best models are fitted by applying the best method and best hyperparameters found previously on the union of *training + validation* data. The produced model is evaluated on a third and final independent *error estimation* portion of the data in order to estimate their error in the general population. Once the error estimation is obtained, a final model is fit-ted on the union of *training + validation + error estimation* data again using the best model family and hyper parameter values found in the model selection stage.

The whole process is nested so that model selection error estimates do not con-taminate the final error estimates, thus avoiding overfitting of the final model's error estimates (see below). The data splits within each cross validation as well as the whole nested analysis is repeated in order to reduce the variance due to the random splitting. This yields the *Repeated Nested N-Fold Cross Validation (RNNFCV)* design [20, 21] depicted in simplified form in Fig. 8.3. As can be seen in the figure, model selection, model fitting, and error estimation are interwoven in the RNNFCV.

It is important to notice that *each and every modeling decision* has to be evalu-ated using the inner (model selection) cross validation. Simon et al. [24] provide a very important illustrative demonstration of how much biased error estimates can be when gene selection is not conducted inside cross validation. What Simon et al. teach, applies to all possible analysis steps however, including normalization, vari-able re-coding, peak detection, etc.

The reader should also be aware of other forms of error estimation, for example Leave One Out (LOO), or Bootsrapping [21, 22]. However these error estimators have problems that render them suboptimal for general use in MP development. Specifically, LOO has higher variance than RNNFCV and is more difficult to com-pute calibration [22]. Bootstrapping is a consistent error estimator but unfortunately a biased one (i.e., has a systematic error that does not vanish as sample size goes to infinity; this bias is generally unknown and needs to be identified for each analysis). Bootstrapping also creates samples with identical instances something that is highly unnatural in omics datasets, further compounding the Bootstrap error by inflating predictivity [21].

The error estimation procedures are estimating a number of *error functions* that are chosen to correspond to the intent of the MP test and the analytics employed. For example, Area under the ROC curve (AUC) is used for binary prediction models [25, 26], Nagelkerke's R^2 [27] is used for survival models (for general model fit), Brier scores [28] are used for general model calibration and for survival analysis, as is probability of concordance. Different metrics have different strengths including interpretability characteristics [29, 30].

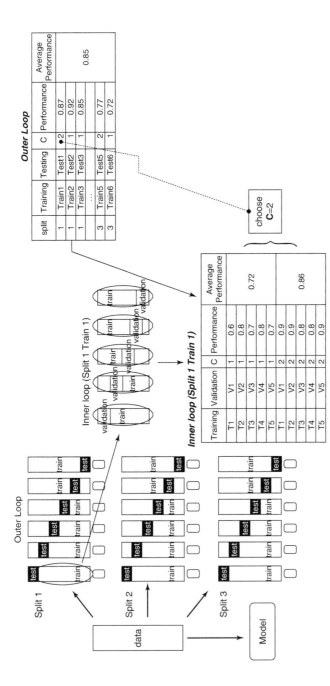

Fig. 8.3 Example of the RNNFCV protocol. Models fitted from data are depicted as unlabeled boxes. A 3-repeat sixfold design is shown for simplicity (typically >50 repeats over ten-fold cross validation (CV) is used in practice, however). For each repeat of the n-fold CV, the data is split randomly in n folds such that the test portions are independently chosen and non-overlapping; and their union forms the original data. Test sets are randomly sampled subject to the constraint that the probability distribution of the response variable values is retained in each train-test sample pair. For each training set of each of the n CV folds, a new $(n - 1)$-fold CV is conducted. Within this nested CV, a fixed set of hyper-parameter values are tested. In the simplified example presented here, only one hyper-parameter ("C") is tuned over two values (C = 1, C = 2). In contrast to hyper-parameters, regular (first-order) parameters are automatically fitted by the learning algorithm employed (e.g., SVM weights, Neural Network weights, Random Forest trees, etc.). The hyper-parameter value C = 2 yields best results in the inner split depicted and thus is used to build a model from the data corresponding to that split. Across the outer loop different values of C are best. Models corresponding to these are built and evaluated in the outer CV loop. The average of these evaluations over each outer CV and then averaged over all repeats provide the expected error of the best model in the general population. Note the actual best model is fitted on all data using the best parameter for C across all repeats and inner loops

Finally an important recent development is protocols that utilize several different types of inputs simultaneously. These so-called "multi-modal" protocols are necessary to effectively combine omic-clinical data types. The reader is referred to Ray et al. [31] for a summary and empirical comparison of cutting-edge multi-modal analysis protocols.

Whenever different data types are employed, *Information content analyses* can be carried out that compare the information content for each class of data input. For example, the analyst can evaluate the unique and shared components of predictivity attributable to gene expression data separately from clinical data and separately from genetic data [31].

Overfitting and Underfitting

As with any multivariate modeling analysis a major danger is that of "overfitting", meaning creating models that describe well the patients in the discovery datasets but fail to generalize equally well to other patients from the same population. The opposite problem is also possible, in the form of "underfitting" where the analyst is creating a model that is not as accurate as the generative function underlying the data [20, 21].

Both overfitting and underfitting are greatly facilitated in data with many variables (as is typical in data used to create MP). In addition, everything else being equal, the complexity of the models we are willing to learn is directly related to underfitting and overfitting: too simple a function yields underfitting and too complex a function yields overfitting. Of course what constitutes "too simple", or "too complex" is entirely an empirical question. *Testing of overfitting* of the overall predictor modeling is commonly done via label reshuffling which also provides p-values for testing the statistical significance of multivariate models [32, 33].

Recent advances in data science have created *methods that prevent overfitting and underfitting* by automatically tailoring the complexity of the learned models to the data at hand. The main methods for preventing overfitting are:

(a) *Feature Selection (FS)*, that is the systematic elimination of input variables that either do not contain information about the response variable we wish to predict, or that contain redundant information [34–37].
(b) *Dimensionality Reduction (DR)*, that is the systematic mapping of the original variables to a smaller set of constructed variables that retain the necessary information about the response variables [21, 22, 37]. In MP, for reasons of cost and convenience, we wish to deploy clinically a test with an as small set of measured variables as possible (and without loss of predictivity for the response variable). Because DR does not eliminate the need to assay the full set of original input variables, it cannot serve these objectives and is that useful only for preliminary analyses. FS has to be brought in at least at the end of the analysis process to obtain the most parsimonious and thus most economical and easiest to deploy MP test.

(c) *Regularization* [22], that is penalizing models for complexity. Regularization has various forms. In Bayesian modeling it manifests as smaller prior probabilities for complex models versus simple models. In "loss plus penalty" learning algorithms, models are evaluated by a combination of how well the describe the data (the "loss" component) and of how complex they are (the "penalty" component) [22]. Other forms of regularization exist, for example in the Random Forest classifier, trees inside the forest model are not allowed to grow beyond a certain size (which is thus a regularization parameter). All successful forms of modern Machine Learning for high-dimensional data employ explicit or subtler forms of regularization.

Common Classifiers and Regressors for MP

Multivariate Predictors for Binary Outcomes. Several large benchmarking studies have yielded important insights about the relative predictivity of modern Machine Learning and statistical methods used for MP in the binary and n-ary prediction case. The studies of Statnikov et al. [38, 39] in particular have demonstrated the advantages of using Support Vector Machines (SVMs). Random Forests (RFs) are also strong methods for MP creation, however they require some external simplification of the production MP because a typical RF is too complex a model with too many variable inputs to be easily and economically deployed in clinical practice.

Multivariate predictors for survival. Survival analyses (i.e., when data is longitudinally observed and observations may be censored) posits a different analytic challenge. Three types of state of the art models are worth referencing: (a) Cox analysis using all molecular, demographic, functional, and clinical lab testing covariates in the model by employing the regularized (elastic net) Cox proportional hazards method of Simon [40]. (b) Causal graph based high-dimensional Cox analysis using the Lagani [41] method which yields the (much more parsimonious but still informative) Markov Boundary around the response variable which will then be fitted with a standard Cox model. (c) Random Survival Forests [42].

Feature Selection Methods Suitable for MP

The Markov Boundary set under broad assumptions is itself the theoretically smallest feature set with maximum predictivity [36, 43]. Importantly for MP, Markov Boundary algorithms employ four distinct regularizers to reduce over-fitting (and in addition the classifiers using the selected features typically employ at least one additional layer of regularization). The combination of the above multi-stage regularization has been empirically shown to provide maximum predictive signal, with maximum parsimony and no overfitting [43, 44]. It has also been shown that additional dimensionality reduction or feature selection can further enhance classification for both Random Forests and regularized regression analyses [38, 43, 44] even though Random Forests [45] and regularized Cox [40] have embedded feature selection. Via nesting in the RNNFCV, the analyst can ensure not to overfit the model selection of hyper parameters [32, 46].

Specialized Downstream Bioinformatics Methods

In some instances the Bioinformaticists in charge of downstream analysis of molecular data for MP construction will have to consider specialized methods applicable to the data at hand. We will provide an example in the domain of miRNA analysis to illustrate the point. Pathway enrichment analysis of the mRNAs discovered is conducted with specialized tools like *DIANA-miRPath* [47]. Gene targets of the sRNAs can be predicted using an array of methods (e.g., see Alexiou et al. [48]). sRNAs can be linked to environmental factors using *miREnvironment* [49], to genetics (SNPs) using *MicroSNiPER* [50], and to known diseases using *OncomiRDB* [51] and *HMDD* [52]. Also because sRNAs are known to often affect genes in a *combinatorial coordinated manner* [53, 54], it is often advisable to consider sRNAs combinatorially. The Triplex RNA database (http://www.sbi.uni-rostock.de/triplexrna/help.html) for example, describes combinatorial triplets (sRNA-sRNA-Gene expression) [54]. We note that other specialized "omics" (e.g., proteomic assays, metabolomics, RNAseq, microbiomics etc.) data usually have their own additional methods that need be considered. These details are outside the scope of a general survey chapter so we refer the reader to the assay specific references covered in the chapter.

Ancillary Analyses for MP

Many additional analytical data science methods can be informative in the process of creating and MP tests. We mention in particular:

(a) *Complex* "Systems" or "integrative biology" *view models of the function and interactions of genes and pathways within cell types and across cell types.* These include both data driven and knowledge-driven "systems" oriented methods. A particularly robust set of methods in that category is *Causal Graph analyses*. Under the assumptions of faithful distributions (i.e., most theoretical distributions including all classical statistical ones belong to this category) as proven, for example, by the results of Pearl and of Spirtes et al. [55, 56], reliable algorithms exist for the discovery of causal relationships by examining observational or quasi experimental data. The FCI method of Spirtes et al. [56] for example, has the capacity to reveal causal relationships, causal direction *and* the presence of confounding (whenever directionality or confounding is impossible to be deciphered without experiments, the algorithm flags the causal arc accordingly). These models can give insights into the complex relationships among these variables. Algorithms like FCI can be made scalable to omics data by learning first a high quality region within which FCI can be effectively applied. Such regions can be obtained using the highly scalable LGL family of methods method [44], which has been shown to be a superior performer when high Positive Predictive Value is sought for local pathway reverse engineering and is applicable with thousands of variables and small samples in relatively sparse or small-world networks [57].

(b) *Knowledge-driven analysis.* These include Gene (set) enrichment analysis (GEA, or GSEA) of the genes and other molecular species discovered as significant. GEA is a form of a "goodness of fit test" where the fundamental hypothesis to be tested is that the biomarkers discovered distribute equally across functional pathways (normalizing for size of each pathway) [58].

(c) *In silico experimentation studies* can be conducted using a Bayesian Network parameterization of the Causal Graph models developed (or far more practically, whenever a fixed set of many input- one output queries are of interest, using regression models with appropriately chosen covariates). These models can be queried to predict qualitative and quantitative effects of silencing or inducing expression of genes individually or in groups using standard Bayesian Network inference algorithms[160] combined with Pearl's "Do Calculous" [55]; the latter identifies an appropriate conditioning set that is given to the inference algorithm to block the influences of extraneous causal paths and ensures that estimation of intervention effects are accurate (we note that whenever such effects can be estimated from observational data, the Do Calculous has been proven to guarantee a correct answer) [59].

(d) *Equivalence class analyses.* In omics data Phenotype-information equivalency (aka "target information equivalency" or "multiplicity") of biomarkers is very common. This means that there are many—not just one—irreducible marker sets that yield optimal predictivity. Whenever the full equivalence class of optimal biomarkers and MPs is of interest, the TIE algorithm [60] that is both theoretically provably sound and successfully tested in multiple datasets and its corresponding theory of information equivalency as described by Statnikov et al. [61, 62] extracts all optimal MP signatures and provides a robust way to address this problem.

Best Practice Guidelines

We close this informatics methods survey section by referring the reader to the informative study by [46] where *best practice guidelines* as given for analysis of molecular data and to the work conducted by the gene expression quality consortia [15] and the clinical proteomics consortia [63] as containing valuable *guidance about MP bioinformatics analysis and the factors that affect it.*

Case Study: Informatics for Molecular Profiling for Use of Bevacizumab in Patients with Ovarian Cancer

We now provide an example of how the above principles are implemented in the context of developing a real-life MP PPM test.

The *Clinical Problem* addressed by this MP is to predict response to platinum-based chemotherapy and anti-angiogenic treatment with bevacizumab using clinical and molecular tumor characteristics in patients with ovarian cancer. This predictive capability can lead to the creation of a clinico-molecular test to guide improved treatment strategies.

Epithelial ovarian cancer (OVCA) has the highest mortality rate of all gynecologic cancers [64] with the majority of patients diagnosed with stage III or IV disease [65]. Additionally, 20–30% of patients will not respond to standard initial treatment consisting of cytoreductive surgery and platinum-based chemotherapy [66]. Patients are considered platinum-refractory if they progress while on treatment or platinum-resistant if their disease recurs less than 6 months from completion of the initial platinum-based chemotherapy. Even in patients who have a complete initial response to chemotherapy, 80% will recur and eventually develop resistance to multiple drugs and die from drug-resistant disease [67]. Efforts are ongoing to study novel, targeted agents, including bevacizumab, an anti-angiogenic monoclonal antibody against vascular endothelial growth factor (VEGF). Two phase III frontline trials in ovarian cancer (ICON7 and GOG 218) showed statistically significant improvements in median progression free survival (PFS) of 2.3 and 3.8 months, respectively, when bevacizumab was added to standard first-line chemotherapy [68, 69]. Bevacizumab was approved by the FDA for unselected frontline use in ovarian cancer in the US in June of 2018. Unfortunately only a subgroup of patients benefits significantly whereas the majority benefit moderately or do not benefit. The problem is further compounded by the high cost of bevacizumab which is currently approx. $400,000 per progression free life saved in the USA, thus making treatment of all patients economically infeasible and the patients who can afford the drug are not necessarily the ones who will benefit from it. This underscores the pressing clinical need for more individualized treatment strategies.

Accordingly, *informatics objectives* were to discover and statistically validate a new clinico-molecular stratification model with sufficient accuracy to be clinically actionable.

The specific questions that drove this case study are:

- Which patients will benefit from bevacizumab?
- Which patients will benefit from conventional platinum based chemotherapy?
- What is the relative information value of clinical and of molecular information and how to optimally combine them?
- How to create viable clinical strategies that incorporate health economics constraints so that all patients who benefit from bevacizumab will receive it, and those who do not will not burden the system?

Informatics and Data Science Methodology and Research Design Considerations

Early feasibility analysis work demonstrated that gene expression analysis of ovarian cancers performed in The Cancer Genome Atlas (TCGA) has led to a molecular classification of four subtypes [70, 71] with prognostic significance [68]. In addition, it was previously demonstrated that differential response to bevacizumab and platinum-based chemotherapy is observed within those four molecular subtypes using formalin-fixed paraffin-embedded (FFPE) tumor samples from the ICON7 clinical trial [72, 73].

To produce clinically actionable models the informatics team worked closely together with clinical scientists and developed predictive and causal models attributing treatment benefit, and predicting benefit from alternate treatment paths.

Tying Modeling to Randomized Clinical Trials (RCTs) Greatly Facilitates Estimating Clinical Benefits of Alternative Treatments

Figure 8.4 shows the methodological benefits of tying the precision medicine tests to RCTs. In designs where treatments are not randomized (left of Fig. 8.4) the effects of the treatment post-surgery are confounded by observed and latent (unmeasured) clinical and genomic factors. Whereas a variety of design and analytic solutions exist (including matching to known confounders, analytical control of known and suspected confounders, propensity scoring, and causal graph-based do-calculous [55, 59]), they leave open the possibility of residual confounding (matching, analytical controls), are subject to bias (propensity scoring), are subject to undetectable latent confounding (all methods), or are not currently practical to apply in genome-wide scale (do-calculous).

In contrast, development of the precision test based on a RCT design eliminates all confounding both from measured and latent variables. The causal effects of post-treatment factors regardless of observed or latent status are incorporated into the total estimated causal effect of the treatment variables. When factors co-determining the outcome are observed, they can be used as covariates in models that individualize the predicted effect on outcome on the basis of these measured factors.

Data, Specimens and Upstream Analysis

Specimens and clinical data for the case study came from the OVAR-11 (German part of the ICON-7 phase III RCT) [68, 69]. Clinical data used for analysis were: age, race, FIGO stage, histology, treatment, PFS, OS, debulking status, ECOG performance status, independent path review diagnosis and visits. Specimens were randomly allocated to RNA extraction and assay run order. In brief, *upstream analysis* was conducted as follows: 200 ng of RNA was analyzed using the Illumina Whole-Genome DASL array with the HumanRef-8 Bead Chip with 29 K gene transcripts or 21 K unique genes according to the manufacturer's protocol [68]. Gene expression data quality was assessed via residual minus vs. average plots, box plots and jitter plots, to detect experimental artifacts such as batch effects. In addition numerical measures such as stress and dfbeta, and measures of the magnitude of change due to normalization, were utilized [68, 72].

Model Selection and Error Estimation Were Conducted with the RNNFCV Protocol [20, 21].

Whereas the importance of nested cross validation for avoiding overfitting error estimates was highlighted in bioinformatics starting from the early 2000s, one aspect of this design that is not widely recognized, but important for our case study, is the ability to perform the analysis in stages as new data and methods become available without overfitting the error estimates of the best models. This is because in each stage of analysis the new models or data compete with the older ones against multiple internal validation tests, without ever accessing the final test set. Only after a winning model

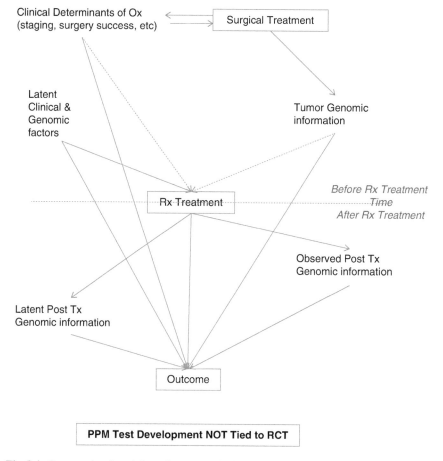

Fig. 8.4 Computational modeling advantages of tying development of precision treatment tests to RCTs. Used with permission from Winterhoff, Boris, et al. "Developing a Clinico-Molecular Test for Individualized Treatment of Ovarian Cancer: The interplay of Precision Medicine Informatics with Clinical and Health Economics Dimensions." AMIA Annual Symposium Proceedings. Vol. 2018. American Medical Informatics Association, 2018, figure 2

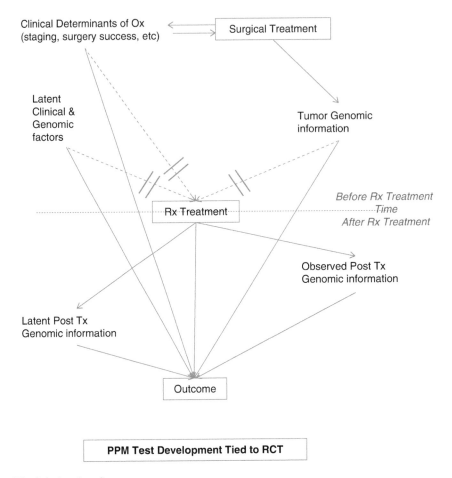

Fig. 8.4 (continued)

has been found, the error estimates are produced up to that round of analysis. This estimate does not affect the choice of best model(s) thus avoiding overfitting. In multi-center, multi-investigator, multi-modality, settings with data obtained in discrete stages, with evolving analytical methods, and with expanding molecular assays, the ability for ongoing, sequential analyses is very important (Fig. 8.5).

Classifiers and Causal Effect Modeling: Supervised Dichotomous Prediction Models for PFS

Whenever a molecular profile is used to predict time-to-event, for example survival in censored data, the data scientist can use time-to-event methods such as survival analysis, and/or methods that discard censored data. Often the choice is an empirical one, especially in high dimensional omics data where survival analyses methods are not yet as fully mature and well-developed as binary outcome ones. In this case study both approaches were followed to create models that were then evaluated for accuracy.

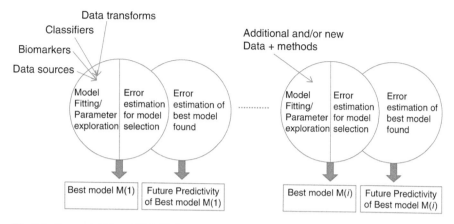

Fig. 8.5 *Sequential* Nested N-Fold Cross-Validation model selection and error estimation design (NNFCV) used for overfitting-resistant *multi-stage analysis* as new methods, and data become available. Used with permission Winterhoff, Boris, et al. "Developing a Clinico-Molecular Test for Individualized Treatment of Ovarian Cancer: The interplay of Precision Medicine Informatics with Clinical and Health Economics Dimensions." AMIA Annual Symposium Proceedings. Vol. 2018. American Medical Informatics Association, 2018, figure 3

First models were created that predict whether patients would relapse within 12, 24, 36, 48, and 60 months from entering the trial and receiving treatment. This analysis excluded patients that dropped out before each prediction point and they were relapse negative. The classifiers of choice were Support Vector Machines (SVMs) [74, 75] with polynomial kernel of degree from 1 to 3, c parameter from 0.1, 1 and 10 optimized with a nested tenfold cross-validation (NNFCV, i.e., inner fold performing grid model selection and outer fold providing unbiased estimates of generalization error measure via ROC AUC). Features entering the analysis included: clinical variables ($n = 20$), and gene expression microarray variables ($n = 29,000$).

Feature Selectors for Binary Prediction Models

The feature selection methods employed in the case study for the dichotomous models were: all features, Markov Boundary induction (via HITON-PC [43, 44] with fixed k parameter to 1), and the 106 ovarian cancer genes from the CLOVAR signature obtained by TCGA analysis and reported in prior literature [73, 76].

Multi-Modal Data Combination Strategies

Multi-modal data combination strategies for clinical+gene expression data included: clinical only, gene expression only and clinical+gene expression in a single input vector. Feature selection and multi-modal combinations evaluation were fully nested in the NNFCV to avoid over-fitting the genes selected to the data. In general, in order to avoid over fitting all data processing steps were always performed and tuned inside the nested cross validation protocol.

Classifiers and Causal Effect Modeling

Classifiers and Causal effect modeling: Time-to-event models that predict risk of relapse under different treatments and identify the patients that will benefit from bevacizumab. In these analyses the informatics steam used Cox modeling [77] combined with Markov Boundary induction [43, 44] for feature selection to model the risk for relapse as a function of treatment and of other measured possible determinants of relapse. Cox modeling uses all available information whereas dichotomous prediction at a fixed time point methods discard information due to censoring [78]. As explained, because the data comes from a randomized trial all possible confounders' effects relating treatment and outcome are eliminating by randomization, thus the estimation of the treatment effect does not require an adjustment for confounders. The multivariate analysis separates the effect of treatment from the effect of other measured co-determinants of relapse, however. The analysis constructed the interaction terms between potential co-determinants of relapse and the treatment. A significant interaction effect indicates a differential treatment effect for different values/levels of a co-determinant, thus results in differential treatment response from patients.

Once a model is fit, one can use the model setting bevacizumab = yes as a prognostic model for the group receiving bevacizumab to estimate the outcome in that group. Similar for bevacizumab = no. It is also straightforward to estimate the difference between the model risk predictions for individual patients setting bevacizumab = yes and then bevacizumab = no in order to estimate the benefit of receiving bevacizumab (i.e., patients for which the estimated risk difference is negative will benefit from bevacizumab). The analysis used 100-repeated 20-fold nested cross-validation. Treatment effects were then estimated for every subject in the testing set. Then different threshold values were applied to the estimated treatment effect to group patients into three groups: (a) predicted to strongly benefit (b) predicted to achieve minor benefit (c) predict to not benefit. For patients in each of the three groups, a comparison is made of the actual observed benefit in terms of relapse between the treated and untreated patients. The relapse outcome was evaluated with Hazard Ratio (HR) and median survival difference between treatment and control [27].

Knowledge-Driven and De Novo Feature Selection for Cox Modeling

Knowledge-Driven and De Novo Feature selection for Cox modeling: to enable the Cox analysis Markov Boundary induction (GLL-PC instantiated with a Cox regression model as the conditional independent test used by the algorithm [43, 44] was used as feature selector; we refer to this feature selector as *GLL-PC-Cox*) *combined with a knowledge-driven gene selection strategy* as follows: genes related to VEGF were selected from the literature and pathway databases strictly based on literature support *without reference to the data in hand (to avoid overfitting)*. The following genes were selected: VEGFA VEGFR2 VEGFB VEGFC VEGFR1 VEGFR3 CLDN6 TUBB2B FGF12 MFAP2 KIF1A. In the current dataset, there are 16 probes measuring 9 of the above genes. A candidate set comprising the 16 gene probes + clinical data variables was formed and Markov Boundary induction was applied on that set using Cox as a conditional independence test when performing feature selection, and then the selected features are fitted with a Cox model. Once more, all steps were fully embedded inside the inner loop of the NNFCV design.

Computational Models

Prognostic Models (Binary Outcomes)

Models predicting Progression Free Survival (PFS) with predictivity and selected feature types/numbers are shown in Table 8.1. In bold are models with sufficient predictivity to be potentially clinically actionable (we operationally set a threshold of .75 AUC, representing the predictivity of current state of the art FDA-approved cancer outcome and other clinically used molecular profiles). As can be seen, the best models have sufficient predictivity to support for clinically actionable prognosis. The de novo feature selection clearly outperforms the predictivity of the 106 genes (CLOVAR signature) previously reported in literature (CLOVAR AUC = 0.63). Also notably for this type of model, just three clinical variables achieve an AUC of .75 A slightly less predictive model can be obtained with gene expression. However the clinical variables are highly subjective e.g. residual disease after surgical cytoreduction is determined by the surgeon, which may not translate to other surgeons and they could also be manipulated or biased to favor decisions towards specific treatment options. This risk can be mitigated by using the objective and tampering-resistant gene expression models. Predictivity after 48 months drops because many patients have exited the trial at that time.

Table 8.1 Dichotomous prognostic models

Time point:		12 month	24 month	36 month	48 month	60 month
Models with clinical features only	AUC	0.71 ± 0.03	**0.75 ± 0.03**	0.73 ± 0.02	**0.75 ± 0.02**	0.71 ± 0.04
	# of features	5	4	4	3	3
Models with gene expression only	AUC	0.56 ± 0.03	0.58 ± 0.03	0.68 ± 0.03	**0.74 ± 0.03**	0.42 ± 0.05
	# of features	149	153	222	215	94
Models with clinical + gene expression	AUC	0.62 ± 0.02	0.65 ± 0.03	0.72 ± 0.03	**0.77 ± 0.02**	0.57 ± 0.03
	# of features	4 + 149	3 + 142	3 + 202	3 + 176	3 + 79
Models with 106 genes from prior work (CLOVAR signature)	AUC	0.62 ± 0.04	0.59 ± 0.03	0.62 ± 0.03	0.62 ± 0.02	0.47 ± 0.06
	# of features	8	4	6	7	2

Used with permission from Winterhoff, Boris, et al. "Developing a Clinico-Molecular Test for Individualized Treatment of Ovarian Cancer: The interplay of Precision Medicine Informatics with Clinical and Health Economics Dimensions." AMIA Annual Symposium Proceedings. Vol. 2018. American Medical Informatics Association, 2018, table 1

Time to Event Model

The final Cox Model (complete model) is shown in Table 8.2. Out of 16 genes + clinical variables and their interaction with the treatment, seven variables remained in the final model after feature selection with GLL-PC-Cox. VEGFA, MFAP2, and ECOG have a significant interaction effect with the treatment, indicating that the effects of these variables on progression free survival depends on if the treatment was administered. For example, MFAP2 show a significant main effect with coefficient of 0.23, a significant interaction with treatment with coefficient of −0.15. In the treatment group, MFAP2 have an overall coefficient of $0.23 + (−0.15) \times 1 = 0.08$ (HR = 1.08). In the control group, MRAP2 have an overall coefficient of $0.23 + (−0.15) \times 0 = 0.23$ (HR = 1.25).

Table 8.2 Time-to-event causal effect and prognostic models

Variables	Coef	exp(Coef)	se exp. (Coef)	z	pval
figo_numeric: figo stage coded as integers, 10 levels, 1 = IA, 2 = IB, …, 9 = IIIC, and 10 = IV	0.31	1.37	0.06	5.58	2.39E-08
surg_outcome: three levels, −1 = suboptimal; 0 = optimal but remaining tissue smaller than 1 cm; +1 = optimal or no macroscopic tissue remaining	−0.35	0.71	0.08	−4.61	3.98E-06
MFAP2: Gene expression level of MFAP2, microfibril associated protein 2, ranges from 6.7 to 15.9 with mean of 13.1	0.23	1.26	0.06	3.70	0.000215
ECOG: ECOG performance status, three levels, 0 = fully active, able to carry on all pre-disease performance without restriction; 1 = restricted in physically strenuous activity but ambulatory and able to carry out work of a light or sedentary nature, 2 = ambulatory and capable of all selfcare but unable to carry out any work activities; up and about more than 50% of waking hours.	0.48	1.61	0.14	3.34	0.000851
VEGFAxrndid *VEGFA*: Gene expression level of MFAP2, vascular endothelial growth factor A, ranges from 4.9 to 13.3 with mean of 10.5 *Rndid*: 1 = bevacizumab+carboplatin; 0 = carboplatin. VEGFAxrndid, MFAP2xrndid,ECOGxrndid indicate interaction effects.	0.19	1.20	0.07	2.76	0.005818
MFAP2xrndid	−0.15	0.86	0.05	−2.83	0.004651
ECOGxrndid	−0.44	0.64	0.19	−2.26	0.023707

Concordance = 0.693 (se = 0.019), Rsquare = 0.281 (max possible = 0.999), likelihood ratio test = 125.2 on 7 df, p = 0, Wald test = 97.88 on 7 df, p = 0, and score (logrank) test = 108.7 on 7 df, p = 0.

Used with permission from Winterhoff, Boris, et al. "Developing a Clinico-Molecular Test for Individualized Treatment of Ovarian Cancer: The interplay of Precision Medicine Informatics with Clinical and Health Economics Dimensions." AMIA Annual Symposium Proceedings. Vol. 2018. American Medical Informatics Association, 2018, table 2

Identifying Subpopulations Who Benefit from Bevacizumab

By exploring different thresholds on the PFS risk produced by the Cox models, individual patients and subpopulations that will benefit the most, the least, and in between can be readily identified. Table 8.3 shows examples of subpopulation identification.

For example, the second row (grey background) depicts separation of a subgroup equal to 20% of the total patient population that will benefit approx. 10 months for survival, or on the other end a subgroup equal to 40% of the total population without benefit (nominal benefit of 1.3 months which is not statistically significant).

Figure 8.6 depicts Kaplan-Meier curves (top) and heatmaps (bottom) corresponding to these subgroups and predictor variables in the reduced model, identifying patients and subgroups that will benefit the most or the least from bevacizumab. Patients that benefit more from the addition of bevacizumab have lower expression level of VEGF-A, higher expression level of MFAP2 and worse EGOC performance

Table 8.3 Examples of using the Cox models to identify patient subgroups that will benefit the most and the least from bevacizumab

		Predict to not benefit				Gray zone				Predict to benefit			
		Median surv diff		HR		Median surv diff		HR		Median surv diff		HR	
Perc.	Thre.	Mean	Sd	Mean	Sd	Mean	Sd	Mean	Sd	Mean	Sd	Mean	Sd
40%	60%	1.28	1.45	0.95	0.07	7.99	4.60	0.82	0.13	7.74	0.86	0.62	0.05
40%	80%	1.28	1.45	0.95	0.07	5.79	2.12	0.77	0.06	9.95	1.53	0.49	0.07
60%	80%	3.34	0.77	0.90	0.04	5.63	2.49	0.73	0.12	9.95	1.53	0.49	0.07

Used with permission from Winterhoff, Boris, et al. "Developing a Clinico-Molecular Test for Individualized Treatment of Ovarian Cancer: The interplay of Precision Medicine Informatics with Clinical and Health Economics Dimensions." AMIA Annual Symposium Proceedings. Vol. 2018. American Medical Informatics Association, 2018, table 3

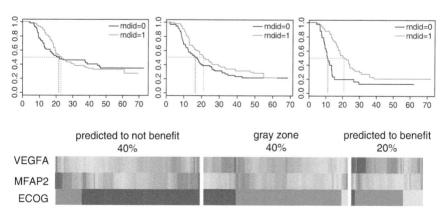

Fig. 8.6 Kaplan-Meier curves (top) and heatmaps (bottom) corresponding to subgroups and predictor variables in the reduced model identifying patients and subgroups that will benefit the most or the least from bevacizumab. Used with permission Winterhoff, Boris, et al. "Developing a Clinico-Molecular Test for Individualized Treatment of Ovarian Cancer: The interplay of Precision Medicine Informatics with Clinical and Health Economics Dimensions." AMIA Annual Symposium Proceedings. Vol. 2018. American Medical Informatics Association, 2018, figure 4

status. Each column indicates a patient. Yellow color indicates higher value, green intermediate value and blue indicates lower value. All variables are scaled between 0 and 1 to assist visualization.

Construction of Treatment Strategies

By using the above analytical models one can construct and evaluate clinical treatment strategies. Two example strategies are depicted in Fig. 8.7. The top strategy identifies a "clear benefit" group that should receive bevacizumab, a "no benefit" group that should receive standard treatment if the dichotomous prognosis models predict good response to Carboplatin or should be routed to experimental therapeutics if predicted response is not good. An intermediate group with "minor/questionable benefit" from bevacizumab may receive standard care plus bevacizumab in case of

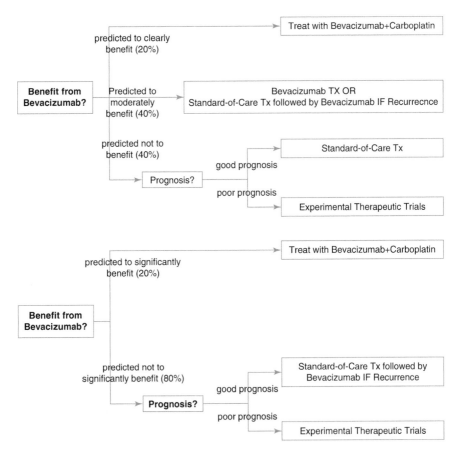

Fig. 8.7 Example of clinical strategies utilizing precision treatment models/tests. Top: benefit-questionable benefit-no benefit subgroups. Bottom: benefit-no/questionable benefit subgroups. Used with permission Winterhoff, Boris, et al. "Developing a Clinico-Molecular Test for Individualized Treatment of Ovarian Cancer: The interplay of Precision Medicine Informatics with Clinical and Health Economics Dimensions." AMIA Annual Symposium Proceedings. Vol. 2018. American Medical Informatics Association, 2018, figure 5

recurrence. An alternative binary strategy is depicted in the lower bottom of Fig. 8.7 where the "no benefit" and "minor/questionable benefit" groups have been merged.

Health Economic Aspects

In a comprehensive study of the cost effectiveness of alternative strategies of using bevacizumab as primary treatment for ovarian cancer, Barnett et al. showed via mathematical modeling that a postulated (i.e., not yet existent at the time of economic analysis) predictive model for benefit from bevacizumab would provide a dominant bevacizumab treatment strategy [79]. The Molecular profile presented in the present case study introduces precisely such a model.

Table 8.4 summarizes the potential for health economic impact of a precision test based on the predictivity of the models discussed and of corresponding clinical strategies outlined in this chapter when treating all patients with bevacizumab com-

Table 8.4 Summary economic impact of precision tests, of data analytics and of coupling R&D to RCTs

Estimated health economic impact of deploying PPM test at full scale –treating all patients with bevacizumab compared to treating only the group predicted to strongly benefit
$96 billion savings over a 10 year horizon.   Assumptions: • 200,000 patients annually globally.   • All patients receive precision medicine test (approx. cost of $2000/test) but only 20% of patients (i.e., those identified to benefit) receive bevacizumab.   • Cost of bevacizumab/patient is $60,000 (lower international cost range used).   • Baseline comparison: all patients receive bevacizumab.
Incremental cost-effectiveness ratio (ICER)
• $40,000–$80,000 per QALY for predictive test—based treatment.   • $180,000–$360,000 per QALY for universal treatment.   Assumptions: • Cost of bevacizumab/patient calculated as $5000 to $10,000/month × 12 month of treatment (depending on US or international costs)   • Average QAL benefit over all patients is 4 months.   • Predictive test accuracy as presented in present work.
Time acceleration and R&D economic impact of RCT tie for development of PPM test
• *5–10 years acceleration* to precision test deployment.   • $50million cost savings.   Assumptions: • Patients number in a RCT is 2000.   • RCT cost per patient is $25,000 (global average).
Economic impact of feature selection to deployment costs of PPM test
• *Maximum of $1.2 billion.*   Assumptions: • Discovery assay cost/patient $3000.   • Deployment assay/model cost/patient = $300.   • 500,000 patients globally over 10 years.

Revised with permission from Winterhoff, Boris, et al. "Developing a Clinico-Molecular Test for Individualized Treatment of Ovarian Cancer: The interplay of Precision Medicine Informatics with Clinical and Health Economics Dimensions." AMIA Annual Symposium Proceedings. Vol. 2018. American Medical Informatics Association, 2018, table 4

pared to treating only the group predicted to benefit the most. Table 8.4 also summarizes other cost savings/economic impact on the R&D side of things (specifically the economic impact of feature selection for reducing the discovery model to a deployment model and costs saved by tying the precision medicine test development to pre-existing RCTs).

As can be seen in Table 8.4, use of the discovered model reported here can save the health system over a projected 10 year lifetime of bevacizumab, a maximum of $96B globally without significant loss of survival/QULY benefit for individual patients.

The *Incremental Cost-Effectiveness Ratio* (ICER) of unselected frontline treatment with bevacizumab is currently >$360,000 per QALY gained, in the USA. The ICR of selective treatment by using the molecular profile in this case study is estimated at $80,000 per QUALY gained, which by current health economic standards in the USA renders it viable. Moreover the selective treatment described renders it a dominant bevacizumab treatment strategy and may also be acceptable in a variety of other willingness-to-pay threshold settings. The test can thus justify reimbursement for patients who do benefit for the drug and can induce payers to cover the medical expenses for those who will benefit. Finally the test can route the patients who will not benefit from either conventional or bevacizumab treatment to alternative experimental treatments with additional life and economic benefits.

Conclusions

The present chapter provided an introduction to key informatics workflows and methods used for molecular profile development. In addition we discussed a case study that showcases how the various principles are implemented together in practice. In combination with Chaps. 7 and 8 the present chapter should give to readers a thorough overview of molecular profiling-based PPM, and how informatics enables it.

Informatics plays a critical role in the development of MPs PPM tests. The research design choice of connecting development of precision medicine tests to RCTs yields extraordinary cost, speed and scientific validity benefits.

The informatics work is most effective when guided by and supporting driving clinical and health economic requirements and objectives, as illustrated.

References

1. Mardis ER. Next-generation DNA sequencing methods. Annu Rev Genom Hum Genet. 2008;9(1):387–402.
2. Mardis ER. The impact of next-generation sequencing technology on genetics. Trends Genet. 2008;24(3):133–41.
3. Schuster SC. Next-generation sequencing transforms today's biology. Nat Methods. 2007;5(1):16.

4. Nuwaysir EF, Huang W, Albert TJ, Singh J, Nuwaysir K, Pitas A, et al. Gene expression analysis using oligonucleotide arrays produced by Maskless photolithography. Genome Res. 2002;12(11):1749–55.
5. Baldi P, Hatfield GW. DNA microarrays and gene expression: from experiments to data analysis and modeling. Cambridge: Cambridge University Press; 2011.
6. Link AJ, Eng J, Schieltz DM, Carmack E, Mize GJ, Morris DR, et al. Direct analysis of protein complexes using mass spectrometry. Nat Biotechnol. 1999;17(7):676–82.
7. Guo Z, Yarasheski K, Jensen MD. High-precision isotopic analysis of palmitoylcarnitine by liquid chromatography/electrospray ionization ion-trap tandem mass spectrometry. Rapid Commun Mass Spectrom. 2006;20(22):3361–6.
8. Syka JE, Coon JJ, Schroeder MJ, Shabanowitz J, Hunt DF. Peptide and protein sequence analysis by electron transfer dissociation mass spectrometry. Proc Natl Acad Sci USA. 2004;101(26):9528–33.
9. Liebler DC. Introduction to proteomics: tools for the new biology. Berlin: Springer; 2001.
10. Chamberlain JS, Gibbs RA, Ranier JE, Nguyen PN, Caskey CT. Deletion screening of the Duchenne muscular dystrophy locus via multiplex DNA amplification. Nucleic Acids Res. 1988;16(23):11141–56.
11. Parmigiani G, Garett ES, Irizarry RA, Zeger SL. The analysis of gene expression data: methods and software. Berlin: Springer; 2006. p. 511.
12. Brown SM. Next-generation DNA sequencing informatics. Harbor Laboratory Press: Cold Spring; 2013.
13. Scherer A. Batch effects and noise in microarray experiments: sources and solutions, vol. 868. Chichester: Wiley; 2009.
14. Zhang W, Shmulevich I, Astola J. Microarray quality control, vol. 158. Hoboken, NJ: Wiley; 2005.
15. Shi L, Campbell G, Jones WD, Campagne F, Wen Z, et al. The MicroArray quality control (MAQC)-II study of common practices for the development and validation of microarray-based predictive models. Nat Biotechnol. 2010;28(8):827–38.
16. Schbath S, Martin V, Zytnicki M, Fayolle J, Loux V, Gibrat J-F. Mapping reads on a genomic sequence: an algorithmic overview and a practical comparative analysis. J Comput Biol. 2012;19(6):796–813.
17. Mandoiu I, Zelikovsky A. Computational methods for next generation sequencing data analysis. Hoboken, NJ: Wiley; 2016. p. 665.
18. Morgan XC, Huttenhower C. Chapter 12: human microbiome analysis. PLoS Comput Biol. 2012;8(12):e1002808.
19. Turroni F, Marchesi JR, Foroni E, Gueimonde M, Shanahan F, Margolles A, et al. Microbiomic analysis of the bifidobacterial population in the human distal gut. ISME J. 2009;3(6):745–51.
20. Statnikov A. A gentle introduction to support vector Machines in Biomedicine: theory and methods. Hardcover: World Scientific Publishing Co; 2011. p. 200.
21. Duda RO, Hart PE, Stork DG. Pattern classification. New York: Wiley; 2012. p. 679.
22. Hastie T, Tibshirani R, Friedman J. The elements of statistical learning: data mining, inference, and prediction. Berlin: Springer; 2013. p. 545.
23. Mitchell TM. Machine learning. Hardcover: McGraw-Hill Education; 1997. p. 414.
24. Simon R, Altman DG. Statistical aspects of prognostic factor studies in oncology. Br J Cancer. 1994;69(6):979–85.
25. Flach PA. The geometry of ROC space: understanding machine learning metrics through ROC isometrics. In: Proceedings of the 20th international conference on machine learning (ICML-03); 2003. p. 194–201.
26. Greiner M, Pfeiffer D, Smith R. Principles and practical application of the receiver-operating characteristic analysis for diagnostic tests. Prev Vet Med. 2000;45(1–2):23–41.
27. Clark TG, Bradburn MJ, Love SB, Altman DG. Survival analysis part I: basic concepts and first analyses. Br J Cancer. 2003;89(2):232–8.
28. Brier GW. Verification of forecasts expressed in terms of probability. Mon Weather Rev. 1950;78(1):1–3.

29. Steyerberg EW, Vickers AJ, Cook NR, Gerds T, Gonen M, Obuchowski N, et al. Assessing the performance of prediction models: a framework for some traditional and novel measures. Epidemiology. 2010;21(1):128–38.
30. Kattan MW. Comparison of Cox regression with other methods for determining prediction models and nomograms. J Urol. 2003;170(Suppl 6):S6–10.
31. Ray B, Henaff M, Ma S, Efstathiadis E, Peskin ER, Picone M, et al. Information content and analysis methods for multi-modal high-throughput biomedical data. Sci Rep. 2014;4:4411.
32. Aliferis CF, Statnikov A, Tsamardinos I. Challenges in the analysis of mass-throughput data: a technical commentary from the statistical machine learning perspective. Cancer Inform. 2007;16(2):133–62.
33. Aliferis CF, Statnikov A, Tsamardinos I, Schildcrout JS, Shepherd BE, Harrell FE. Factors influencing the statistical power of complex data analysis protocols for molecular signature development from microarray data. PLoS One. 2009;4(3):e4922.
34. Guyon I, Elisseeff A. An introduction to variable and feature selection. J Mach Learn Res. 2003;3:1157–82.
35. Liu H, Motoda H. Computational methods of feature selection. Boca Raton, FL: CRC Press; 2007. p. 437.
36. Tsamardinos I, Aliferis CF. Towards principled feature selection: relevancy, filters and wrappers; 2003. p. AISTATS.
37. Guyon I, Gunn S, Nikravesh M, Zadeh LA. Feature extraction: foundations and applications. Berlin: Springer; 2008. p. 765.
38. Statnikov A, Wang L, Aliferis CF. A comprehensive comparison of random forests and support vector machines for microarray-based cancer classification. BMC Bioinformatics. 2008;9:319.
39. Statnikov A, Aliferis CF, Tsamardinos I, Hardin D, Levy S. A comprehensive evaluation of multicategory classification methods for microarray gene expression cancer diagnosis. Bioinformatics. 2005;21(5):631–43.
40. Simon N, Friedman J, Hastie T, Tibshirani R. Regularization paths for Cox's proportional hazards model via coordinate descent. J Stat Softw. 2011;39(5):1–13.
41. Lagani V, Tsamardinos I. Structure-based variable selection for survival data. Bioinformatics. 2010;26(15):1887–94.
42. Ishwaran H, Kogalur UB, Blackstone EH, Lauer MS. Random survival forests. Ann Appl Stat. 2008;2(3):841–60.
43. Aliferis CF, Statnikov A, Tsamardinos I, Mani S, Koutsoukos XD. Local causal and Markov blanket induction for causal discovery and feature selection for classification part i: algorithms and empirical evaluation. J Mach Learn Res. 2010;11:171–234.
44. Aliferis CF, Statnikov A, Tsamardinos I, Mani S, Koutsoukos XD. Local causal and Markov blanket induction for causal discovery and feature selection for classification part ii: analysis and extensions. J Mach Learn Res. 2010;11:235–84.
45. Breiman L. Random forests. Mach Learn. 2001;45(1):5–32.
46. Dupuy A, Simon RM. Critical review of published microarray studies for cancer outcome and guidelines on statistical analysis and reporting. J Natl Cancer Inst. 2007;99(2):147–57.
47. Vlachos IS, Zagganas K, Paraskevopoulou MD, Georgakilas G, Karagkouni D, Vergoulis T, et al. DIANA-miRPath v3.0: deciphering microRNA function with experimental support. Nucleic Acids Res. 2015;43(Web Server issue):W460–6.
48. Alexiou P, Maragkakis M, Papadopoulos GL, Reczko M, Hatzigeorgiou AG. Lost in translation: an assessment and perspective for computational microRNA target identification. Bioinformatics. 2009;25(23):3049–55.
49. Yang Q, Qiu C, Yang J, Wu Q, Cui Q. miREnvironment database: providing a bridge for microRNAs, environmental factors and phenotypes. Bioinformatics. 2011;27(23):3329–30.
50. Barenboim M, Zoltick BJ, Guo Y, Weinberger DR. MicroSNiPer: a web tool for prediction of SNP effects on putative microRNA targets. Hum Mutat. 2010;31(11):1223–32.
51. Wang D, Gu J, Wang T, Ding Z. OncomiRDB: a database for the experimentally verified oncogenic and tumor-suppressive microRNAs. Bioinformatics. 2014;30(15):2237–8.
52. Huang Z, Shi J, Gao Y, Cui C, Zhang S, Li J, et al. HMDD v3.0: a database for experimentally supported human microRNA-disease associations. Nucleic Acids Res. 2019;47(D1):D1013–7.

53. Lanceta J, Prough RA, Liang R, Wang E. MicroRNA group disorganization in aging. Exp Gerontol. 2010;45(4):269–78.
54. Schmitz U, Lai X, Winter F, Wolkenhauer O, Vera J, Gupta SK. Cooperative gene regulation by microRNA pairs and their identification using a computational workflow. Nucleic Acids Res. 2014;42(12):7539–52.
55. Pearl J. Causality: models, reasoning and inference. New York, NY: Cambridge University Press; 2009. p. 478.
56. Spirtes P, Glymour CN, Scheines R. Causation, prediction, and search [Internet], vol. xxi. 2nd ed. Cambridge, MA: MIT Press; 2000. p. 543. http://cognet.mit.edu/book/causation-prediction-and-search
57. Narendra V, Lytkin NI, Aliferis CF, Statnikov A. A comprehensive assessment of methods for de-novo reverse-engineering of genome-scale regulatory networks. Genomics. 2011;97(1):7–18.
58. Subramanian A, Tamayo P, Mootha VK, Mukherjee S, Ebert BL, Gillette MA, et al. Gene set enrichment analysis: a knowledge-based approach for interpreting genome-wide expression profiles. Proc Natl Acad Sci U S A. 2005;102(43):15545–50.
59. Huang Y, Valtorta M. Pearl's Calculus of intervention is complete. arXiv:12066831 [cs] [Internet]. 2012 Jun 27 [cited 2018 Oct 27]. http://arxiv.org/abs/1206.6831.
60. Statnikov A, Lytkin NI, Lemeire J, Aliferis CF. Algorithms for discovery of multiple Markov boundaries. J Mach Learn Res. 2013;14:499–566.
61. Statnikov A, Lytkin NI, McVoy L, Weitkamp J-H, Aliferis CF. Using gene expression profiles from peripheral blood to identify asymptomatic responses to acute respiratory viral infections. BMC Res Notes. 2010;3:264.
62. Statnikov A, Alekseyenko AV, Li Z, Henaff M, Perez-Perez GI, Blaser MJ, et al. Microbiomic signatures of psoriasis: feasibility and methodology comparison. Sci Rep. 2013;3:2620.
63. Ellis MJ, Gillette M, Carr SA, Paulovich AG, Smith RD, Rodland KK, et al. Connecting genomic alterations to cancer biology with proteomics: the NCI clinical proteomic tumor analysis Consortium. Cancer Discov. 2013;3(10):1108–12.
64. Cancer Facts & Figures 2016 | American Cancer Society [Internet]. [cited 2018 Mar 7]. https://www.cancer.org/research/cancer-facts-statistics/all-cancer-facts-figures/cancer-facts-figures-2016.html
65. Barnholtz-Sloan JS, Schwartz AG, Qureshi F, Jacques S, Malone J, Munkarah AR. Ovarian cancer: changes in patterns at diagnosis and relative survival over the last three decades. Am J Obstet Gynecol. 2003;189(4):1120–7.
66. Friedlander ML, Stockler MR, Butow P, King MT, McAlpine J, Tinker A, et al. Clinical trials of palliative chemotherapy in platinum-resistant or -refractory ovarian cancer: time to think differently? JCO. 2013;31(18):2362.
67. Baker VV. Salvage therapy for recurrent epithelial ovarian cancer. Hematol Oncol Clin North Am. 2003;17(4):977–88.
68. Kommoss S, Winterhoff B, Oberg AL, Konecny GE, Wang C, Riska SM, et al. Bevacizumab may differentially improve ovarian Cancer outcome in patients with proliferative and mesenchymal molecular subtypes. Clin Cancer Res. 2017;23(14):3794–801.
69. Perren TJ, Swart AM, Pfisterer J, Ledermann JA, Pujade-Lauraine E, Kristensen G, et al. A phase 3 trial of bevacizumab in ovarian Cancer. N Engl J Med. 2011;365(26):2484–96.
70. Cancer Genome Atlas Research Network. Integrated genomic analyses of ovarian carcinoma. Nature. 2011;474(7353):609–15.
71. Tothill RW, Tinker AV, George J, Brown R, Fox SB, Lade S, et al. Novel molecular subtypes of serous and endometrioid ovarian cancer linked to clinical outcome. Clin Cancer Res. 2008;14(16):5198–208.
72. Winterhoff B, Hamidi H, Wang C, Kalli KR, Fridley BL, Dering J, et al. Molecular classification of high grade endometrioid and clear cell ovarian cancer using TCGA gene expression signatures. Gynecol Oncol. 2016;141(1):95–100.
73. Konecny GE, Wang C, Hamidi H, Winterhoff B, Kalli KR, Dering J, et al. Prognostic and therapeutic relevance of molecular subtypes in high-grade serous ovarian cancer. J Natl Cancer Inst. 2014;106(10):dju249.

74. Vapnik V. The nature of statistical learning theory. 2nd ed. New York: Springer; 2000. [cited 2018 Mar 8]. (Information Science and Statistics). //www.springer.com/us/book/9780387987804

75. Boser BE, Guyon IM, Vapnik VN. A training algorithm for optimal margin classifiers. In: Proceedings of the fifth annual workshop on computational learning theory. New York, NY: ACM; 1992. [cited 2018 Mar 8], (COLT '92). p. 144–52. https://doi.org/10.1145/130385.130401.

76. Verhaak RGW, Tamayo P, Yang J-Y, Hubbard D, Zhang H, Creighton CJ, et al. Prognostically relevant gene signatures of high-grade serous ovarian carcinoma. J Clin Invest. 2013;123(1):517–25.

77. Cox DR. Regression models and life-tables. In: Breakthroughs in statistics, Springer Series in Statistics. New York, NY: Springer; 1992. [cited 2018 Mar 8]. p. 527–41. https://doi.org/10.1007/978-1-4612-4380-9_37.

78. Efron B. The efficiency of Cox's likelihood function for censored data. J Am Stat Assoc. 1977;72(359):557–65.

79. Barnett JC, Alvarez Secord A, Cohn DE, Leath CA III, Myers ER, Havrilesky LJ. Cost effectiveness of alternative strategies for incorporating bevacizumab into the primary treatment of ovarian cancer. Cancer. 2013;119(20):3653–61.

Chapter 9
Constructing Software for Cancer Research in Support of Molecular PPM

Richard Simon and Yingdong Zhao

Introduction

Collaboration between biostatisticians or bioinformaticists and clinical investigators has been effective and important for the improvements in cancer treatment achieved over the past two decades. This model, however, has not scaled successfully when utilizing whole genome data to understand biological mechanisms or discover new therapeutic targets. Collaborations between clinical investigators and biostatisticians typically address problems of hypothesis testing. These problems may be large and complex, but they are generally well defined.

For problems of exploratory biological discovery, we have tried to pair basic biomedical investigators with bioinformaticists. This provides the biomedical investigators with access to the data, but the collaboration is often not synergistic unless the bioinformaticist has detailed knowledge of the biological areas under investigation. This type of interaction can either be "inter-disciplinary" or "trans-disciplinary". The former means that each collaborator knows his or her own field, but not much about the field of the other collaborator. Only with "trans-disciplinary" collaboration, where each collaborator knows both his or her own field and a lot about the collaborator's field, do we usually see the type of synergy that leads to discovery. Bioinformaticists with a strong background in biology but lacking sufficient qualifications in data analysis will often fail to make the collaboration truly synergistic. The bioinformaticist needs the expertise to inform the biological investigator about weaknesses in the proposed exploratory and hypothesis-free research that may render it sterile, lest he or she may be serving as a technician. The biomedical

R. Simon (✉) · Y. Zhao
Computational and Systems Biology Branch, Biometric Research Program,
Division of Cancer Treatment and Diagnosis, National Cancer Institute, Rockville, MD, USA
e-mail: rsimon@mail.nih.gov; zhaoy@mail.nih.gov

© Springer Nature Switzerland AG 2020
T. Adam, C. Aliferis (eds.), *Personalized and Precision Medicine Informatics*,
Health Informatics, https://doi.org/10.1007/978-3-030-18626-5_9

investigator must be sufficiently insightful to devise an approach that is scientifically sound and creative and not just a blind tabulation of results. Although this type of collaboration can work effectively, there is a dearth of bioinformaticists with expertise in both biology and data analysis.

In the Biometric Research Program at the National Cancer Institute we have tried the structuring of several types of collaborative teams. The Program consists of both a Biostatistics Branch and a Systems & Computational Biology Branch and we have trained a large number of post-doctoral fellows in bioinformatics and computational biology. We have found that for exploratory and hypothesis-free problems it can be effective to develop software that empowers the biomedical scientist to perform discovery analysis on his or her own. The software must have built-in easy access to data sources, biological annotations, statistical analyses and biologically sophisticated types of analyses. We have generally found that this software must be focused on specific areas of discovery; general software lacks the biological sophistication needed for deep analysis. In this chapter we will describe one software system we have developed for this purpose.

Data for NCI Transcriptional Pharmacodynamics Workbench

The National Cancer Institute has over many years screened compounds for anti-cancer activity against 60 human tumor cell lines [1, 2]. The cell lines are very well characterized with regard to exome sequencing, micro-array gene expression profiling, copy number alterations, etc. The cell lines represent multiple tumor histologies [3]. What is most unique about these cell lines is the tens of thousands of compounds that have been screened for growth modifying effects [4, 5].

There are other sets of human tumor cell lines that have also been characterized in various ways. The characterizations are almost always of the un-treated cell lines [6, 7]. There are not good examples of human tumor cell lines which are expression profiled after treatment with a cancer drug. Although the NIH Library of Integrated Network-based Cellular Signatures (LINCS) project and the Connectivity Map have collected the after-treatment gene expression data for thousands of compounds, the data are restricted to less than 10 cancer cell lines and the vast majority are using L1000 assay that only measures expression of around 1000 "landmark" genes [8–10]. The NCI set out to perform micro-array gene expression profiling to the NCI-60 after treatment with one of 15 anti-cancer drugs [11]. The drugs were selected for a spectrum of mechanism of actions; both DNA damaging agents, kinase inhibitors and receptor antagonists: azacytidine, bortezomib, cisplatin, dasatinib, doxorubicin, erlotinib, geldanamycin, gemcitabine, lapatinib, paclitaxel, sirolimus, sorafenib, sunitinib, topotecan, and vorinostat. Each drug was studied at low and high concentrations as well as a control of zero concentration. Expression profiling was performed at 2, 6 and 24 h after drug administration.

This experiment involved 7652 micro-array assays with 12,704 transcripts represented per array. It is the type of experiment that no single laboratory can typically afford. It provided a discovery data-set that would be unlikely to be funded by ordinary grant mechanisms. In addition to the gene expression profiles, there were 1227 genes with mutation data, and GI50 data on all cell lines and drugs. It was hoped that cancer biologists, pharmacologists and therapeutics developers could use the data to understand mechanisms that tumors use in response to drug insults, in order to understand the mechanisms of resistance and to discover therapeutic targets.

NCI Transcriptional Pharmacodynamics Workbench Software

Methods

Raw CEL files were background-subtracted and normalized using the Robust Multi-array Average (RMA) algorithm [12] for all cell lines treated by the same drug. There were 170,463,604 data points in 7652 Affymetrix array experiments. The data containing 22,227 probe sets was then summarized into 12,704 genes by taking the average of log base 2 measurements of probe sets for each gene (gene list obtained from Affymetrix U133A). The data matrix for NCI60 cell lines treated by each of the 15 drugs at different time points and different dose levels, including baseline experiments (zero concentration), were then stored in backend SQLite tables. Data analysis and graphic display were all performed under R 2.15.0 package.

There are 50 tables total in the backend SQLite database. These tables include: 15 tables for gene expression profiles in cell lines treated by 15 different drugs, respectively; 15 tables for the sample information in 15 gene expression profiles, respectively; 15 tables for the phenotypes (logGI50, doubling time, and multidrug resistance) information, each of which is related to a specific drug; one table for 1227 gene mutation data in cell lines; one table for 154 protein expression data in cell lines; one table for 65 BioCarta pathways and the genes involved in these pathways, one table for 256 experimentally verified transcription factors and their targeted genes, and one table for 53 groups of receptors. Details of the data set used in this web application are summarized in Table 9.1. Table 9.2 shows the actual dosage for each of the 15 drugs at high or low concentration used in gene expression experiments. Table 9.3 lists 9 tissue types of cell lines and cell line names in each tissue type.

We needed the website to be able to provide on-the-fly detailed analyses of the data in ways directed by the user. Where possible, we performed analyses in advance and saved the results in order to expedite response times but in many cases this was not possible. The website was programmed using Perl, JavaScript, the R statistical programming language, and SQLite database. All analyses were menu driven by the user.

Figure 9.1a shows the architecture of the NCI TP Workbench. The six main modules are characterized as shown on the right panel of Fig. 9.1a: Query for a single gene; Correlation analysis; Time course graphs; Pathway analyses; Transcription factors and targets, and Receptor analysis. We will provide a summary of each of these modules.

Table 9.1 Summary table for NCI60 drug treated gene expression data set

Drugs	Azacytidine, bortezomib, cisplatin, dasatinib, doxorubicin, erlotinib, geldanamycin, gemcitabine, lapatinib, paclitaxel, sirolimus, sorafenib, sunitinib, topotecan, vorinostat
Concentration	Baseline, low dose, high dose
Time point	2 h, 6 h, 24 h
Number of data points in gene expression experiments	169,817,571
Number of arrays	7623
Number of probe sets per chip	22,277
Number of genes per chip	12,704
Number of GI50 measurements	866
Number of gene mutations	1227
Number of protein expression	154
Number of pathways	65
Number of transcription factors	256
Number of groups of receptors	53

Table 9.2 Dosage used at high and low concentrations for each drug

Drug	High concentration (nM)	Low concentration (nM)
Azacytidine	5000	1000
Bortezomib	100	10
Cisplatin	15,000	3000
Dasatinib	2000	100
Doxorubicin	1000	100
Erlotinib	10,000	1000
Geldanamycin	1000	100
Gemcitabine	2000	200
Lapatinib	10,000	1000
Paclitaxel	100	10
Sirolimus	100	10
Sorafenib	10,000	5000
Sunitinib	2000	200
Topotecan	1000	10
Vorinostat	5000	1000

Query for Single Gene

Having a gene of interest in mind, the first thing a user may want to know is a general picture of how the expressions of this gene change when treated by a specific drug. By entering a gene symbol (e.g., MYC) and selecting one of the 15 drugs from the drop-down menu (e.g., bortezomib), this query function will return a series of graphs that show the expression of the gene MYC in cell lines treated with bortezomib relative to the untreated baseline cell lines. These increments are shown in bar graphs, one bar for each cell line and one graph for each drug concentration (Fig. 9.1b). In the bar plots, right bars indicate elevated gene expression and left

Table 9.3 NCI60 cell lines stratified in nine tissue types

Tissue type	Cell line
Breast	BT-549, HS-578T, MCF7, MDA-MB-231, MDA-MB-468, T-47D
CNS	SF-268, SF-295, SF-539, SNB-19, SNB-75, U251
Colon	COLO-205, HCC-2998, HCT-116, HCT-15, HT29, KM12, SW-620
Leukemia	CCRF-CEM, HL-60, K-562, MOLT-4, RPMI-8226, SR
Lung	A549, EKVX, HOP-62, HOP-92, NCI-H226, NCI-H23, NCI-H322M, NCI-H460, NCI-H522
Melanoma	LOX, M14, MALME-3M, MDA-MB-435, SK-MEL-2, SK-MEL-28, SK-MEL-5, UACC-257, UACC-62
Ovarian	IGR-OV1, NCI-ADR-RES, OVCAR-3, OVCAR-4, OVCAR-5, OVCAR-8, SK-OV-3
Prostate	DU-145, PC-3
Renal	786-0, A498, ACHN, CAKI-1, RXF-393, SN12C, TK-10, UO-31

bars depressed expression. Each bar stands for a cell line. Cell lines are grouped and color coded by tissue type in these graphs. The analysis also provides two scatter plots that show the change in gene expression as related to the basal growth rate (log(GI50)) of the untreated cell lines (Fig. 9.1c). In the scatter plots, each point represents a cell line; vertical axis shows the relative (compared to no treatment) gene expression value and horizontal axis shows log(GI50) of the drug against cell lines. The points above line $y = 0$ denote elevated gene expression and the points below it denote depressed expression relative to cell lines untreated by drugs. Pearson correlation coefficients are calculated and shown in each of the above scatter plots. In addition, the output page also displays scatter plots that show the relative expression of the gene versus doubling time or multidrug resistance protein expression in cell lines treated by high and low dose of drug, respectively. At the bottom of the page, there is a link to save the data by creating output graphs in a comma-separated values (CSV) format file, which can be opened by excel.

The Single gene query module also enables the user to see the effects of each of the 15 drugs on the selected gene. There are static and dynamic types of graph options. Figure 9.2 shows a static output of 15 time course line plots for BRAC1 when treated by each of the 15 drugs at high concentration. In each line plot, each line stands for the log(2) fold change in gene expression for a specific cell line across three time points (i.e., 2, 6, and 24 h). Time profiles under high dose levels are shown by default. The user can also click the link at the bottom on the page to see the time profiles under low dose levels. The graphs can further be stratified by tissue types by checking "Also display the figures stratified by tissue type". The user can then click on each graph in the output page to get the time profiles grouped by tissue type.

To boost the processing speed, the TP Workbench also provides a dynamic way to generate time course line plots. After the user enters a gene name, the system uses a powerful D3 library JavaScript function to load the data into the client side and displays the line plots dynamically. On the screenshot shown in Fig. 9.3a, 15 time course line plots for BRAF are shown, each one corresponding to cell lines treated by one of the 15 drugs. When moving the mouse cursor on each of the nine tissue types color coded on the top panel, only cell lines for the specified tissue type are highlighted. The highlighted lines can be fixed by clicking on one of the tissue types. On the top

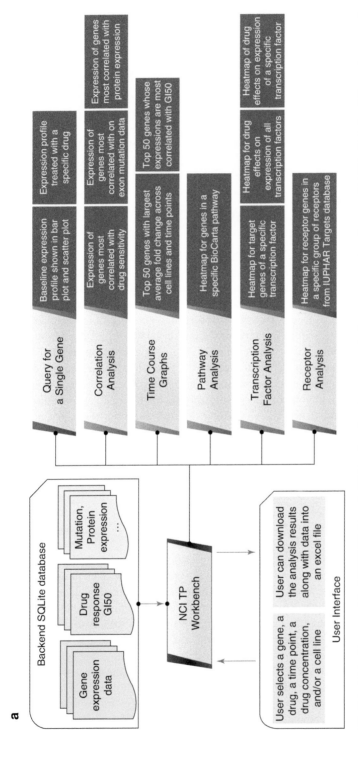

Fig. 9.1 (**a**) Architecture of the NCI TP Workbench. (**b**) Bar plots showing query results for gene expression changes of MYC in NCI 60 cell lines when treated with bortezomib at high dose (100 nM, top panel) and low dose (10 nM, bottom panel). (**c**) Scatter plots show gene expression changes of MYC vs. GI50 when treated with bortezomib at high dose (100 nM, top panel) and low dose (10 nM, bottom panel) at time points 2, 6, and 24 h

b Query Result for Expression of A Specific Gene in NCI-60 Cell Lines Treated with Drug

Note: all cell lines are categorized by colors which represent different tissue origins of them.

Expression of MYC in NCI-60 cell lines treated with high concentration of bortezomib (100nM)

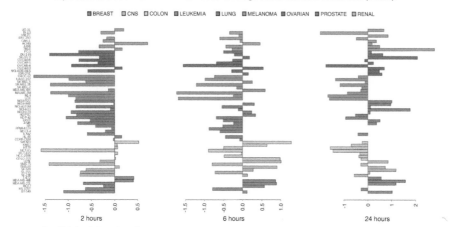

Note: Right bars indicate elevated gene expression and left bars depressed expression relative to cell lines untreated by drug.

Expression of MYC in NCI-60 cell lines treated with low concentration of bortezomib (10nM)

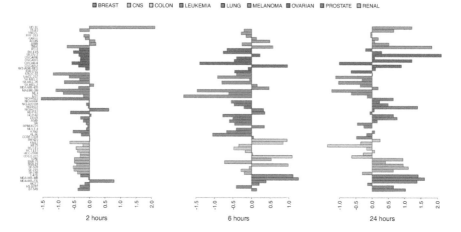

Fig. 9.1 (continued)

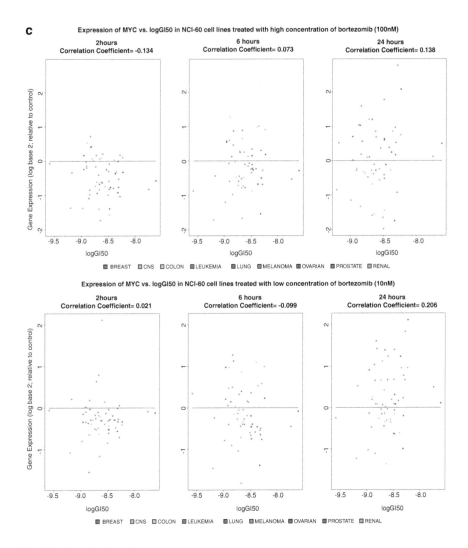

Fig. 9.1 (continued)

left side of the display, the dosage level is selected. When clicking on any of the 15 drug time course line plots, the user sees a pop-up window which shows enlarged line plots for that drug. Figure 9.3b shows an example of time course line plots for cisplatin. Each line in the plot represents a cell line, which is color coded according to nine different tissue types (Table 9.3). When moving the mouse cursor on any of the lines, the cell line name, tissue type, log(GI50) and its quartile are shown on top of the page. When clicking on "melanoma" on the top color panel stands for tissue types, only melanoma cell lines in orange are highlighted as shown in Fig. 9.3b. There are four drug sensitivity buttons at the bottom panel of the pop-up window. NCI60 cell lines are sorted into quartiles by their drug sensitivity, i.e., log(GI50) value, from the most sensitive (first quartile) to the most resistant (fourth quartile). Hovering the mouse over the GI50 Quartile buttons highlights only cell lines with

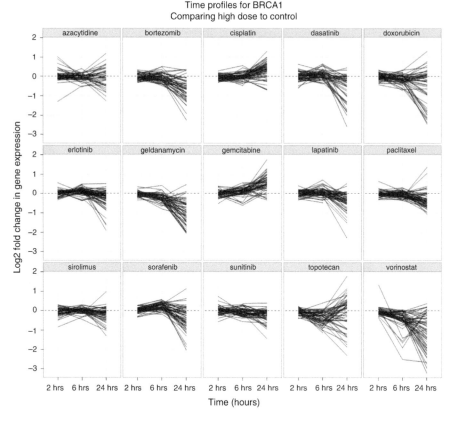

Fig. 9.2 Static time course line plots for BRCA1 treated with 15 drugs at high concentration. Each line plot represents gene expression fold changes of BRCA1 treated with one drug at high concentration, while each line in the plot represents gene expression fold changes of BRCA1 in one cell line at 2, 6, and 24 h

drug sensitivity in the selected quartile. When clicking on top left bar "View Stratified Tissue Types", a second pop-up window shows nine time-course line plots for this drug, each representing cell lines in one of the nine tumor tissue types (Fig. 9.3c). Similarly as in the previous pop-up window, hovering on each line shows the cell line name, tissue type, and log(GI50) value for the highlighted cell lines. Again, the GI50 Quartile buttons are located at the bottom panel of the window, allowing the user to move the mouse to highlight or to click to isolate the cell lines by drug sensitivity.

Correlation Analyses for a Group of Genes

This functional module provides a heat map for a group of genes whose gene expressions are most correlated with a user-selected cell line characteristic: either logGI50, doubling time, multidrug resistance, gene mutation data, or protein expression data. The user selects the drug, the dose level, the time point, and the number of most

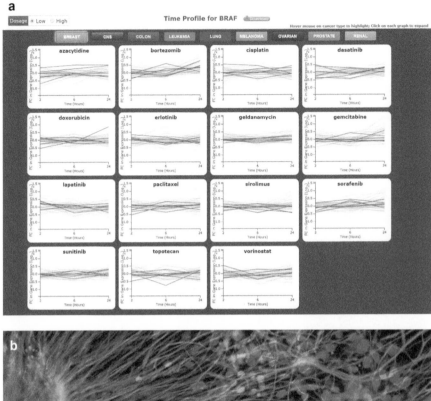

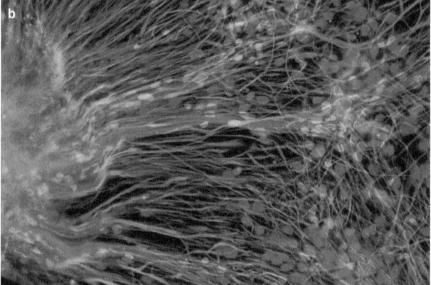

Fig. 9.3 (**a**) Dynamic time course line plots for BRAF treated with 15 drugs with breast cancer cell lines highlighted. (**b**) Pop-up window shows an enlarged time profile for BRAF treated with cisplatin. (**c**) Pop-up window shows tissue stratified time profile for BRAF treated with cisplatin. In the graph, the most sensitive cell lines (dark red) are highlighted

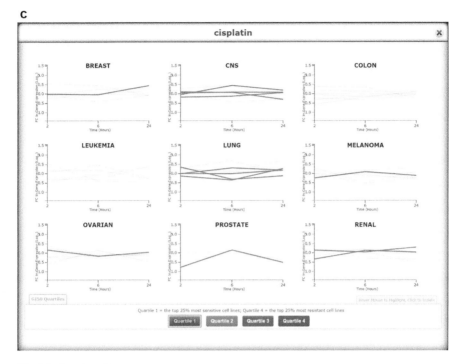

Fig. 9.3 (continued)

significant genes (maximum 100 genes) (Fig. 9.4a). For the gene mutation "phenotype", the n genes with the largest absolute t-statistics of gene expression in gene-mutant versus wild-type cell lines are selected. The t-statistics are calculated based on Welch's two sample t-test for unequal variances. For the other phenotypes, the n genes with the largest absolute correlation of gene expression and phenotype in cell lines are selected. The correlation is calculated based on the Pearson method. In the output page, as shown in Fig. 9.4b, a heat map is displayed with cell lines on the y-axis and genes on the x-axis. The top color key legend indicates the ranges for log ratio data, when compared to the base line data. The genes are clustered using the hierarchical clustering method implemented in the R function heat map, while the cell lines are ordered by log(GI50) from the most sensitive to the most resistant (from left to right). The color legend for log(GI50) is located at the bottom panel of the heat map. A JavaScript magnifier is provided to zoom in when moving the mouse cursor on the heat map, making it easy for user to see the graph detail (e.g., gene names). There are two data tables listed below the heat map. The top table lists genes that are positively correlated with GI50. Those genes are sorted by the mean log folder changes in resistant cell lines, with gene names hyperlinked to the corresponding GENECARD website entry. Pearson correlation coefficients, mean log fold changes in sensitive cell lines, mean log fold changes in resistant cell lines, and the differences of the above two fold changes between sensitive and resistant cell lines are also listed in this table. The bottom table lists genes that are negatively

a

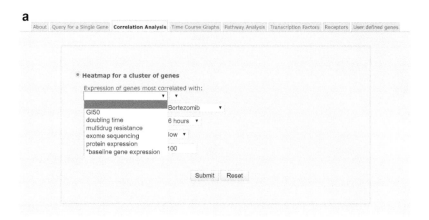

b

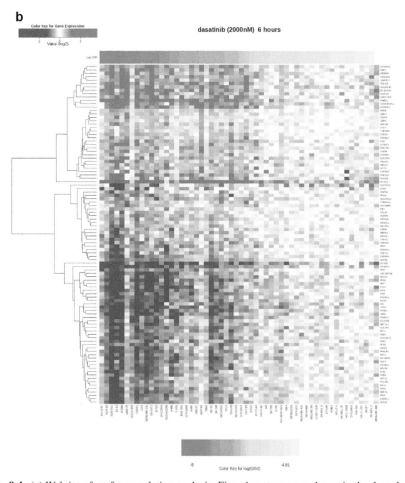

Fig. 9.4 (**a**) Web interface for correlation analysis. Five phenotypes are shown in the drop down menu: GI50, doubling time, multi-drug resistance, exome sequencing, and protein expression. (**b**) Heat map shows one hundred genes whose gene expression changes are most correlated with log(GI50) for NCI60 treated with dasatinib at 2000 nM at 6 h

correlated with drug sensitivity using the same indexes as in table one. Resistant cell lines are defined as cell lines whose growth inhibition for this drug are in the top 25th percentile of NCI60 cell lines when ordered by log(GI50). Sensitive cell lines are defined as cell lines whose growth inhibition for this drug are in the bottom 25th percentile of NCI60 cell lines when ordered by log(GI50). By studying the two data tables, the user can easily identify genes that are over- or under-expressed in resistant cell lines. At the bottom of the page, a link is provided for the user to download the raw data used to generate the heat map and the tables.

Time Profiles

This analysis module enables the user to generate for a selected drug a series of time profiles of gene expression changes for the genes with the largest average fold changes across cell lines (Fig. 9.5). The second option is to generate expression changes for the genes that are most correlated with drug sensitivity (i.e., GI50). For

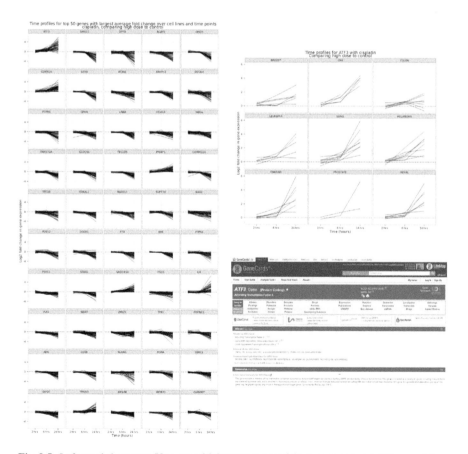

Fig. 9.5 Left panel shows top 50 genes with largest average fold change across cell lines and time points when treated with cisplatin. Right panel top is the tissue stratified time course line plots for gene ATF, while right panel bottom display gene information of ATF on GENECARD website

each gene, correlation coefficients between gene expression and GI50 for three time points are calculated. The genes are sorted by the maximum absolute value of the correlation coefficients among the three time points. The program outputs time profiles for the 50 genes with the largest correlations. Clicking on each individual time profile will display the tissue stratified figure for that gene while clicking on the gene name will direct the user to the gene annotation page in the GENECARD website. In order to boost the speed for the function, all gene lists and graphs are pre-generated and stored in the server.

Pathway Analysis

This module contains two parts: a heat map display for genes in user specified pathways and a pathway analysis. The gene lists for 65 BioCarta pathways were obtained from the Cancer Genome Anatomy Project (CGAP) website. By default, six heat maps are displayed in the output html page for three time points and two concentrations, respectively. The genes and cell lines are both clustered by default (Fig. 9.6). The user can click on "View larger image" to get an enlarged heat map in better quality. Users can also choose to sort the cell line by drug sensitivity (GI50) so that the orders of cell lines across all six heat maps are identical, making it easy to compare the difference among different concentrations and time points.

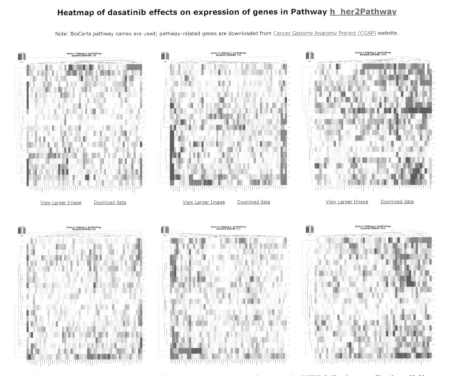

Fig. 9.6 Heat map of dasatinib effects on expression of genes in HER2 Pathway. Both cell lines and genes are clustered

Transcription Factors and TF Targets

We obtained data for 256 transcription factors relevant to cancer research and their experimentally verified gene targets from the website developed and managed by Dr. Michael Zhang's lab. There are three options to generate the heat maps.

Heat map for target genes of a specific transcription factor (Fig. 9.7). By defining the transcription factor and drug name, the user can generate six heat maps of drug effects on expression of target genes of the specified transcription factor at three time points and two concentrations, respectively. By default, the cell lines on the x-axis and the target genes on y-axis are all clustered. The user has the option to disable the cell line clustering and sort the cell lines on the x-axis by drug sensitivity (GI50).

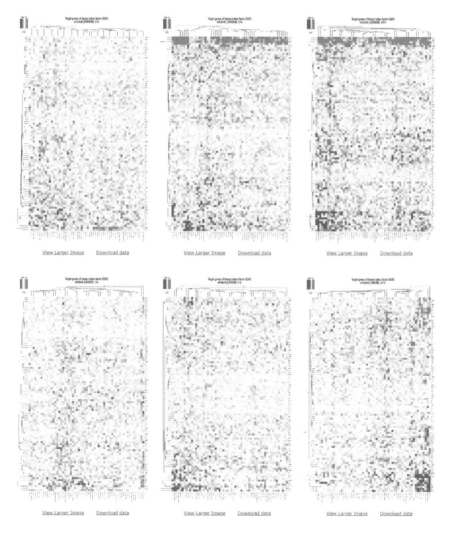

Fig. 9.7 Heat map of erlotinib effect on target genes of transcription factor EGR1. Both cell lines and genes are clustered

Heat map on drug effects on expression of all transcription factors. By selecting a drug name, the program will generate six heat maps for all 256 transcription factors in three time points and two concentrations, respectively. The transcription factor genes on the y-axis and cell lines on the x-axis are clustered by default.

Heat map of drug effects on gene expression of a specific transcription factor. By selecting one of the 256 transcription factors from the pull down menu, the system will generate a heat map with cell lines on y-axis and drugs on x-axis at three time points and two concentrations, respectively. By default, cell lines and drugs are all clustered at each axis.

Receptors Analysis

Abnormal expression of receptors and their ligands can lead to tumorgenesis by disruption of cell cycle, apoptosis, and DNA repair. Over-expressed receptors may also serve as drug targets. Discovery and development of mechanism-based therapies targeting cancer-related receptors have improved outcome for many cancer patients. Examining the expression pattern of genes in certain receptor groups treated with anti-cancer agents may provide better understanding of mechanisms of action and resistance to these drugs. We include 53 receptor groups from the IUPHAR Targets database. By selecting a receptor group and a drug name, the program will generate six heat maps for all genes in the chosen receptor group in three time points and two concentrations, respectively. The cell lines on x-axis and genes on y-axis are clustered by default.

User Defined Gene Sets

This option gives users flexibility to generate a heat map of expression modulation by treatment for any set of genes of interest. Users can simply copy the gene symbol list to the "Enter gene symbol" field. For the drug selected, six heat maps of gene expressions are generated for the three time points and two concentrations, respectively. By default, the cell lines on the x-axis and the user-defined genes on the y-axis are all clustered. It is optional to disable the cell line cluster and sort the cell lines on the x-axis by drug sensitivity (GI50). All data used to generate these heat maps can be downloaded as a CSV format file by clicking "download data".

Discussion

Developments of high-throughput genome-wide assays have created important opportunities for biological and translational research. There are, however, significant challenges in transforming "big data" to the biological and translational knowledge that is essential for PPM. These challenges are based on the complexity of biological systems, the difference between hypothesis-driven and discovery research, and limitations of current models for inter-disciplinary research.

Biological systems, particularly mammalian systems are complex, and finding a set of genes that are induced or repressed following an experimental intervention often does not go very far toward a biological understanding of the underlying mechanisms. Developing such understanding is often an iterative process involving the analysis of different types of data and the conducting of new experiments.

Discovery research is, in many ways, more complex than hypothesis-driven research. New assays may provide a first ever look at biological samples akin to looking through a new kind of microscope. Distinguishing important biological information from randomly generated patterns and technical artifacts depends heavily on the expertise, experience, and creativity of the investigator doing the examination. Hypothesis-driven research is often amenable to analysis using analytic statistical tools whereas exploratory biological discovery based on high-dimensional assays often benefits from data visualization tools.

In clinical therapeutics research, there has been a history of success with interdisciplinary collaborations between professional data analysts and biomedical scientists. The data analysts (e.g., statisticians) take responsibility for data management, quality control, and analysis based on testing hypotheses specified by clinical protocols. Statisticians are often less comfortable where there are no pre-stated hypotheses and sometimes dismiss such attempts at discovery as "data dredging". For biological discovery using genome-wide assays in basic or translational research laboratories, such interdisciplinary research is often difficult because few data analysts have the training, experience, and detailed biological knowledge needed. At the same time, the biological investigators usually do not have the computational and statistical knowledge and tools needed for in-depth data analysis.

In this chapter, we described our experience in developing a web-based system of powerful visualization tools for use by biologists and pharmacologists for understanding the transcriptional response of 60 genomically characterized human tumor cell lines to treatment by 15 different oncologic agents. For each of the 60 cell lines and 15 drugs, whole genome transcriptomes were assayed at three time points following treatment with three concentrations of each drug, a total of more than 7000 genome-wide transcriptomes of 10,000 plus genes. The database we built also included genomic mutation data based on whole exome sequencing of the 60 tumor cell lines and drug sensitivity data for the 15 drugs against each of the 60 tumor cell lines.

We found that this dataset was too complex to be used efficiently for biological discovery in the traditional ways by either statisticians, computational biologists, biologists, or pharmacologists. We thus tried to build a system that would empower biologists and pharmacologists to interrogate this data in deep ways to formulate hypotheses about mechanisms of resistance, pharmacodynamic and predictive biomarkers of response, and for discovery of molecular targets and candidate drug combinations.

Effective knowledge discovery systems must be tailored to the knowledge domain. Consequently, we have integrated gene annotations, pathway maps, and analyses based on pathways and transcription factor targets into the system. We have also provided analysis tools that focus on receptors. Because the system is domain-focused, the power of its visualization tools surpasses many web-based systems that provide only simple queries or full data downloads. This system is focused on visual data analysis that facilitates integration of multiple data sources and a graphical interface that makes it easy for the user to use the tools in an adaptive manner.

In this chapter, we described the data on which the system is based, the analysis tools, the software architecture and an example analysis. The NCI TP Workbench will be serving as a powerful web tool for researchers to interrogate such essential underpinnings of molecular PPM as the time-course data on genome-wide response to treatment with drugs and their relation to mechanisms of resistance, pharmacodynamics and predictive biomarkers of response, and for discovery of molecular targets and candidate drug combinations.

References

1. Alley MC, Scudiero DA, Monks A, Hursey ML, Czerwinski MJ, Fine DL, et al. Feasibility of drug screening with panels of human tumor cell lines using a microculture tetrazolium assay. Cancer Res. 1988;48:589–601. http://www.ncbi.nlm.nih.gov/pubmed/3335022.
2. Monks A, Scudiero D, Skehan P, Shoemaker R, Paull K, Vistica D, et al. Feasibility of a high-flux anticancer drug screen using a diverse panel of cultured human tumor cell lines. J Natl Cancer Inst. 1991;83:757–66. http://www.ncbi.nlm.nih.gov/pubmed/2041050.
3. Stinson SF, Alley MC, Kopp WC, Fiebig HH, Mullendore LA, Pittman AF, et al. Morphological and immunocytochemical characteristics of human tumor cell lines for use in a disease-oriented anticancer drug screen. Anticancer Res. 1992;12:1035–53. http://www.ncbi.nlm.nih.gov/pubmed/1503399.
4. Grever MR, Schepartz SA, Chabner BA. The National Cancer Institute: cancer drug discovery and development program. Semin Oncol. 1992;19:622–38. http://www.ncbi.nlm.nih.gov/pubmed/1462164.
5. Boyd MR, Paull KD. Some practical considerations and applications of the national cancer institute in vitro anticancer drug discovery screen. Drug Dev Res. 1995;34:91–109. https://doi.org/10.1002/ddr.430340203.
6. Barretina J, Caponigro G, Stransky N, Venkatesan K, Margolin AA, Kim S, et al. The cancer cell line encyclopedia enables predictive modelling of anticancer drug sensitivity. Nature. 2012;483:603–7. http://www.nature.com/articles/nature11003.
7. Yang W, Soares J, Greninger P, Edelman EJ, Lightfoot H, Forbes S, et al. Genomics of Drug Sensitivity in Cancer (GDSC): a resource for therapeutic biomarker discovery in cancer cells. Nucleic Acids Res. 2012;41:D955–61. http://academic.oup.com/nar/article/41/D1/D955/1059448/Genomics-of-Drug-Sensitivity-in-Cancer-GDSC-a.
8. Duan Q, Flynn C, Niepel M, Hafner M, Muhlich JL, Fernandez NF, et al. LINCS Canvas Browser: interactive web app to query, browse and interrogate LINCS L1000 gene expression signatures. Nucleic Acids Res. 2014;42:W449–60. http://academic.oup.com/nar/article/42/W1/W449/2438294/LINCS-Canvas-Browser-interactive-web-app-to-query.
9. Koleti A, Terryn R, Stathias V, Chung C, Cooper DJ, Turner JP, et al. Data Portal for the Library of Integrated Network-based Cellular Signatures (LINCS) program: integrated access to diverse large-scale cellular perturbation response data. Nucleic Acids Res. 2018;46:D558–66. http://academic.oup.com/nar/article/46/D1/D558/4621325.
10. Subramanian A, Narayan R, Corsello SM, Peck DD, Natoli TE, Lu X, et al. A next generation connectivity map: L1000 platform and the first 1,000,000 profiles. Cell. 2017;171:1437–1452.e17. https://www.sciencedirect.com/science/article/pii/S0092867417313090?via%3Dihub.
11. Monks A, Zhao Y, Hose C, Hamed H, Krushkal J, Fang J, et al. The NCI transcriptional pharmacodynamics workbench: a tool to examine dynamic expression profiling of therapeutic response in the NCI-60 cell line panel. Cancer Res. 2018;78(24):6807–17. http://www.ncbi.nlm.nih.gov/pubmed/30355619.
12. Irizarry RA, Bolstad BM, Collin F, Cope LM, Hobbs B, Speed TP. Summaries of Affymetrix GeneChip probe level data. Nucleic Acids Res. 2003;31:e15. http://www.ncbi.nlm.nih.gov/pubmed/12582260.

Chapter 10
Platform-Independent Gene-Expression Based Classification-System for Molecular Sub-typing of Cancer

Yingtao Bi and Ramana V. Davuluri

Molecular Sub-classification of Cancers as a Prelude to Personalized Medicine

Traditionally, tumors have been categorized based solely on tumor histological features. The large-scale genomics studies from The Cancer Genome Atlas (TCGA) project, initiated by NIH (http://cancergenome.nih.gov), have found that molecular signatures can be used to classify these tumors into sub-types that predict patient outcome more effectively. These promising studies are providing unprecedented understanding of the molecular basis of cancer, the key to developing effective diagnostic and therapeutic strategies, which eventually lead to personalized treatment. Molecular profiling of gene expression, using microarrays, and more recently using NextGen sequencing methods, has shown that heterogeneity in outcome and survival in cancer can be explained, in part, by genomic variation within the primary tumor. These technologies have helped identify changes in the genome (in DNA) and epigenome (changes other than in the underlying DNA sequence), which are involved in the initiation and progression of various cancers. Furthermore, novel drugs (e.g. Dasatinib [1], Nilotinib [2], Imatinib [3], Avastin (bevacizumab) [4]), have been developed to target some of the molecular pathways underlying the carcinogenic processes and maintenance of cancer phenotypes. In almost all cases, the intent is to inhibit or shut down a specific molecular pathway. Yet, these drugs provide limited survival benefits to only a small subset of cancer patients, and furthermore, only a small number of practically useful biomarkers are presently available. Therefore, molecular classification of cancers is essential to identify highly sensitive and specific biomarkers and therapeutic targets that reflect the molecular

Y. Bi · R. V. Davuluri (✉)
Division of Health and Biomedical Informatics, Department of Preventive Medicine, Feinberg School of Medicine, Northwestern University, Evanston, IL, USA
e-mail: yingtao.bi@northwestern.edu; ramana.davuluri@northwestern.edu

© Springer Nature Switzerland AG 2020
T. Adam, C. Aliferis (eds.), *Personalized and Precision Medicine Informatics*,
Health Informatics, https://doi.org/10.1007/978-3-030-18626-5_10

mechanisms that dictate tumor type-specific survival, drug resistance, tumor relapse and patient outcome [5, 6]. However, despite numerous gene-expression studies conducted on tumor subgrouping, few of the published gene signatures derived from high-throughput platforms (e.g., microarrays) were successfully transitioned to low-content clinically useful platforms (e.g., RT-qPCR). While the assessment of molecular subtyping accuracy based on data from a specific analytical platform has received much attention in cancer research, the extent of variability in classification accuracy based on gene-expression estimates of the same gene-set from different platforms (e.g., NGS and RT-qPCR) remains poorly understood. Moreover, most of the tumor subtyping studies have ignored the complexity of human transcriptome and focused the analyses mainly on gene-level expression profiles.

Alternative Transcription and Alternative Splicing in Cancer

With each successive discovery in genetics, the true dynamic complexity of the genome has become increasingly apparent, requiring relatively consistent updates to the technical definition of the word "gene" [7]. It is now understood that the majority of human genes produce multiple functional products, or isoforms, primarily through alternative transcription and alternative splicing [8–10]. Different isoforms within the same gene have been shown to participate in different functional pathways [11, 12], and the altered expression of specific isoforms has been associated with numerous diseases [13–17]. For example, specific isoforms for numerous genes are linked with cancer and its prognosis, as cancer cells manipulate regulatory mechanisms to express specific isoforms that confer drug resistance and survival advantages [18]. Moreover, cancer-associated alterations in alternative exons and splicing machinery have been identified in cancer samples [19–21]. In a recent study, we discovered that the majority of genes associated with neurological diseases expressed multiple transcripts through alternative promoters by performing integrative ChIP-seq, RNA-seq and bioinformatics analysis in developing mouse cerebellum. We also observed aberrant use of alternative promoters in medulloblastoma, a cancer arising in the cerebellum [8]. Therefore, specific transcript-variants could be more effective as cancer diagnostic and prognostic markers than corresponding genes.

Isoform-Level Cancer Gene Signatures

Cancer-associated alternative splicing variants may be new tools for the diagnosis and classification of cancers and could be the targets for innovative therapeutic interventions based on highly selective splicing correction approaches or design of isoform-specific antibodies. With the availability of multiple genome sequence and high-throughput techniques, it is feasible to study alternative transcription and splicing on a genomic scale. Genome-wide approaches have revealed that tumorigenesis often involves large-scale alterations in transcription and splicing [22]. Such approaches have been valuable in providing insight into the regulation of splicing in cancer, and have even proven useful in the classification of tumors [23–25]. Indeed, we have demonstrated that cancer cell lines, regardless of their tissue of origin, can be effectively discriminated from non-cancer cell lines at the isoform-level, but not at the gene-level [26]. Furthermore, the isoform-level transcriptome changes could provide better patient stratification in terms of overall prognosis and classification accuracy for glioblastoma [27]. Therefore, computational methods and bioinformatics tools for comprehensive genomic analyses of cancer must be designed to detect, estimate and model the gene isoform-level alterations stemming from the biological complexity and heterogeneity of human tumors and subtypes; otherwise, we risk ignoring important dynamics that are not discernible at lower resolutions of gene-level analyses.

Platform-Independent Isoform-Level Gene-Expression Based Classification System (PIGExClass)

In this section, we describe a general purpose informatics workflow for deriving a tumor subtyping classifier (or gene-signature), using transcriptome data from a high-dimensional platform and translating the derived signature to a clinically adaptable low-dimensional platform. PIGExClass was developed to derive numerically comparable measures of gene expression between different platforms and to translate the gene-panel (from the classifier) across platforms by combining a data-discretization [28] procedure with "variable selection", a Random Forest-based variable selection algorithm [29]. The algorithm was first implemented for Glioblastoma multiforme (GBM) subtyping [27] and recently has been used for high-grade serous ovarian cystadenocarcinoma (HGSOC) [30]. The PIGExClass algorithm involves both model building and validation on independent patient cohorts and two different platforms (Fig. 10.1). The key steps in the workflow are explained as follows.

Step 1: Data preparation: This step performs three main tasks:

- *Calculate the gene-level or isoform-level expression estimates*: For example, for Affymetrix exon-array data, the gene-level and isoform-level expression estimates can be obtained using Multi-Mapping Bayesian Gene expression for Affymetrix whole-transcript arrays (MMBGX) [31] using the latest version of Ensembl database as the reference genome. The expression estimates are normalized across the samples using a locally weighted scatter plot smoothing algorithm (LOESS) [32]. Similarly, for RNA-seq data, estimate the gene/isoform-level expression by the best performing algorithm (e.g., RSEM [33], IsoformEx [34] or Kallisto [35]) based on our recent benchmarking study [36]. Transform the gene expression data to log-count per million and calculate associated precision weights by voom [37].

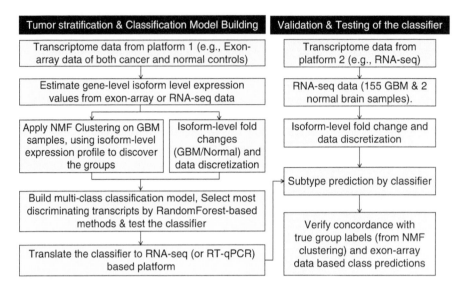

Fig. 10.1 PIGExClass workflow to perform transcriptome analysis and build a gene- or isoform-level classifier

- *Calculate fold-change (FC)* as a measure of a quantitative change of gene expression, defined by FC = $\log_2$ (*T/N*), where *T* is the estimated expression values of a tumor sample and *N* is the median expression of normal (or matched control) samples.
- *Retrieve clinical information* relevant to survival (e.g., vital status, days to death, etc.). Samples with no such information will be removed.

Step 2: Data filtering: The purpose of this step is to eliminate highly correlated isoforms from selected isoforms of a gene. If two or more isoforms of a gene are highly correlated ($r \geq 0.8$) in their expression patterns across the tumor samples, retain only the isoform with the highest mean absolute deviation (MAD), measuring variability across patients, and eliminate the other.

Step 3: Clustering analysis: Consensus clustering approaches along with methods for interpretation and validation of the robustness of the derived clusters are implemented in this step. It contains the following tasks:

- *Perform consensus clustering* [38]. In general, consensus clustering is an effective and robust technique in discovering unsupervised class membership of heterogeneous cancer data where intrinsic subgroups may exist sharing biological features. Consensus clustering assesses stability of the clustering results by multiple runs of the clustering algorithm (e.g., *k*-means, Non-negative Matrix factorization (NMF) clustering) on resampled data, which we and others have successfully applied in previous studies [27].
- *Evaluate the groupings* by using the cophenetic correlation coefficient and silhouette width methods [39]. The larger silhouette width of a sample indicates higher similarity to its own group than any other group members. These methods are available in the R packages 'ConsensusClusterPlus' and 'cluster.'

Step 4: Classification analysis: Implement four functions in order to group the samples into different molecular subgroups and evaluate the survival differences between the derived patient groups.

- *Data discretization*: The goal of this module is to transform the continuous FC data matrix into a discretized data format. Our recent studies [27, 40] have shown that data discretization, in particular the equal frequency binning (Equal-F), increased the correlation of gene expression FC values across different platforms, such as RNA-Seq, exon-array, and RT-qPCR. Moreover, the classifiers trained on discretized fold-change data provided platform-independent gene signatures with a high degree of concordance and prediction accuracy. Therefore, the Equal-F data discretization is implemented in this step. However, other data-discretization methods could be explored and compared here.
- *Feature Selection*: The Random Forest (RF) based feature selection algorithm uses both backward elimination strategy and the importance spectrum to search a set of important variables [41]. Multiple random forests are iteratively constructed to search for a set of variables in each forest that yields the smallest out-of-bag (OOB) error rate. The main advantage of this method is that it returns a very small set of genes while retaining high accuracy.
- *Classification*: We implemented RF [42], an ensemble learning method that builds decision trees with binary splits, which we have successfully applied in our previous studies [4, 43–45]. Each tree is grown randomly in two steps. First, a subset of predictors is chosen at random from all the predictors. Second, a bootstrap sample of the data is randomly drawn with replacement from the original sample. For each RF tree, observations not used for training are utilized to calculate the classification accuracy.
- *Survival analysis*: Kaplan–Meier survival curves are plotted to show the survival differences. Log-rank test is applied to determine p-values for the statistical significance. The functions available in the R package 'survival' [46] are implemented in this step.

Application of PIGExClass GBM Subtyping

GBM or grade IV gliomas are molecularly heterogeneous and are the most lethal of the malignant adult brain tumors. The GBM disease prognosis remains dismal, even with aggressive combination therapies, with median survival of 15 months after diagnosis [47]. Molecular subtyping by TCGA consortium, based on gene-level expression profiles, has led to the identification of four molecular subgroups (namely, neural-N, proneural-PN, mesenchymal-M, and classical-CL), but the derived subgroups did not show any significant survival and prognostic stratification unless lower histopathological grade glioma patients were included [48].

The clustering and classification modeling steps of the workflow were performed by analyzing the unprocessed exon-array and clinical data for 419 GBM and 10 normal brain samples downloaded from TCGA data portal. Clustering of the GBM samples, based on isoform-level gene-expression profiles, recaptured the four known molecular subgroups but switched the subtype for 19% of the samples, resulting in significant (p = 0.0103) survival differences among the refined subgroups. A four-class classifier, which requires only 121 transcript variants, assigned GBM patients' molecular subtype with 92% accuracy. In the validation phase, the transition of the classifier from exon-array to an independent platform was first successfully evaluated by applying on 155 RNA-seq TCGA samples. An RT-qPCR assay was designed to profile the gene expression patterns of the transcripts in the gene-signature and validated in an independent cohort of 206 GBM samples.

Application of PIGExClass High-Grade Serous Ovarian Carcinoma (HGSOC) Subtyping

HGSOC accounts for 70–80% of ovarian cancer deaths, with little improvement in overall survival in recent years [49]. The majority of HGSOC patients respond to initial standard therapy, which includes maximal cytoreductive surgery followed by platinum and taxane chemotherapy. However, most tumors recur and become increasingly resistant to chemotherapy, with an overall five-year survival rate of approximately 30% [50]. As a heterogeneous disease, the molecular subtyping of HGSOC tumors may serve as a useful clinical tool to predict response to therapy and guide novel personalized medicine treatment plans.

Indeed, four molecular subtypes of ovarian cancer were first identified by the Australian Ovarian Cancer Study (AOCS) via microarray-based gene expression profiling of a cohort of 285 serous and endometrioid tumors of the ovary, peritoneum, and fallopian tube [51]. Using 489 HGSOC tumor samples, TCGA consortium similarity identified four molecular subgroups—Mesenchymal (M), Immunoreactive (I), Differentiated (D) and Proliferative (P)—which largely overlap with the AOCS subtypes [52]. Similar to GBM gene-based subtyping, HGSOC molecular subtypes published by the TCGA consortium did not show statistically significant survival differences. Therefore, an important question is whether the unsupervised clustering of samples based on gene-level expression estimates, which largely ignores the isoform-level expression changes, is still the best approach to identify clinically relevant subtypes that associate with prognosis.

We, therefore, applied the PIGExClass algorithm to derive a novel platform-independent classification system for molecular subtyping with the goal of identifying subgroups of HGSOC with differential survival outcomes. The model development and validation phases were performed using the unprocessed Affymetrix exon-array (569 tumor and 9 normal) and RNA-seq (376 tumor) datasets, respectively. TCGA HGSOC datasets along with the clinical annotations were downloaded from the GDC portal. Clustering of the HGSOC samples recaptured the four TCGA molecular subgroups (namely, Differentiated—D; Proliferative—P,

Mesenchymal—M, and Immunoreactive—I) but switched the subtype for 22% of the samples, resulting in significant (p = 0.006) survival differences among the refined subgroups. Both gene-level and isoform-level classifiers achieved more than 92% prediction accuracy when tested on independent samples profiled on the exon-array platform. When the platform translatability was tested by applying the isoform-level classifier on RNA-seq data, the subtyping calls were in agreement with the predictions made from exon-array data for 95% of the 279 samples that were profiled by both of the platforms.

In both examples, we found that the classification models, trained and tested on data from the same platform, yielded similar accuracies in predicting the cancer subgroups. However, when dealing with cross-platform data, from exon-array to RNA-seq, the classifiers yielded stable models with the highest classification accuracies only on data transformed by equal frequency binning data discretization. Without the data-discretization step, the accuracies of the classifiers dropped to unsatisfactory levels. In machine learning, data discretization is mainly used as a data pre-processing step for various reasons. Examples include, (1) classification methods that can handle only discrete variables, (2) improving the human interpretation, (3) faster computation process with a reduced level of data complexity, (4) handling non-linear relations in the data (e.g., very highly and very lowly expressed genes are more relevant to cancer subtype), and (5) harmonizing the heterogeneous data. In the PIGExClass workflow, we found that simple unsupervised discretization indeed improved the classification accuracy by harmonizing the data that come in different scale and magnitude from different gene expression platforms. The data-discretization step is critical to derive numerically comparable measures of gene expression between different platforms and to translate the classification models (consisting of multiple transcript variables) across platforms.

These published results demonstrated the efficacy of PIGExClass in the design of clinically adaptable molecular subtyping assay, either using RT-qPCR or NGS based assay for GBM and HGSOC molecular sub-typing, see the publications [27, 30] for further details. In summary, the gene- or isoform-level classifiers derived from PIGExClass workflow provide a quantitative and reproducible stratification of cancer patients with prognostic significance, with the potential to improve precision therapy and the selection of drugs with subtype-specific efficacy [53, 54]. The PIGExClass workflow described here can be applied to other cancer types for molecular classification and identification of subgroups with better prognostic and diagnostic value.

The workflow involves both development and validation phases of molecular subtyping assay design and translation of the derived classifier to a clinically applicable diagnostic assay.

Acknowledgments This work was supported by the National Library of Medicine of the National Institutes of Health [Award Number R01LM011297 to RD]. The content is solely the responsibility of the authors and does not necessarily represent the official views of the National Institutes of Health.

References

1. Steinberg M. Dasatinib: a tyrosine kinase inhibitor for the treatment of chronic myelogenous leukemia and philadelphia chromosome-positive acute lymphoblastic leukemia. Clin Ther. 2007;29:2289–308. http://www.ncbi.nlm.nih.gov/entrez/query.fcgi?cmd=Retrieve&db=PubMed&dopt=Citation&list_uids=18158072.
2. Deremer DL, Ustun C, Natarajan K. Nilotinib: a second-generation tyrosine kinase inhibitor for the treatment of chronic myelogenous leukemia. Clin Ther. 2008;30:1956–75. http://www.ncbi.nlm.nih.gov/entrez/query.fcgi?cmd=Retrieve&db=PubMed&dopt=Citation&list_uids=19108785.
3. Saglio G, Baccarani M. First-line therapy for chronic myeloid leukemia: new horizons and an update. Clin Lymphoma Myeloma Leuk. 2010;10:169–76. http://www.ncbi.nlm.nih.gov/entrez/query.fcgi?cmd=Retrieve&db=PubMed&dopt=Citation&list_uids=20511160.
4. Qin H, Chan MW, Liyanarachchi S, Balch C, Potter D, Souriraj IJ, et al. An integrative ChIP-chip and gene expression profiling to model SMAD regulatory modules. BMC Syst Biol. 2009;3:73. http://www.ncbi.nlm.nih.gov/pubmed/19615063.
5. Vitucci M, Hayes DN, Miller CR. Gene expression profiling of gliomas: merging genomic and histopathological classification for personalised therapy. Br J Cancer. 2010;104:545–53. http://www.ncbi.nlm.nih.gov/entrez/query.fcgi?cmd=Retrieve&db=PubMed&dopt=Citation&list_uids=21119666.
6. Yeghiazaryan K, Peeva V, Shenoy A, Schild HH, Golubnitschaja O. Chromium-picolinate therapy in diabetes care: molecular and subcellular profiling revealed a necessity for individual outcome prediction, personalised treatment algorithms and new guidelines. Infect Disord Drug Targets. 2011;11:188–95. http://www.ncbi.nlm.nih.gov/entrez/query.fcgi?cmd=Retrieve&db=PubMed&dopt=Citation&list_uids=21470100.
7. Gerstein MB, Bruce C, Rozowsky JS, Zheng D, Du J, Korbel JO, et al. What is a gene, post-ENCODE? History and updated definition. Genome Res. 2007;17:669–81. http://www.ncbi.nlm.nih.gov/pubmed/17567988.
8. Pal S, Gupta R, Kim H, Wickramasinghe P, Baubet V, Showe LC, et al. Alternative transcription exceeds alternative splicing in generating the transcriptome diversity of cerebellar development. Genome Res. 2011;21:1260–72. http://www.ncbi.nlm.nih.gov/pubmed/21712398.
9. Pan Q, Shai O, Lee LJ, Frey BJ, Blencowe BJ. Deep surveying of alternative splicing complexity in the human transcriptome by high-throughput sequencing. Nat Genet. 2008;40:1413–5. http://www.ncbi.nlm.nih.gov/pubmed/18978789.
10. Wang ET, Sandberg R, Luo S, Khrebtukova I, Zhang L, Mayr C, et al. Alternative isoform regulation in human tissue transcriptomes. Nature. 2008;456:470–6. http://www.ncbi.nlm.nih.gov/entrez/query.fcgi?cmd=Retrieve&db=PubMed&dopt=Citation&list_uids=18978772.
11. Khoury MP, Bourdon JC. p53 isoforms: an intracellular microprocessor? Genes Cancer. 2011;2:453–65. http://www.ncbi.nlm.nih.gov/pubmed/21779513.
12. Grabowski P. Alternative splicing takes shape during neuronal development. Curr Opin Genet Dev. 2011;21:388–94. http://www.ncbi.nlm.nih.gov/pubmed/21511457.
13. Tazi J, Bakkour N, Stamm S. Alternative splicing and disease. Biochim Biophys Acta. 2009;1792:14–26. http://www.ncbi.nlm.nih.gov/pubmed/18992329.
14. Botta A, Malena A, Tibaldi E, Rocchi L, Loro E, Pena E, et al. MBNL142 and MBNL143 gene isoforms, overexpressed in DM1-patient muscle, encode for nuclear proteins interacting with Src family kinases. Cell Death Dis. 2013;4:e770. http://www.ncbi.nlm.nih.gov/pubmed/23949219.
15. Twine NA, Janitz K, Wilkins MR, Janitz M. Whole transcriptome sequencing reveals gene expression and splicing differences in brain regions affected by Alzheimer's disease. PLoS One. 2011;6:e16266. http://www.ncbi.nlm.nih.gov/pubmed/21283692.
16. Birzele F, Voss E, Nopora A, Honold K, Heil F, Lohmann S, et al. CD44 isoform status predicts response to treatment with anti-CD44 antibody in Cancer patients. Clin Cancer Res. 2015;21:2753–62. http://www.ncbi.nlm.nih.gov/pubmed/25762343.

17. Zhang Y, Chen K, Sloan SA, Bennett ML, Scholze AR, O'Keeffe S, et al. An RNA-sequencing transcriptome and splicing database of glia, neurons, and vascular cells of the cerebral cortex. J Neurosci. 2014;34:11929–47. http://www.ncbi.nlm.nih.gov/pubmed/25186741.

18. Pal S, Gupta R, Davuluri RV. Alternative transcription and alternative splicing in cancer. Pharmacol Ther. 2012;136:283–94. http://www.ncbi.nlm.nih.gov/pubmed/22909788.

19. Lapuk A, Marr H, Jakkula L, Pedro H, Bhattacharya S, Purdom E, et al. Exon-level microarray analyses identify alternative splicing programs in breast cancer. Mol Cancer Res. 2010;8:961–74. http://www.ncbi.nlm.nih.gov/entrez/query.fcgi?cmd=Retrieve&db=PubMed&dopt=Citation&list_uids=20605923.

20. Misquitta-Ali CM, Cheng E, O'Hanlon D, Liu N, McGlade CJ, Tsao MS, et al. Global profiling and molecular characterization of alternative splicing events misregulated in lung cancer. Mol Cell Biol. 2010;31:138–50. http://www.ncbi.nlm.nih.gov/entrez/query.fcgi?cmd=Retrieve&db=PubMed&dopt=Citation&list_uids=21041478.

21. Ebert B, Bernard OA. Mutations in RNA splicing machinery in human cancers. N Engl J Med. 2011;365:2534–5. http://www.ncbi.nlm.nih.gov/pubmed/22150007.

22. Venables JP, Klinck R, Koh C, Gervais-Bird J, Bramard A, Inkel L, et al. Cancer-associated regulation of alternative splicing. Nat Struct Mol Biol. 2009;16:670–6. http://www.ncbi.nlm.nih.gov/pubmed/19448617.

23. Omenn GS, Yocum AK, Menon R. Alternative splice variants, a new class of protein cancer biomarker candidates: findings in pancreatic cancer and breast cancer with systems biology implications. Dis Markers. 2010;28:241–51. http://www.ncbi.nlm.nih.gov/pubmed/20534909.

24. Skotheim RI, Nees M. Alternative splicing in cancer: noise, functional, or systematic? Int J Biochem Cell Biol. 2007;39:1432–49. http://www.ncbi.nlm.nih.gov/pubmed/17416541.

25. Venables JP. Unbalanced alternative splicing and its significance in cancer. BioEssays. 2006;28:378–86. http://www.ncbi.nlm.nih.gov/pubmed/16547952.

26. Zhang Z, Pal S, Bi Y, Tchou J, Davuluri R. Isoform-level expression profiles provide better cancer signatures than gene-level expression profiles. Genome Med. 2013;5:33. http://www.ncbi.nlm.nih.gov/pubmed/23594586.

27. Pal S, Bi Y, Macyszyn L, Showe LC, O'Rourke DM, Davuluri RV. Isoform-level gene signature improves prognostic stratification and accurately classifies glioblastoma subtypes. Nucleic Acids Res. 2014;42:e64. http://www.ncbi.nlm.nih.gov/pubmed/24503249.

28. Liu H, Hussain F, Tan CL, Dash M. Discretization: an enabling technique. Data Min Knowl Disc. 2002;6:393–423.

29. Diaz-Uriarte R, Alvarez de Andres S. Gene selection and classification of microarray data using random forest. BMC Bioinformatics. 2006;7:3. http://www.ncbi.nlm.nih.gov/pubmed/16398926.

30. Shilpi A, Kandpal M, Ji Y, Seagle BL, Shahabi S, Davuluri RV. Platform-independent classification system for predicting high-grade serous ovarian carcinoma molecular subtypes. JCO Clin Cancer Inform. 2019;3:1–9.

31. Turro E, Lewin A, Rose A, Dallman MJ, Richardson S. MMBGX: a method for estimating expression at the isoform level and detecting differential splicing using whole-transcript Affymetrix arrays. Nucleic Acids Res. 2010;38:e4. https://www.ncbi.nlm.nih.gov/pubmed/19854940.

32. Workman C, Jensen LJ, Jarmer H, Berka R, Gautier L, Nielser HB, et al. A new non-linear normalization method for reducing variability in DNA microarray experiments. Genome Biol. 2002;3:research0048. http://www.ncbi.nlm.nih.gov/pubmed/12225587.

33. Li B, Dewey CN. RSEM: accurate transcript quantification from RNA-Seq data with or without a reference genome. BMC Bioinformatics. 2011;12:323. http://www.ncbi.nlm.nih.gov/pubmed/21816040.

34. Kim H, Bi Y, Davuluri RV. Estimating the expression of transcript isoforms from mRNA-Seq via nonnegative least squares. In: Proceedings of the 10th IEEE International Conference Bioinformatics and Bioengineering, Philadelphia, PA, USA; 2010. p. 296–7. http://ieeexplore.ieee.org/stamp/stamp.jsp?tp=&arnumber=5521668.

35. Bray NL, Pimentel H, Melsted P, Pachter L. Near-optimal probabilistic RNA-seq quantification. Nat Biotechnol. 2016;34:525–7. https://www.ncbi.nlm.nih.gov/pubmed/27043002.
36. Dapas M, Kandpal M, Bi Y, Davuluri RV. Comparative evaluation of isoform-level gene expression estimation algorithms for RNA-seq and exon-array platforms. Br Bioinform. 2016;18:260–9. https://www.ncbi.nlm.nih.gov/pubmed/26944083.
37. Law CW, Chen Y, Shi W, Smyth GK. Voom: precision weights unlock linear model analysis tools for RNA-seq read counts. Genome Biol. 2014;15:R29. http://www.ncbi.nlm.nih.gov/pubmed/24485249.
38. Wilkerson MD, Hayes DN. ConsensusClusterPlus: a class discovery tool with confidence assessments and item tracking. Bioinformatics. 2010;26:1572–3. http://www.ncbi.nlm.nih.gov/pubmed/20427518.
39. Rousseeuw PJ. Silhouettes: a graphical aid to the interpretation and validation of cluster analysis. Comput Appl Math. 1987;20:53–65.
40. Jung S, Bi Y, Davuluri RV. Evaluation of data discretization methods to derive platform independent gene expression signatures for multi-class tumor subtyping. BMC Genomics. 2015;11(16 Suppl):S3.
41. Diaz-Uriarte R. GeneSrF and varSelRF: a web-based tool and R package for gene selection and classification using random forest. BMC Bioinformatics. 2007;8:328. http://www.ncbi.nlm.nih.gov/pubmed/17767709.
42. Breiman L. Random forests. Mach Learn. 2001;45:5–32.
43. Jung S, Bi Y, Davuluri RV. Evaluation of data discretization methods to derive platform independent isoform expression signatures for multi-class tumor subtyping. BMC Genomics. 2015;16(Suppl 1):S3. http://www.ncbi.nlm.nih.gov/pubmed/26576613.
44. Liu Q, Sung AH, Chen Z, Liu J, Chen L, Qiao M, et al. Gene selection and classification for cancer microarray data based on machine learning and similarity measures. BMC Genomics. 2011;12(Suppl 5):S1. http://www.ncbi.nlm.nih.gov/pubmed/22369383.
45. Gupta R, Wikramasinghe P, Bhattacharyya A, Perez FA, Pal S, Davuluri RV. Annotation of gene promoters by integrative data-mining of ChIP-seq pol-II enrichment data. BMC Bioinformatics. 2010;11(Suppl 1):S65. http://www.ncbi.nlm.nih.gov/pubmed/20122241.
46. Therneau TM, Grambsch PM. Modeling survival data: extending the cox model. New York, NY: Springer; 2000.
47. Dunn GP, Rinne ML, Wykosky J, Genovese G, Quayle SN, Dunn IF, et al. Emerging insights into the molecular and cellular basis of glioblastoma. Genes Dev. 2012;26:756–84. http://www.ncbi.nlm.nih.gov/pubmed/22508724.
48. Verhaak RG, Hoadley KA, Purdom E, Wang V, Qi Y, Wilkerson MD, et al. Integrated genomic analysis identifies clinically relevant subtypes of glioblastoma characterized by abnormalities in PDGFRA, IDH1, EGFR, and NF1. Cancer Cell. 2010;17:98–110. http://www.ncbi.nlm.nih.gov/pubmed/20129251.
49. Siegel RL, Miller KD, Jemal A. Cancer statistics, 2016. CA Cancer J Clin. 2016;66:7–30. https://www.ncbi.nlm.nih.gov/pubmed/26742998.
50. Reid BM, Permuth JB, Sellers TA. Epidemiology of ovarian cancer: a review. Cancer Biol Med. 2017;14:9–32. https://www.ncbi.nlm.nih.gov/pubmed/28443200.
51. Tothill RW, Tinker AV, George J, Brown R, Fox SB, Lade S, et al. Novel molecular subtypes of serous and endometrioid ovarian cancer linked to clinical outcome. Clin Cancer Res. 2008;14:5198–208. https://www.ncbi.nlm.nih.gov/pubmed/18698038.
52. Cancer Genome Atlas Research N. Integrated genomic analyses of ovarian carcinoma. Nature. 2011;474:609–15. https://www.ncbi.nlm.nih.gov/pubmed/21720365.
53. Tanaka S, Louis DN, Curry WT, Batchelor TT, Dietrich J. Diagnostic and therapeutic avenues for glioblastoma: no longer a dead end? Nat Rev Clin Oncol. 2013;10:14–26. http://www.ncbi.nlm.nih.gov/pubmed/23183634.
54. Huse JT, Holland E, DeAngelis LM. Glioblastoma: molecular analysis and clinical implications. Annu Rev Med. 2013;64:59–70. http://www.ncbi.nlm.nih.gov/pubmed/23043492.

Chapter 11
Tumor Sequencing: Enabling Personalized Targeted Treatments with Informatics

Jinhua Wang

Introduction

Recent progress in next-generation sequencing (NGS) technologies and parallel innovations in informatics methods have enabled the analysis of whole genome sequencing (WGS), whole exome sequencing (WES), and RNA transcriptome sequencing (RNA-Seq), leading to the identification of a huge number and diversity of genomic and genetic abnormalities in tumor samples [1]. Several large-scale investigations using the NGS sequencing platforms, such as The Cancer Genome Atlas (TCGA), have profiled tumor genomes in reasonably sized cohorts in 33 different tumor types including breast [2], central nervous system [3], endocrine [4], gastrointestinal [5], gynecologic [6], head neck [7], hematologic [8], skin [9], soft tissue [10], thoracic [11] and urologic system [12] cancer tissues. The TCGA dataset encompassing 2.5 petabytes of data describing tumor tissue and matched normal tissues from more than 11,000 patients, is publically available and has been used widely by the research community [11, 13–16].

Initial analyses of these sequencing efforts have determined and archived cancer type-specific mutations, mutation allele frequencies, transcriptional or epigenetic signatures of cancer subtypes and mutational signatures of cancer genomes. Many clinically actionable gene mutations were identified and annotated in different tumor types [17]. Gene mutations or transcription signatures that might be predictive biomarkers for targeted therapy and prognostic biomarkers have also been identified.

These targetable mutations, tumor specific transcription signatures and other genomics features acquired by NGS sequencing lay the foundation for targeted and

J. Wang (✉)
Institute for Health Informatics, University of Minnesota, Minneapolis, MN, USA

Cancer Bioinformatics, Masonic Cancer Center, University of Minnesota,
Minneapolis, MN, USA
e-mail: wangjh@umn.edu

© Springer Nature Switzerland AG 2020
T. Adam, C. Aliferis (eds.), *Personalized and Precision Medicine Informatics*,
Health Informatics, https://doi.org/10.1007/978-3-030-18626-5_11

personalized cancer treatments [18]. We will elaborate on tumor transcriptome profiling, exome and gene panel sequencing below to discuss technologies and informatics involved in groundbreaking targeted cancer treatments. We will also provide an introduction to the current tumor genomics data sharing networks.

Cancer Transcriptome Profiling: From Transcriptomics to Precision Oncology

With the growing availability of NGS technologies, information resources on gene expression profiles of normal and tumor tissues have grown significantly. With the availability of large, annotated compendia of gene expression profiles across normal tissues from data sources such as GTEx [19, 20], tumor tissue transcription profiles from the efforts of TCGA and the International Cancer Genome Consortium (ICGC), and cell lines transcription data sets of ENCODE [21] cell lines and NCI-60 [22], scientists now have a much clearer and more comprehensive understanding of the structure of global gene function in normal tissues and tumor tissues.

Many products have been developed and commercialized based on transcription profiles of tumor tissues. The clinical validations of these products are among the great achievements of precision oncology. For example, prognostic panels are now available and are clinically used for many major cancer types, including breast (MammaPrint [23], Oncotype DX [24] and Prosigna [25]), lung (GeneFx [26]), prostate (Oncotype Dx, Prolaris [27]) and colon (ColoPrint [28]). Similarly, the prediction analysis of microarray (PAM50 [29]) signatures has been developed to classify breast cancer into molecular subtypes. The four intrinsic subtypes of breast cancer (luminal A, luminal B, Her2 positive and basal-like) were shown to be independently associated with clinical outcomes and harbor a different set of genetic aberrations. The PAM50 expression test is among the most widely known and clinically successful cancer diagnostics. These panels measure gene expression levels and make fairly accurate diagnostic and prognostic predictions with high specificity and sensitivity.

With rapid NGS technology development and a significant decline in the costs of whole-transcriptome sequencing, embedding multiple panels within a single assay has become viable. Comprehensive whole transcriptome profiling will be particularly advantageous in areas where gene expression signatures are not yet established and for retrospective clinical trials. For example, RNA-seq profiling of Philadelphia chromosome-like acute lymphoblastic leukemia (ALL) identified its phenotypic similarity to IKZF1-deleted ALL and many actionable kinase fusions, provided potential gene signatures to identify subgroups of patients for potential tailored targeted therapy [30].

Core analytical informatics methods for transcriptome analysis include *quality control and sequence reads alignment* processing pipelines developed for RNA-seq transcriptome analysis, *differential expression analysis* and *predictive modeling*.

The actual analysis of transcriptome RNA-seq data starts with quality control, read alignment with and without a reference genome, summarize mapped read counts and deduce gene and transcript expression. The second step is to select optimal approaches for detecting differential gene expression. The differential expressed gene list will facilitate the following feature gene selection for predictive modelling.

Quality control for the raw sequence reads involves the analysis of sequence quality, GC content, the presence of adaptors, overrepresented k-mers and duplicated reads in order to detect sequencing errors, PCR artifacts or contaminations. Acceptable duplication, k-mer or GC content levels are experiment- and organism-specific, but these values should be homogeneous for samples in the same experiments. Fastqc [31] is a popular tool to perform these analyses on Illumina reads, whereas NGSQC [32] can be applied to a variety of platforms. As a general rule, read quality decreases towards the $3'$ end of reads, and if it becomes too low, bases should be trimmed to improve mappability. Software tools such as the FASTX-Toolkit [33] and Trimmomatic [34] can be used to discard low-quality reads, trim adaptor sequences, and eliminate poor-quality bases.

Sequence reads passing quality control are typically aligned to either a genome or transcriptome gene sets. An important mapping quality parameter is the percentage of mapped reads, which reflects the overall sequencing accuracy and the potential presence of contaminating DNA. For example, the normal range of RNA-seq reads mapped onto the reference genome sequence fall between 70% and 90% depending on the read mapper used, with a significant fraction of reads mapping to a limited number of identical regions equally well ('multi-mapping reads'). When reads are mapped against the transcribed gene sets, the mapping percentages will be slightly lower because reads coming from unannotated transcripts will not be mapped, and we will also see significantly more multi-mapping reads because of reads falling onto exons that are shared by different transcript isoforms of the same gene.

Other important parameters are the uniformity of read coverage on exons and the mapped strand. If reads primarily accumulate at the $3'$ end of transcripts in poly(A)-selected samples, this might indicate low RNA quality in the starting material. The GC content of mapped reads may reveal PCR biases. Tools for quality control in mapping include Picard [35], RSeQC [36] and Qualimap [37].

After transcript quantification values are calculated using the mapped reads count, normalization methods are applied to adjust for the biases caused by GC content, gene length, and sequence depth. The normalization procedure is essential for comparisons across samples. So far there is not clear consensus on how to choose the right normalization methods. Various bench marking studies conclude that the widely used methods, RPKM, and FPKM, (reads/fragments per kilobase per million mapped) normalize away the most important factor for comparing samples, which is sequencing depth, whether directly or by accounting for the number of transcripts, which can differ significantly between samples [38, 39]. These approaches rely on normalizing methods that are based on total or effective counts, and tend to perform poorly when samples have heterogeneous transcript distributions, that is, when highly and differentially expressed features can skew the count distribution. While the TPM (Transcripts per kilobase per million mapped) measure seems to be more appropriate in dealing with this issue since the sums of normalized reads of each sample are the same across all samples, making it more suitable to compare samples, another option is the TMM (trimmed mean of M values) normalization method, which shows better performance in simulation studies [40].

Many statistical methods have been developed and are used widely in detecting differential gene or transcript expression from RNA-seq data, and the major practical challenge is how to choose the most suitable tool for a particular RNA-seq data analysis task. There are various benchmark results comparing the performance of different methods. Some methods, such as the popular edgeR [41], use raw sequence read counts and introduce possible bias sources into the statistical model to perform an integrated normalization as well as a differential expression analysis. In other methods, the differential expression requires the data to be previously normalized using the method as just described. DESeq2 [42], like edgeR, uses the Negative Binomial as the reference distribution and provides its own normalization approach. BaySeq [43] and EBSeq [44] are Bayesian approaches, also based on the negative binomial model, that define a collection of models to describe the differences among experimental groups and to compute the posterior probability of each one of them for each gene. While some of the differential expression tools can only perform uni-variant comparison, others such as edgeR, limma-voom [45], DESeq, DESeq2, and maSigPro [46] can perform multiple variant comparisons, include different covariates or analyze time-series data.

In the applications of cancer transcriptome profiling, sequencing coverage and depth are key factors in determining analytical strategies. The depth that an RNA-seq library should be sequenced depends mostly on the goal of the application and is often limited by the sequencing platform. In general, if RNA-seq is used for the detection of genetic variants, such as mutations or fusion genes, higher sequencing depth above 40 million reads is warranted. On the other hand, if the use of RNA-seq is only for transcriptional profiling, moderate amounts of sequencing from 10 million to 15 million reads will generate good results. Including more replicates in the experimental design is a substantially better strategy than including more reads. However, much higher read depths (100 million paired-end reads or more) are required for the study of alternative splicing or allele-specific expression [47].

The clinical utility of RNA-seq transcriptome profiling for personalized immunotherapy has been demonstrated in a landmark longitudinal study that demonstrated signatures of adaptive immunity are predictive of response to immune checkpoint blockade treatment [48]. As both prognostic and predictive approaches require the expression levels of hundreds of genes, their clinical translation will depend on the routine use of whole-transcriptome RNA-seq profiling or custom-targeted panels. It has been shown that comprehensive immune-phenotypic data can be obtained from RNA-seq transcriptomes and that they provide unique insights into the immunological heterogeneity of metastatic tumors across all major primary tissue types. RNA-seq data are also particularly valuable for the development of personalized cancer vaccines, where they can be used to identify chimeric fusion proteins that contain putative mutant epitopes and help in the selection of potentially highly abundant neoantigens [49].

Single cell RNA-seq has been proven to be an efficient strategy to dissect tumor heterogeneity in order to understand tumor micro-environment. Customized treatment of tumor based on the single cell RNA-seq analysis of cancer tissues promises to provide more accurate treatment strategy to target tumor subclones and predict response to immunotherapies [50]. Single cell assays also hold great promise for improving the accuracy of conventional treatment selection.

Cancer Exome/Panel Sequencing: From DNA Variants Detection to Targeted Cancer Treatment

Whole genome sequencing (WGS) and whole exome sequencing (WES) of tumors have identified numerous genetic variants, including DNA mutations, small insertion and deletions, and copy number variations. Many of those genetic abnormalities are potential targets for new targeted treatment. Targeted therapy against certain actionable gene mutations shows a significantly higher response rate as well as longer survival compared to conventional chemotherapy, and has become a standard therapy for many cancer types. Based on sequencing results of certain mutations or mutation load, patients can get recommendations to undergo targeted therapy or immunotherapy. In cases where there are no available FDA approved drugs for the genetic mutations detected in the patients, patients can be routed to genetic variants-based clinical trials. For that purpose, a NGS-based sequencing panel that can simultaneously target multiple genes in a single investigation has been used in daily clinical practice. To date, a variety of sequencing panels focused on cancer related genes or specific tumors have been developed to investigate genetic aberrations with tumor somatic variants, high-level copy number alterations, and gene fusions through comprehensive bioinformatics analysis. Because sequencing panels are efficient and cost-effective, they are quickly being adopted outside the lab, in hospitals and clinics, in order to identify personal targeted therapy for individual cancer patients [51].

The predesigned panel covers the most commonly mutated genes or candidate actionable genes in various cancers. A gene panel may contain anywhere from a single digit number of genes to a few thousand genes. Many gene panels also cover genetic regions with high copy number variations. On one hand, custom panels or tumor-specific predesigned panels are developed to investigate the genes that are specifically focused on or found in a tumor-specific mutation. While *TP53* mutations are broadly identified in various cancers, most actionable gene mutations are identified differently among cancer types. For colorectal cancer, genetic testing of *KRAS*, *NRAS*, and *BRAF* mutations are necessary, while on the other hand, for lung adenocarcinoma, testing of *EGFR*, *KRAS*, *BRAF* and *HER2* mutations and *ALK*, *RET*, and *ROS1* fusions are necessary. It has been reported that gene mutation profiles differ even in different histological cancer subtypes. Therefore, it is necessary to select the appropriate sequencing panel for patients with different types of cancers, in order to determine actionable gene mutations to develop personalized targeted therapy.

Several cancer centers all over the world have developed their own in-house sequence panels. Most notably, the Memorial Sloan Kettering (MSK) Cancer Center developed MSK-IMPACT (Integrated Mutation Profiling of Actionable Cancer Targets) [52], a hybridization capture-based NGS panel that can detect protein-coding mutations, copy number alterations, selected promoter mutations, and structural rearrangement in 468 cancer-associated genes. In 2017, the MSK-IMPACT panel test was approved by the US Food and Drug Administration (FDA) for in vitro diagnostic tests for tumor profiling and was recommended CMS coverage status [53]. To date, MSK-IMPACT has sequenced tumors from more than 20,000 patients with advanced cancer. According to a recent study that sequenced tumors from more than 10,000 patients using MSK-IMPACT, nearly 37% of patients had at least one actionable gene mutation and 11% were able to participate in clinical trials of treatments that directly targeted their genetic alterations [54]. One impressive feature of MSK-IMPACT is that this panel can be used to analyze both tumor and matched normal tissue and blood, and it identifies both somatic and germline mutations. Therefore, MSK-IMPACT results in accurate somatic mutation calls due to the elimination of germline variants. MSK-IMPACT also accurately determines mutational signatures to reveal multiple mutational processes and tumor mutation burden which can identify patients who can receive the most benefit from immunotherapy. In addition, germline variants can provide therapeutic opportunity as well as cancer susceptibility information. The FDA approved a PARP inhibitor for the germline BRCA1/2-mutant ovarian cancer. Furthermore, the PARP inhibitor is also approved for maintenance therapy in both germline and somatic BRCA-mutant ovarian cancer. The FDA has also approved the Oncomine Dx Target test [55], which targets gene mutations in non-small cell lung cancer (NSCLC). This test is used as a companion diagnosis to aid in the selection of specific drugs for individual NSCLC patients with EGFR mutations, BRAF mutations or ROS1 fusions.

The Foundation Medicine panel FoundationOne [56] and the Caris [57] panel are also among the FDA approved gene panels. There are many companies that offer similar products as will be described in the following section. With the panel sequencing result, a report with detailed bioinformatics analysis of the gene mutations, the potential targeted therapies, clinical trials, and other mutation-related metrics are generated to facilitate clinical decision making.

Cancer Genomics Data Sharing: Large Genomic Datasets Realize the Full Impact of Precision Oncology

Precision oncology involves the analysis of a person's tumor genome and the use of this analysis to inform diagnosis, prognosis, disease management, and eventually personalized treatment, tailor-made to the individual's germline or somatic genomic profile. To realize the full impact of genomic medicine, genomic and clinical data must be interoperable across traditional geographic, jurisdictional, sectorial and domain boundaries. Extremely large and diverse data sets are needed to provide a context for the interpretation of genetic information and the annotation of genetic variants. No single research group, institute or company will be able to collect a sufficiently large genomic dataset; it is only through cooperation, together with super computing power that we can truly understand how genotypes and phenotypes relate. Various cancer genomics data sharing networks have been formed and many of these are building large patient cohorts through the participation of partner institutes to harness the power of big sample size and population diversity. The following four major cancer genomics data sharing networks are important examples and will be summarized below along with a brief appraisal of strengths and weaknesses (as of the time of the writing of this book),

Additional details about these networks are provided in Table 11.1.

1. Oncology Research Information Exchange Network (ORIEN) [58]
   ORIEN is a research partnership started in May 2014 by Moffitt and The Ohio State University's The James Comprehensive Cancer Centers. Fifteen current members are part of the network as of February 2017. Notable members include: Moffitt, Ohio State, City of Hope, Iowa, Colorado, and the University of South California. It is the oldest network and currently has the most active members. It is driven by a Total Cancer Care protocol that all members are required to implement, which standardizes the data collection process across member organizations.

   - Strengths: Comprehensive, stringent and well thought out, detailed protocols, strong bioinformatics infrastructure for clinical trials.
   - Weaknesses: Clinical reports still in development, implementation procedure may prove to be difficult and risky given the different biorepository standards in different institutes.

2. Caris Centers of Excellence
   A collective effort started 2 years ago, led by Caris Life Sciences and chaired by Dr. John Marshall at the Lombardi Georgetown Comprehensive Cancer Center (CCC). There are currently 15 members. Notable members include Georgetown CCC, USC CCC, and Fox Chase CCC. The network objective is to capture and track protein and genomic information with matched clinical data across member sites to advance the delivery of molecular testing and establish standards of care for profiling tumors.

   - Strengths: Well-supported and balances research and clinical applications. Well-developed clinical report for targeted therapy and genetic risk assessment. Participating maintenance costs are minimal. Valuable tumor boards—with emphasis on research.
   - Weaknesses: The implementation of C.O.D.E. umbrella protocol could be challenging, but not uniquely. Tissue sample requirements are high (4–6 18 gauge cores).

Table 11.1 Cancer genomic data sharing initiatives

Data exchange initiative	Inception	Platform, how to scale up to the latest seq tech/capacity/partner with seq powerhouse?	Allow multiple memberships?	Data sharing/ clinical data integration	Database/number of profiled cases/ projected increase	Value add to clinical trial, research, proven utility	Data ownership**	Data compliance	Sample ownership**	Initial costs?*	Ongoing costs?*	Costs to patients?	Current notable members	Other notes
ORIEN	May 2014	300x WES, 100m reads RNA-seq, 100x germline.	Not restricted on initiatives, however, the pooling of the ORIEN member data is done through M2Gen (Contract language: "Members shall not engage in Pooling of Cancer Patient Data for Commercial Purposes during the Term.")	Share limited data; project-specific additional data sharing	159,000 patients consented, clinical data, tissue; future- contact available	Avatar, physician portal, NCI-Match, $1500/patient that are TCC-consented, and enrolled in avatar (need tumor, normal specimens, high-risk/late stage cancers)	Contractual alliance with a federated data model. Participants own their data. Members license data collected under the TCC protocol to M2Gen.	Developing cloud capacity for data compliant security and storage	Tissue collected under TCC protocol stays and is owned by UMN (Addendum to master agreement: ORIEN avatar—large clinical trial matching initiative under TCC protocol—specimens collected in high risk/rare disease—are shipped to Hudson Alpha molecular lab—CLIA lab—data comes back to parent inst. @ no cost, $900 per patient reimbursement to participant org)	$30,000 annual fee; Tissue bank in place; Protocol Implementation; Need to cover costs for consenting patients to TCC protocol, PA in pathology, Specimen runners, Operation of central bioreposititory, etc.	$30,000 fee & ongoing support of added infrastructure for TCC protocol, free tier 1 data for patients enrolled in Avatar	None. Patient consents to collect residual tissue from clinical specimens	Moffitt (co-founder), OSU (cofounder), City of Hope, UVA, Colorado, New Mexico, Rutgers, UNC Norris, Huntsman Cancer Ctr, Emory	Implementation of Total Cancer Care protocol = partnership w/ patient (big difference btw. ORIEN and others) Needs: Centralized biobanking entity either A) needs to be part of the Total Cancer Care protocol, or B) use TCC as the basis for central biobanking efforts

CARIS centers of excellence	January 2015	NGS, 592 gene panel, RNA seq fusion gene detection, DNA copy number, IHC, FA, CISH	Caris does not restrict or require exclusivity with participation.	Provide clinical data to complement the genomic database, CODE to match genomics with clinical outcome	>10K consented eligible for retrospective data collection 500 patients/month (goal 1 K) 3M Biomarkers 50K individual assays	Two studies show "patients treated according to CMI results in one year longer survival." publications on molecular profiling of various tumors.	"Provider acknowledges and agrees that, as between the Parties, all right, title and interest in and to Clinical Molecular Data and Warehouse Data is solely and exclusively owned by Caris. Caris acknowledges and agrees that, as between the Parties, all right, title and interest in and to Clinical Data is solely and exclusively owned by Provider"	For all Clinical Data provided to Caris, Provider shall also provide to Caris all corresponding enrollment data and outcomes data and any other related health information related to patients requested under the Protocol in accordance with all applicable state and federal human subject and data protection laws and regulations	Sample clinical data owned by provider	Free to opt in	Unclear; possible additional costs for tissue collection	$550/ patient max out of pocket	Fox Chase, Georgetown, Wayne State, USC	Implementation of CODE consent protocol
AACR Genie	November 2015	n/a	GENIE does not restrict or require exclusivity with participation	Share SNVs, Indels, Path report, Diagnosis, CNVs and structural changes when available Genomic data: gender, age, ethnicity, cancer type, date of histopath diagnosis, primary/ metastasis, etc.	19,000 records in first release (3K lung, 2K breast)	Registry effort, ~$440/case reimbursement for data abstraction	Members retain access to own data; sharing only fully de-identified	HIPAA compliant	n/a	Cost to establish CLIA certified infrastructure	Minimal administrative, coordination effort ($440/ case reimbursement for data abstraction)	3rd party billing, depends on insurace	Dana-Farber Vanderbilt Sidney Kimmel Kettering International: Ctr for Personalized Cancer Treatment, Utrecht, NL, Institut Gustave Roussy, Princess Margaret CC, Toronto	Requires CLIA certified data 'Rolling' applications, but w a letter of intent before the deadline"

(continued)

Table 11.1 (continued)

Data exchange initiative	Inception	Platform, how to scale up to the latest seq tech/capacity/partner with seq powerhouse?	Allow multiple memberships?	Data sharing/clinical data integration	Database/number of profiled cases/projected increase	Value add to clinical trial, research, proven utility	Data ownership*	Data compliance	Sample ownership*	Initial costs?*	Ongoing costs?*	Costs to patients?	Current notable members	Other notes
Foundation medicine PMEC	September 2015			Shared de-identified, matched clinical outcomes and genomic data contributed by members		utility	n/a		n/a	n/a	n/a	3rd party billing, depends on insurace	Vanderbilt, Sidney Kimmel, Cleveland Clinic; Hackensack University, Northwestern, UC Davis, UNC, Wake Forest	
Tempus	July 2016	n/a	No restriction	Anonymized data about patient survival rates and other information	5K (estimated)	Relatively unknown	Members retain data ownership	Unclear	Sample clinical data owned by provider	Relatively unknown	Relatively unknown	3rd party billing, depends on insurace	Northwestern, Michigan, Rush, Mayo Clinic, Penn, U of Chicago	

* Cost of participation
** Key factors for final decision making

3. AACR's Genomics Evidence Neoplasia Information Exchange (GENIE) [59]
   This international data-sharing project seeks to create a real-world set of registry data that aggregates and links clinical-grade cancer genomic data with limited clinical data (tumor staging, treatment, outcome data not currently available) from cancer patients treated at multiple international institutions. Annually, they plan to publicly release de-identified data. There are currently 12 members. Notable members include: Sloan Kettering, Vanderbilt, Dana Farber, MD-Anderson, Sidney Kimmel.

   - Strengths: Clear focus on research value. Data abstraction reimbursement of $100/case. 10% IDC could prove valuable. Easy access to shared datasets, excellent open source software environment.
   - Weaknesses: Very limited clinical data. No current, ready-to-use clinical report forms. Would need to be accompanied by a membership with another network to support local clinical usage. Requires application submission process.

4. Tempus [60]

   - A company developed by Eric Lefkofsky to streamline the integration of genomic data with clinical decision-making. The group specializes in storing big data and they have enlisted institutions like Mayo Clinic, Michigan Cancer Center, and Lurie CC (Northwestern), to build the necessary infrastructure to be successful. Strengths: Resource-rich environment that can arguably adapt as needed; data management and visualization tools are very strong compared to similar offerings in other environments.
   - Weaknesses: This is a relatively new initiative and time will tell the degree of adoption and success. Development of a clear and compelling business model will be a pre-requisite of success.

References

1. Goodwin S, McPherson JD, McCombie WR. Coming of age: ten years of next-generation sequencing technologies. Nat Rev Genet. 2016;17:333–51. http://www.nature.com/articles/nrg.2016.49.
2. Koboldt DC, Fulton RS, McLellan MD, Schmidt H, Kalicki-Veizer J, McMichael JF, et al. Comprehensive molecular portraits of human breast tumours. Nature. 2012;490:61–70. https://doi.org/10.1038/nature11412.
3. Brennan CW, Verhaak RGW, McKenna A, Campos B, Noushmehr H, Salama SR, et al. The somatic genomic landscape of glioblastoma. Cell. 2013;155:462–77. https://www.sciencedirect.com/science/article/pii/S0092867413012087?via%3Dihub.
4. Getz G, Gabriel SB, Cibulskis K, Lander E, Sivachenko A, Sougnez C, et al. Integrated genomic characterization of endometrial carcinoma. Nature. 2013;497:67–73. https://doi.org/10.1038/nature12113.
5. Bass AJ, Thorsson V, Shmulevich I, Reynolds SM, Miller M, Bernard B, et al. Comprehensive molecular characterization of gastric adenocarcinoma. Nature. 2014;513:202–9. https://doi.org/10.1038/nature13480.

6. Cancer Genome Atlas Research N. Integrated genomic analyses of ovarian carcinoma. Nature. 2011;474:609–15. https://www.ncbi.nlm.nih.gov/pubmed/21720365.

7. Agrawal N, Akbani R, Aksoy BA, Ally A, Arachchi H, Asa SL, et al. Integrated genomic characterization of papillary thyroid carcinoma. Cell. 2014;159:676–90. https://www.science-direct.com/science/article/pii/S0092867414012380?via%3Dihub.

8. The Cancer Genome Atlas Research Network, Ley T, Miller C, Ding L, Raphael B, Mungall A, et al. Genomic and epigenomic landscapes of adult de novo acute myeloid leukemia. N Engl J Med. 2013;368:2059–2074. https://doi.org/10.1056/NEJMoa1301689

9. Hoadley KA, Yau C, Wolf DM, Cherniack AD, Tamborero D, Ng S, et al. Multiplatform analysis of 12 cancer types reveals molecular classification within and across tissues of origin. Cell. 2014;158:929–44. https://www.sciencedirect.com/science/article/pii/S0092867414008769?via%3Dihub.

10. The Cancer Genome Atlas Research Network, Hammerman P, Lawrence M, Voet D, Jing R, Cibulskis K, et al. Comprehensive genomic characterization of squamous cell lung cancers. Nature. 2012;489:519–25. http://www.ncbi.nlm.nih.gov/pubmed/22960745

11. Verhaak RGW, Hoadley KA, Purdom E, Wang V, Qi Y, Wilkerson MD, et al. Integrated genomic analysis identifies clinically relevant subtypes of glioblastoma characterized by abnormalities in PDGFRA, IDH1, EGFR, and NF1. Cancer Cell. 2010;17:98–110. http://www.ncbi.nlm.nih.gov/pubmed/20129251.

12. The Cancer Genome Atlas Research Network, Weinstein J, Akbani R, Broom B, Wang W, Verhaak R, et al. Comprehensive molecular characterization of urothelial bladder carcinoma. Nature. 2014;507:315–22. http://www.nature.com/articles/nature12965.

13. Davis CF, Ricketts CJ, Wang M, Yang L, Cherniack AD, Shen H, et al. The somatic genomic landscape of chromophobe renal cell carcinoma. Cancer Cell. 2014;26:319–30. https://www.sciencedirect.com/science/article/pii/S1535610814003043?via%3Dihub.

14. Network TCGAR. Comprehensive molecular characterization of clear cell renal cell carcinoma. Nature. 2013;499:43–9. http://www.nature.com/articles/nature12222.

15. Noushmehr H, Weisenberger DJ, Diefes K, Phillips HS, Pujara K, Berman BP, et al. Identification of a CpG Island Methylator phenotype that defines a distinct subgroup of glioma. Cancer Cell. 2010;17:510–22. https://www.sciencedirect.com/science/article/pii/S15356 1081000108X?via%3Dihub.

16. McLendon R, Friedman A, Bigner D, Van Meir EG, Brat DJ, Mastrogianakis GM, et al. Comprehensive genomic characterization defines human glioblastoma genes and core pathways. Nature. 2008;455:1061–8. https://doi.org/10.1038/nature07385.

17. Forbes SA, Bhamra G, Bamford S, Dawson E, Kok C, Clements J, et al. The Catalogue of Somatic Mutations in Cancer (COSMIC). Curr Protoc Hum Genet. Hoboken, NJ: Wiley; 2008. p. 10.11.1–10.11.26. https://doi.org/10.1002/0471142905.hg1011s57.

18. Yeang C-H, McCormick F, Levine A. Combinatorial patterns of somatic gene mutations in cancer. FASEB J. 2008;22:2605–22. https://doi.org/10.1096/fj.08-108985.

19. National Institutes of Health- Office of Strategic Coordination. Genotype-Tissue Expression (GTEx). 2018. https://commonfund.nih.gov/gtex.

20. Stranger BE, Brigham LE, Hasz R, Hunter M, Johns C, Johnson M, et al. Enhancing GTEx by bridging the gaps between genotype, gene expression, and disease. Nat Genet. 2017;49:1664–70. https://doi.org/10.1038/ng.3969.

21. Stanford University. ENCODE: Encyclopedia of DNA Elements – ENCODE. 2018. https://www.encodeproject.org/.

22. Shoemaker RH. The NCI60 human tumour cell line anticancer drug screen. Nat Rev Cancer. 2006;6:813–23. http://www.nature.com/articles/nrc1951.

23. Cardoso F, van't Veer LJ, Bogaerts J, Slaets L, Viale G, Delaloge S, et al. 70-Gene signature as an aid to treatment decisions in early-stage breast Cancer. N Engl J Med. 2016;375:717–29. https://doi.org/10.1056/NEJMoa1602253.

24. Gianni L, Zambetti M, Clark K, Baker J, Cronin M, Wu J, et al. Gene expression profiles in paraffin-embedded core biopsy tissue predict response to chemotherapy in women with locally advanced breast cancer. J Clin Oncol. 2005;23:7265–77. https://doi.org/10.1200/JCO.2005.02.0818.

25. Wallden B, Storhoff J, Nielsen T, Dowidar N, Schaper C, Ferree S, et al. Development and verification of the PAM50-based Prosigna breast cancer gene signature assay. BMC Med Genomics. 2015;8:54. https://doi.org/10.1186/s12920-015-0129-6.

26. Castellanos J, Liu Q, Beauchamp R, Zhang B. Predicting colorectal cancer recurrence by utilizing multiple-view multiple-learner supervised learning. Ann Surg Oncol Soc Surg Oncol 70th Annu Cancer Symp. 2017;24:S7–8. http://www.surgonc.org/docs/default-source/pdf/sso-2017-annals-edition-of-abstracts-final.pdf?sfvrsn=2.

27. Myriad Genetic Laboratories Inc. Prolaris [Internet]. https://myriad.com/products-services/prostate-cancer/prolaris/.

28. Kopetz S, Tabernero J, Rosenberg R, Jiang Z-Q, Moreno V, Bachleitner-Hofmann T, et al. Genomic classifier ColoPrint predicts recurrence in stage II colorectal cancer patients more accurately than clinical factors. Oncologist. 2015;20:127–33. http://www.ncbi.nlm.nih.gov/pubmed/25561511.

29. Liu MC, Pitcher BN, Mardis ER, Davies SR, Friedman PN, Snider JE, et al. PAM50 gene signatures and breast cancer prognosis with adjuvant anthracycline- and taxane-based chemotherapy: correlative analysis of C9741 (Alliance). NPJ Breast Cancer. 2016;2:15023. http://www.ncbi.nlm.nih.gov/pubmed/28691057.

30. Rusch M, Nakitandwe J, Shurtleff S, Newman S, Zhang Z, Edmonson MN, et al. Clinical cancer genomic profiling by three-platform sequencing of whole genome, whole exome and transcriptome. Nat Commun. 2018;9:3962. http://www.nature.com/articles/s41467-018-06485-7.

31. Illumina. FastQC [Internet]. 2018. https://www.illumina.com/products/by-type/informatics-products/basespace-sequence-hub/apps/fastqc.html.

32. Mendoza-Parra MA, Saleem M-AM, Blum M, Cholley P-E, Gronemeyer H. NGS-QC generator: a quality control system for ChIP-Seq and related deep sequencing-generated datasets. New York, NY: Humana Press; 2016. p. 243–65. http://link.springer.com/10.1007/978-1-4939-3578-9_13.

33. Hannon GJ. FASTX-Toolkit [Internet]. 2018. http://hannonlab.cshl.edu/fastx_toolkit/index.html.

34. Bolger AM, Lohse M, Usadel B. Trimmomatic: a flexible trimmer for Illumina sequence data. Bioinformatics. 2014;30:2114–20. https://doi.org/10.1093/bioinformatics/btu170.

35. Broad Institute. Picard Tools [Internet]. https://broadinstitute.github.io/picard/.

36. Wang L, Nie J, Sicotte H, Li Y, Eckel-Passow JE, Dasari S, et al. Measure transcript integrity using RNA-seq data. BMC Bioinformatics. 2016;17:58. http://www.biomedcentral.com/1471-2105/17/58.

37. Okonechnikov K, Conesa A, García-Alcalde F. Qualimap 2: advanced multi-sample quality control for high-throughput sequencing data. Bioinformatics. 2015;36:btv566. https://doi.org/10.1093/bioinformatics/btv566.

38. Mortazavi A, Williams BA, McCue K, Schaeffer L, Wold B. Mapping and quantifying mammalian transcriptomes by RNA-Seq. Nat Methods. 2008;5:621–8. http://www.nature.com/articles/nmeth.1226.

39. Wagner GP, Kin K, Lynch VJ. Measurement of mRNA abundance using RNA-seq data: RPKM measure is inconsistent among samples. Theory Biosci. 2012;131:281–5. https://doi.org/10.1007/s12064-012-0162-3.

40. Robinson MD, Oshlack A. A scaling normalization method for differential expression analysis of RNA-seq data. Genome Biol. 2010;11:R25. https://doi.org/10.1186/gb-2010-11-3-r25.

41. McCarthy DJ, Chen Y, Smyth GK. Differential expression analysis of multifactor RNA-Seq experiments with respect to biological variation. Nucleic Acids Res. 2012;40:4288–97. https://academic.oup.com/nar/article/40/10/4288/2411520.

42. Love MI, Huber W, Anders S. Moderated estimation of fold change and dispersion for RNA-seq data with DESeq2. Genome Biol. 2014;15:550. https://doi.org/10.1186/s13059-014-0550-8.

43. Hardcastle TJ. baySeq: empirical Bayesian analysis of patterns of differential expression in count data. R package version 2.14.0. 2012.

44. Leng N, Kendziorski C. EBSeq: an R package for gene and isoform differential expression analysis of RNA-seq data. R package version 1.20.0. 2015.

45. Law CW, Chen Y, Shi W, Smyth GK. Voom: precision weights unlock linear model analysis tools for RNA-seq read counts. Genome Biol. 2014;15:R29. http://www.ncbi.nlm.nih.gov/pubmed/24485249.
46. Conesa A, Nueda MJ. maSigPro: significant gene expression profile differences in time course gene expression data. R package version 1.52.0. 2018.
47. Sims D, Sudbery I, Ilott NE, Heger A, Ponting CP. Sequencing depth and coverage: key considerations in genomic analyses. Nat Rev Genet. 2014;15:121–32. http://www.nature.com/articles/nrg3642.
48. Auslander N, Zhang G, Lee JS, Frederick DT, Miao B, Moll T, et al. Robust prediction of response to immune checkpoint blockade therapy in metastatic melanoma. Nat Med. 2018;24:1545–9. http://www.nature.com/articles/s41591-018-0157-9.
49. Cieślik M, Chinnaiyan AM. Cancer transcriptome profiling at the juncture of clinical translation. Nat Rev Genet. 2017;19:93–109. https://doi.org/10.1038/nrg.2017.96.
50. Schelker M, Feau S, Du J, Ranu N, Klipp E, MacBeath G, et al. Estimation of immune cell content in tumour tissue using single-cell RNA-seq data. Nat Commun. 2017;8:2032. http://www.nature.com/articles/s41467-017-02289-3.
51. Allegretti M, Fabi A, Buglioni S, Martayan A, Conti L, Pescarmona E, et al. Tearing down the walls: FDA approves next generation sequencing (NGS) assays for actionable cancer genomic aberrations. J Exp Clin Cancer Res. 2018;37:47. https://doi.org/10.1186/s13046-018-0702-x.
52. Cheng DT, Mitchell TN, Zehir A, Shah RH, Benayed R, Syed A, et al. Memorial sloan kettering-integrated mutation profiling of actionable cancer targets (MSK-IMPACT). J Mol Diagnostics. 2015;17:251–64. http://www.ncbi.nlm.nih.gov/pubmed/25801821.
53. Hyman DM, Solit DB, Arcila ME, Cheng DT, Sabbatini P, Baselga J, et al. Precision medicine at memorial Sloan Kettering Cancer center: clinical next-generation sequencing enabling next-generation targeted therapy trials. Drug Discov Today. 2015;20:1422–8. https://www.sciencedirect.com/science/article/pii/S1359644615003219?via%3Dihub.
54. Cheng DT, Prasad M, Chekaluk Y, Benayed R, Sadowska J, Zehir A, et al. Comprehensive detection of germline variants by MSK-IMPACT, a clinical diagnostic platform for solid tumor molecular oncology and concurrent cancer predisposition testing. BMC Med Genomics. 2017;10:33. https://doi.org/10.1186/s12920-017-0271-4.
55. U.S. Food and Drug Administration. Premarket Approval (PMA). 2018. https://www.accessdata.fda.gov/scripts/cdrh/cfdocs/cfpma/pma.cfm?id=P160045.
56. U.S. Food and Drug Administration. Recently-approved devices – FoundationOne CDx – P170019. 2017. https://www.fda.gov/medicaldevices/productsandmedicalprocedures/deviceapprovalsandclearances/recently-approveddevices/ucm590331.htm.
57. Caris Life Sciences. Precision Oncology Alliance. https://www.carislifesciences.com/precision-oncology-alliance/.
58. ORIEN- Oncology Research Information Exchange Network. ORIEN- Oncology Research Information Exchange Network [Internet]. 2015. http://oriencancer.org/#about.
59. Micheel CM, Sweeney SM, LeNoue-Newton ML, André F, Bedard PL, Guinney J, et al. American Association for Cancer Research project genomics evidence neoplasia information exchange: from inception to first data release and beyond—lessons learned and member institutions' perspectives. JCO Clin Cancer Informatics. 2018;2:1–14. https://doi.org/10.1200/CCI.17.00083.
60. Tempus. Tempus – Data-Driven Precision Medicine. 2018. https://www.tempus.com/.

Chapter 12
Largescale Distributed PPM Databases: Harmonizing and Standardizing PPM Cohorts and Clinical Genomics Data Sharing Consortia

Deanna Cross and Catherine A. McCarty

Introduction

As the era of "omic" (genomics, proteomics, metabolomics, etc) medicine proceeds, there is a need for larger cohorts to be created in order to test hypotheses and generate and validate discoveries. This is a particularly acute need when the events and outcomes being collected and investigated are rare. In an effort to establish these large cohorts, both disease-specific and general population biobanks and associated databases have been combined to form super-cohorts to answer questions of interest. This combination of several different cohorts into one larger cohort for data analysis is most often performed with distributed data analysis methods where samples are held within local repositories and data elements are collected and harmonized within a central analysis center.

This method of cohort combination presents a number of unique challenges. Initial decisions need to be made regarding how data elements will be collected and shared. In some cohorts, data elements are static and samples are shipped with a preset metadata file for a single sample extraction and analysis. In other cohorts, the samples are kept within the site and both phenotypic and biological biomarker data are sent to the central analysis center. In this chapter, we will discuss the strengths and challenges of these types of cohort creation.

D. Cross
Department of Microbiology, Immunology, and Genetics, Health Science Center,
University of North Texas, Denton, TX, USA
e-mail: deanna.cross@unthsc.edu

C. A. McCarty (✉)
Department of Family Medicine and Biobehavioral Health, University of Minnesota Duluth,
Duluth, MN, USA
e-mail: cathy@d.umn.edu

© Springer Nature Switzerland AG 2020
T. Adam, C. Aliferis (eds.), *Personalized and Precision Medicine Informatics*,
Health Informatics, https://doi.org/10.1007/978-3-030-18626-5_12

   Whether samples are collected for analysis from different biobanks or individual level data from previous analyses are used, there are a number of universal steps that must occur prior to analysis. Before combination, all of the existing data elements need to be harmonized. Data harmonization is the process in which data variables measuring the same type of entity from different sources are transformed into a standardized data format across all samples and populations. Data harmonization efforts have a number of challenges that must be addressed in order to have a successful outcome. All aspects of the data must be harmonized and standardized in order for an assessment to be valid. This includes quantitative laboratory tests, clinical outcomes and social measures used for data analysis (Fig. 12.1).

   In order to determine appropriate analysis and to harmonize biological samples, data elements from collection and analytic analysis need to be evaluated.

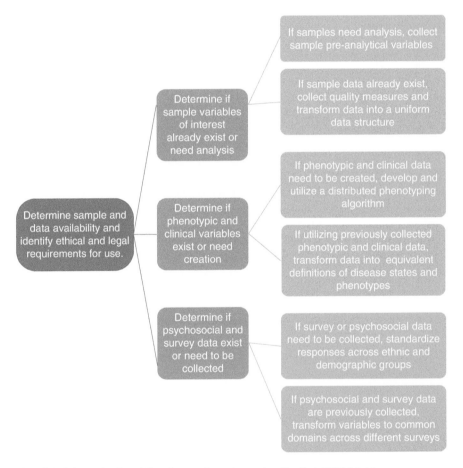

Fig. 12.1 Schematic of workflow for creating cohort using distributed PPM databases

Pre-analytical variables related to sample collection and storage and data elements that explain the methods and equipment used for previous testing need to be considered. As an example, prior to analysis for protein, RNA, DNA or methylation assays, there needs to be a clear understanding of the testing performed and any uncertainties or biases within the test. Each sample needs to be associated with a set of metadata elements that include preclinical features such as sample storage and collection methods. For data elements such as genotyping, the data need to be converted to a single build number within the human genome, and genotyping, data cleaning and conversion need to be transparent.

Clinical data can be harmonized using a number of different methods, including providing a distributed phenotyping algorithm to sample sites or defining a clinical phenotype by combining or equilibrating previously collected elements. To harmonize clinical data elements such as diagnosis through a distributed algorithm, there needs to be a defined algorithm that is tested for diagnosis fidelity across multiple cohorts in order to achieve accurate categorization. When using previously collected data, data must be standardized through either shared data elements or through the creation of equivalency tables. It is also important to recognize the limitations and strengths of any disease or condition definition.

When harmonizing social measures, it is important to define the social domains that are being measured in any survey and to determine whether values from different instruments can be cross-validated for data set combinations. This can be done either through providing all relevant survey instruments to a smaller cohort for validation or through statistical methodologies based on the construct being measured. Furthermore when collecting and analyzing social measures across different cultural and economic backgrounds, different correlation factors may need to be utilized to standardize the data.

Finally, it is important to understand the ethical and legal implications of combining a diverse set of samples. Samples were likely collected with different IRB frameworks, and there must be a clear understanding of what research question or questions are allowable under each consent. In general, consent for the proposed research project can be provided either site-by- site or through a centralized clearinghouse. The nature of the consent will depend on both the proposed study as well as the biobank(s) being queried.

Different biobank consortia and distributed databases have approached each of these problems differently. In this chapter we will determine what types of clinical problems are best approached using a distributed PPM database and how different research groups have tackled the challenges presented in harmonizing disparate sources. We will discuss the workflows and data distribution challenges that need to be addressed prior to establishing a large cohort and the benefits and limitations of a distributed database. Furthermore, we will discuss the current tools available for data harmonization and the standardized elements that are currently available for planning future amalgamation into large distributed networks.

Clinical Problems that May Be Addressed with Distributed PPM Databases

In general, rare events or outcomes need large sample sizes in order to have enough power for analysis. It is only through coordination of genotyping and phenotyping of many different individuals in multiple databases that rare variants that affect disease can be found. Examples of disease-specific consortia being used for rare variant detection include diabetic kidney disease [1], Alzheimer's disease [2] and age-related macular degeneration [3]. It has been demonstrated that distributed PPM databases can be used to ascertain enough samples to create a cohort large enough to investigate a rare outcome, such as a rare disease. The eMERGE consortium developed and validated electronic algorithms to classify phenotypes across multiple biobanks in order to ensure that enough individuals were available to provide power for disease specific studies [4]. Currently the NIH All of Us study is enrolling over a million participants across the country with different disease states and electronic health records that will be used to create cohorts of individuals with similar disease states across the population [5].

Even for common diseases, there is often a need to use a large distributed cohort in order to achieve a sample size large enough for analysis of certain disease outcomes or disease subtypes. An example of this is the use of multiple distributed sample banks for diseases, such as EyeGENE, an NEI administered biorepository and database for subjects' clinical eye exam data and family history [6] (https://eyegene.nih.gov/).

Challenges and Tools for Identifying Distributed Cohorts Available for Analysis and Further Data Collection

Unfortunately, there is no central clearing house for previously collected cohorts, and each disease type and individual biobank may have different requirements for access and rules for sample and data utilization. There are a number of websites that list individual cohorts that could be used by investigators in future research endeavors. Table 12.1 lists a few examples of broad cohort collections.

It is important to remember that each cohort may have different ethical and legal restrictions for use. Some of the websites with cohort information include details about the cohort, such as contact information, IRB consents, and sample availability, while other sites may list only the cohort and the contact information. In addition to listed biobanks, there may be disease-specific consortia available with samples stored either in a single site like the PLCO EEMS biobank (https://prevention.cancer.gov/major-programs/prostate-lung-colorectal/etiology-and-early-marker) [7] or at each individual clinical site.

Table 12.1 Websites that list different types of cohorts that could be used for research

http://www.birthcohorts.net	Lists available birth cohorts
https://epi.grants.cancer.gov/Consortia/members	Lists members in the NCI cohort consortium
https://biolincc.nhlbi.nih.gov/home	NHLBI biospecimen and data coordinating center
https://repository.niddk.nih.gov/home	NIDDK repository
https://www.nia.nih.gov/research/dab/nia-virtual-repository	NIA list of repositories with available data and biospecimens
https://emerge.mc.vanderbilt.edu	NHGRI biobank list of eMERGE collaborators and link to tools for harmonizing data
https://commonfund.nih.gov/gtex	Genotype-tissue expression data and sample availability
https://neurobiobank.nih.gov	Brain tissue and data inventory
http://specimencentral.com/biobank-directory/#North%20American%20Biobanks	List of North American biobanks
https://www.ncbi.nlm.nih.gov/gap?db=gap	dbGAP repository for genomic data and associated phenotype measures

Challenges and Tools for Samples that Have Not Been Genotyped or Do Not Have Analytical Data Already Attached

There are a number of sample sources that do not have analytical data attached prior to requesting access to the data. In these instances, pre-analytical variables may need to be collected from the PPM distributed databases to ensure that accurate sample analysis is achieved. As an example, the quality of results with expression analysis will vary based on the tissue of interest, the sample preparation and fixation methodology and the sample collection date in relation to the disease course. All these variables may be important to have a valid analysis. A list of necessary requirements needed to ensure accurate and repeatable analytic testing of samples has been created [8]. For immunohistochemistry experiments, the minimum standards are outlined in the MYFISHE specifications [9]. For RNA analysis, there are several different standards– a comprehensive review is provided by Castel et al. [10]. Other tools can be found outlined on the NCI genome harmonization website [11]. Knowing these pre-analytical variables allows individual investigators to determine whether a sample is suitable for a planned analysis and makes results more likely to be repeatable. In some instances, the time between phenotypic data collection and sample collection may be important, particularly when using samples for RNA analysis and disease categorization.

Challenges and Tools for PPM Databases that Have Genotyped Data

Distributed databases may or may not have samples that have been genotyped previously; however, one of the advantages of using PPM databases is that combining biobanks that have genotypes readily available may reduce the costs of a study. Previously genotyped samples will need additional data cleaning and harmonization prior to creating a combined dataset. Because there are a variety of genotyping platforms and genotyping chips within each platform, it is necessary to capture informative data elements prior to any analysis. Three important data elements that are necessary in order for any combined database to be utilized are the genotyping quality measures, the platform and chip used, and the build number of the human genome that the genotyping references. A discussion of the challenges and steps for data harmonization can be found in Turner et al.'s paper [12].

Quality measures include the quality of the sample, the platform and the genotype. This is often captured in information such as missingness, that is, the frequency of missing values. In general, samples and genotypes with large missingness are excluded from final analysis. While the exact genotyping efficiency can vary from study to study, this threshold is generally set prior to analysis, with typical range for missingness between 1 and 2%. Another quality measure that may be available is the concordance rate, i.e., the rate at which duplicate samples have the same genotype. Generally concordance rates of less than 99% indicate poor quality genotyping either for the particular marker or the entire chip. Information on the platform used for genotyping as well as the standardized error curves are needed to ensure that batch-to-batch variability within the genotypes are not carried into the final database. There may also be batch effects as the genotypes being combined may have been done at different times and on different platforms. Therefore, it is advisable to determine whether the allele frequencies of the genotypes being used are different in different cohorts (accounting for the potential for population substructure in any cohort).

Beyond quality control, it is important to know which platform and which particular chip were used and which build number of the human genome was used to build the chip. This information is necessary because different platforms code alleles differently; they can be in ACGT format, TOP format or AB format, which makes harmonization difficult and data analysis impossible until all data are in the same format. There are a number of tools that can be used to convert the genotypes to the same format. One good source for this is the converting tool available at the GenGen website [13] (gengen.openbioinformatics.org). Prior to analysis, the format and the human genome build need to be the same for all genotypes utilized.

All alleles need to be aligned with a single build number, because with each build number, the reference sequence and position could change. Polymorphisms have been combined, and even chromosome mapping of the polymorphism can change with different build numbers; therefore, it is important to ensure that all genotypes are aligned with the same build number to ensure that comparisons are valid. It is possible to change genotypes to a common build number, using tools such as GACT [14] and Liftover [15]. Given that not every genotyping platform has the same geno-types within every chip, there may be a need to use tools to obtain the genotypes of interest. In order to utilize different genotyping platforms, it may be necessary to impute genotypes for analysis. In general, two different methods of imputation can be used: local imputation, which uses the genetic information directly sur-rounding the imputed genotype to make an inference, or global imputation, which is computationally intensive and uses all of the genetic information available for imputation. There are a number of bioinformatics tools that are available for impu-tation. SHAPEIT [16] and Impute2 [17] are two programs that are widely used. It is important to remember that imputation is a probabilistic genotype, and it may be necessary to set thresholds for the call probability and to carry forward the call probability into the analysis.

For samples with next generation sequencing, the reference sequence used for sequence alignment is important information as different reference sequence ver-sions will need harmonization prior to analysis. In addition, the depth of sequence coverage within both the entire batched sequence and any particular sequences of interest is important information, as next generation sequencing coverage may vary for different parts of the genome. Hart et al. [18] describe the technical challenges of harmonizing data from different sequencing platforms and times and, they outline the necessary steps to ensure accuracy for data analysis.

Challenges and Tools for Phenotyping Samples from Diverse Datasets

Accurate phenotypic data are important for any analysis. When utilizing distrib-uted databases there are a number of challenges that can occur when determining the phenotype. Some databases are static, with no ability to phenotype individuals beyond previously defined and collected variables. In this case, it is important to include the metadata that defines all of the phenotypic characteristics and to deter-mine if the definitions are compatible. Fortunately, there are tools available for har-monizing data sets that are not static. In some cases, this may mean scoring a small standard dataset across different cohort definitions as was done with the AMD consortium [3]. After the scoring is completed there will be a cross walk table for different variables. This type of data harmonization also will allow a researcher to determine if there are accuracy differences in the desired phenotype. The i2b2 data ontology was created so that different sample and patient banks could be queried with the same terminology, and so that sample banks that utilize the i2b2 ontology could be harmonized [19]. The PhenX toolkit is also a set of phenotypic tools that have created consensus-guided phenotypes [20]. The BioShare project created a suite of tools for phenotypic harmonization with each data set residing in a local environment [21].

If, however, the phenotype of interest is not contained within a previously defined variable, there are methods for creating a phenotype. One validated method is through using a distributed algorithm [22]. This method has been extensively utilized within large biobank consortia such as the eMERGE network [23]. Briefly, a single cohort is used to develop an algorithm using clinical data such as laboratory values, diagnoses, and medications. The positive and negative predictive values (PPV and NPV) of the algorithm are calculated. In general a 70% or greater PPV is needed to test the algorithm on other cohorts. A test cohort from another biobank is then used to score the PPV and NPV. If the second cohort is also reliably classified accurately, then the algorithm can be used on all of the distributed biobanks. The eMERGE website [24] has a number of previously developed phenotyping algorithms and has been used as a model for development of distributed phenotyping, including both a PheKB [25] tool and the eleMAP tool (https://victr.vanderbilt.edu/eleMAP/) (see Chap. 15 for a more thorough discussion of the eMERGE network).

Challenges and Tools for Harmonizing Survey and Psychosocial Data in Diverse Datasets

On some occasions, the data elements of interest are not clinical data but rather patient-collected data. Surveys such as food frequency or dietary questionnaires, such as those used in the PLCO study [7], and environmental questionnaires, such as those used in the ECHO child health study [26], are often used to collect data within a cohort. Even when validated questionnaires are used, it may be difficult to harmonize data between cohorts because different questionnaires may not have exact equivalency measures. Fortunately there are a number of strategies that can be used to harmonize these data elements. One of the methods for creating equivalency between previously collected survey data is to collect data on a small subset of all of the cohorts using multiple survey instruments. For example, the quality of life scores for the PROMIS 29 measures can be mapped to the EQ5-D responses to provide a quality of life equivalency score based on Revicki et al.'s work [27]. Another method of harmonizing data in surveys is to use item response theory. An example of this method can be found in Chan et al.'s harmonization of cognitive aging measures [28].

In conclusion, largescale distributed PPM databases will continue to be developed and enhanced as sequencing data and additional phenotypic data become available. Data harmonization is a major key to unlocking the research potential in these databases.

References

1. van Zuydam NR, Ahlqvist E, Sandholm N, Deshmukh H, Rayner NW, Abdalla M, et al. A genome-wide association study of diabetic kidney disease in subjects with type 2 diabetes. Diabetes. 2018;67:1414–27. http://www.ncbi.nlm.nih.gov/pubmed/29703844.
2. Bis JC, Jian X, Kunkle BW, Chen Y, Hamilton-Nelson KL, Bush WS, et al. Whole exome sequencing study identifies novel rare and common Alzheimer's-associated variants involved in immune response and transcriptional regulation. Mol Psychiatry. 2018. http://www.nature.com/articles/s41380-018-0112-7.
3. Klein R, Meuer SM, Myers CE, Buitendijk GHS, Rochtchina E, Choudhury F, et al. Harmonizing the classification of age-related macular degeneration in the three-continent AMD Consortium. Ophthalmic Epidemiol. 2014;21:14–23. https://doi.org/10.3109/09286586.2013.867512.
4. Mosley JD, Feng Q, Wells QS, Van Driest SL, Shaffer CM, Edwards TL, et al. A study paradigm integrating prospective epidemiologic cohorts and electronic health records to identify disease biomarkers. Nat Commun. 2018;9:3522. http://www.nature.com/articles/s41467-018-05624-4.
5. Precision Medicine Initiative (PMI) Working Group, Hudson K, Lifton R, Patrick-Lake B, Burchard EG, Collins R, et al. The Precision Medicine Initiative Cohort Program– Building a Research Foundation for 21st Century Medicine Precision Medicine Initiative (PMI) Working Group Report to the Advisory Committee to the Director, NIH [Internet]. https://www.nih.gov/sites/default/files/research-training/initiatives/pmi/pmi-working-group-report-20150917-2.pdf.
6. National Eye Institute NI of H. The National Ophthalmic Disease Genotyping and Phenotyping Network eyeGENE. https://eyegene.nih.gov/.
7. Hayes RB, Sigurdson A, Moore L, Peters U, Huang W-Y, Pinsky P, et al. Methods for etiologic and early marker investigations in the PLCO trial. Mutat Res Mol Mech Mutagen. 2005;592:147–54. https://www.sciencedirect.com/science/article/pii/S0027510705002472?via%3Dihub.
8. True LD. Methodological requirements for valid tissue-based biomarker studies that can be used in clinical practice. Virchows Arch. 2014;464:257–63. https://doi.org/10.1007/s00428-013-1531-0.
9. Deutsch EW, Ball CA, Berman JJ, Bova GS, Brazma A, Bumgarner RE, et al. Minimum information specification for in situ hybridization and immunohistochemistry experiments (MISFISHIE). Nat Biotechnol. 2008;26:305–12. http://www.nature.com/articles/nbt1391.
10. Castel SE, Levy-Moonshine A, Mohammadi P, Banks E, Lappalainen T. Tools and best practices for data processing in allelic expression analysis. Genome Biol. 2015;16:195. http://genomebiology.com/2015/16/1/195.
11. National Cancer Institute NI of H. Genomic Data Harmonization | NCI Genomic Data Commons [Internet]. https://gdc.cancer.gov/about-data/data-harmonization-and-generation/genomic-data-harmonization-0.
12. Turner S, Armstrong LL, Bradford Y, Carlson CS, Crawford DC, Crenshaw AT, et al. Quality control procedures for genome-wide association studies. Curr Protoc Hum Genet. 2011;68:1.19.1–1.19.18. https://doi.org/10.1002/0471142905.hg0119s68.
13. Wang K, Li M, Hakonarson H. Analysing biological pathways in genome-wide association studies. Nat Rev Genet. 2010;11:843–54. http://www.nature.com/articles/nrg2884.
14. Sulovari A, Li D. GACT: a genome build and allele definition conversion tool for SNP imputation and meta-analysis in genetic association studies. BMC Genomics. 2014;15:610. https://doi.org/10.1186/1471-2164-15-610.

15. Hickey G, Paten B, Earl D, Zerbino D, Haussler D. HAL: a hierarchical format for storing and analyzing multiple genome alignments. Bioinformatics. 2013;29:1341–2. https://doi.org/10.1093/bioinformatics/btt128.

16. O'Connell J, Gurdasani D, Delaneau O, Pirastu N, Ulivi S, Cocca M, et al. A general approach for haplotype phasing across the full spectrum of relatedness. Gibson G, editor. PLoS Genet. 2014;10:e1004234. https://doi.org/10.1371/journal.pgen.1004234.

17. Howie BN, Donnelly P, Marchini J. A flexible and accurate genotype imputation method for the next generation of genome-wide association studies. Schork NJ, editor. PLoS Genet. 2009;5:e1000529. https://doi.org/10.1371/journal.pgen.1000529

18. Hart SN, Maxwell KN, Thomas T, Ravichandran V, Wubberhorst B, Klein RJ, et al. Collaborative science in the next-generation sequencing era: a viewpoint on how to combine exome sequencing data across sites to identify novel disease susceptibility genes. Brief Bioinform. 2016;17:672–7. https://doi.org/10.1093/bib/bbv075.

19. Klann JG, Abend A, Raghavan VA, Mandl KD, Murphy SN. Data interchange using i2b2. J Am Med Informatics Assoc. 2016;23:909–15. https://doi.org/10.1093/jamia/ocv188.

20. Hendershot T, Pan H, Haines J, Harlan WR, Marazita ML, CA MC, et al. Using the PhenX toolkit to add standard measures to a study. Curr Protoc Hum Genet. 2015;86:1.21.1–1.21.17. https://doi.org/10.1002/0471142905.hg0121s86.

21. Doiron D, Burton P, Marcon Y, Gaye A, Wolffenbuttel BHR, Perola M, et al. Data harmonization and federated analysis of population-based studies: the BioSHaRE project. Emerg Themes Epidemiol. 2013;10:12. https://doi.org/10.1186/1742-7622-10-12.

22. Xu J, Rasmussen LV, Shaw PL, Jiang G, Kiefer RC, Mo H, et al. Review and evaluation of electronic health records-driven phenotype algorithm authoring tools for clinical and translational research. J Am Med Informatics Assoc. 2015;22:ocv070. https://doi.org/10.1093/jamia/ocv070.

23. Pacheco JA, Rasmussen LV, Kiefer RC, Campion TR, Speltz P, Carroll RJ, et al. A case study evaluating the portability of an executable computable phenotype algorithm across multiple institutions and electronic health record environments. J Am Med Informatics Assoc. 2018;25(11):1540–6. https://doi.org/10.1093/jamia/ocy101/5075388.

24. eMerge network electronic medical records and genomics. eMerge tools [internet]. 2014. https://emerge.mc.vanderbilt.edu/tools/.

25. Kirby JC, Speltz P, Rasmussen LV, Basford M, Gottesman O, Peissig PL, et al. PheKB: a catalog and workflow for creating electronic phenotype algorithms for transportability. J Am Med Informatics Assoc. 2016;23:1046–52. https://doi.org/10.1093/jamia/ocv202.

26. Jacobson LP, Lau B, Catellier D, Parker CB. An environmental influences on child health outcomes viewpoint of data analysis centers for collaborative study designs. Curr Opin Pediatr. 2018;30:269–75. http://insights.ovid.com/crossref?an=00008480-201804000-00019.

27. Revicki DA, Kawata AK, Harnam N, Chen W-H, Hays RD, Cella D. Predicting EuroQol (EQ-5D) scores from the patient-reported outcomes measurement information system (PROMIS) global items and domain item banks in a United States sample. Qual Life Res. 2009;18:783–91. https://doi.org/10.1007/s11136-009-9489-8.

28. Chan KS, Gross AL, Pezzin LE, Brandt J, Kasper JD. Harmonizing measures of cognitive performance across international surveys of aging using item response theory. J Aging Health. 2015;27:1392–414. https://doi.org/10.1177/0898264315583054.

Chapter 13
Redefining Disease Using Informatics

Glenn N. Saxe

Introduction

Two critical questions are at the center of efforts to pursue Personalized and Precision Medicine (PPM) for specific diseases [1–3]:

1. How do we build a model of a disease that will use all relevant information available, to accurately predict disease-related events (e.g., disease onset, prognosis, emergencies, intervention response) for a specific patient?
2. How do we use such a model for disease classification and diagnosis that will enable the accurate prediction of disease-related events?

An appropriate model of a given disease for PPM will be able to: (1) integrate information from and about an individual patient to inform the prediction of disease-related events the patient will encounter by virtue of the patient's classification within the disease category; and (2) inform decisions on interventions for the patient based on accurate prediction of the patient's disease response, to an intervention that is considered.

In this chapter, I will review the integral relationship between disease conceptualization, modeling, and theory with disease classification and diagnosis, and the challenges and opportunities to these processes for PPM, entailed by the informational revolution that now affects all medical fields. This informational revolution concerns both the availability of vast amounts of new information relevant for PPM and the informatics and computational tools that enable the use of this information. The chapter will illustrate these ideas with particular reference to the field of psychiatry, with which this author is intimately familiar however the relevant principles apply across medical fields.

G. N. Saxe (✉)
Department of Child and Adolescent Psychiatry, School of Medicine, New York University, New York, NY, USA
e-mail: glenn.saxe@nyumc.org

© Springer Nature Switzerland AG 2020   185
T. Adam, C. Aliferis (eds.), *Personalized and Precision Medicine Informatics*,
Health Informatics, https://doi.org/10.1007/978-3-030-18626-5_13

The genomic revolution has unlocked a previously unfathomable treasure of personal information that can be used to predict disease-related events. The value of this information will increase many-fold when it is used with other domains of information (e.g., social, developmental, molecular, physiological, disease expression) to predict disease-related events based on the conditional dependencies between variables. To use this information will require refinements in the way diseases are typically conceptualized and classified, in order to integrate the breadth and depth of the conditional dependencies that would determine the occurrence of disease-related events for individual patients. Medical fields are now in the process of re-conceptualizing and reclassifying diseases for these purposes.

Disease Theory, Disease Classification, and the Prediction of Disease-Related Events

A theory of a disease (which when sufficiently mature can be made operational via a computational model encoding this theory) is an accepted understanding of the causal processes underlying the disease, shared by a community of clinicians and scientists with professional expertise in the disease. Disease classification concerns the way a medical field places patients into groups based on its theory/model of disease, in order to facilitate the prediction of disease-related events. A theory/model of a disease is essentially based on understood conditional dependencies between causal processes for disease-related events and therefore the greater the number of causal processes and interactions between them included in the model, the more categories and subcategories will be available to classify patients for accurate prediction. The informational revolution makes available for consideration, vastly increased numbers of possible causes and interactions for disease-related events, and this state-of-affairs has prompted many medical fields to pursue updates to their disease classification approaches. These refinements can therefore lead to vastly improved capacity for prediction concerning individual patients.

Theory building is an exercise in causal inference and is also highly related to the process of classification [4]. This is true for how individual humans learn to understand and predict their world, and for how communities of humans (including scientists and clinicians) learn to understand and predict their worlds via communally accepted theory and classification [5–7]. The integral relationship between the way a medical field may arrive at a causal model or theory of the processes underlying disease expression and the way it creates disease classification is not often recognized. Accordingly, it is important to understand that the information available to clinicians and scientists concerning an underlying pathological state comes from the signs and symptoms expressed from patients that may be caused by underlying pathologic processes. The clinician or scientist makes sense of the information received (in the form of signs and symptoms) by putting this information into meaningful categories that presumably reflect the underlying causal processes that generated this data. Thus, disease classification and diagnosis is a result of a causal inferential process [8–10].

Briefly, causal inference concerns the application of a reasoning process to identify causal factors that have produced the data that one seeks to understand. In a fundamental way this reasoning concerns the result of actions on the world (*if my action on entity X serves to change the likelihood of event Y, then entity X is a cause of event Y*). When applied in scientific research such a causal inference exercise often takes the form of *an experiment*. In most cases, however, when causal inference is needed, experimental actions cannot be conducted for a variety of reasons: ethical considerations, cost, long time horizons to observe effects, or simple inability to affect certain entities with available experimental technology.

In such cases, the powerful process of counterfactual reasoning supports causal inference (*given my model of the world: if I were to act to change entity X, it would change the likelihood of event Y in a way that differs from the likelihood of event Y, if I do not act. Therefore my action on X will cause a change in the likelihood of event Y*). Powerful and well-validated methods that enable causal inference with observational data sets employ versions of such counterfactual reasoning processes [11–13].

Such causal inference as applied to medicine serves to establish a causal model of the patient's disease that integrates the clinician's or scientist's understanding of the causal processes (and conditional dependencies between processes[1]) for generating the data (i.e., the signs and symptoms) that are observed. Once such a model is established, it is then used to predict disease-related events from data that has not been previously encountered. Such new data can come from the same patient(s) upon which the model of the disease was generated, or, if the model is believed to be a more generalized account of the conditional dependencies between the causal process, for a wider set of patients or in all patients with the underlying disease, the model is used to predict disease-related events with this wider set of patients. The quality (i.e. performance) of the model is determined by the resulting predictive accuracy for disease-related events for the population the model is intended to describe, under a variety of interventions or passive data observations.

The process just described is known as causal reasoning, is based on *generative models*. A generative model is a model of the inferred causal processes that *generated* the data that comes to us from the world. When such data is in the form of the signs and symptoms of disease, as well as causes and mediators of disease, the application of causal reasoning is immediately relevant to clinical care and clinical science [8–10]. Causal reasoning has far more general application and likely underlies the fundamental processes by which humans understand their world (and predict relevant events in the world) [5, 6]. This process is always bidirectional. First,

---

[1] Editors' comment: underlying the author's emphasis on conditional independencies is that there is a close relationship between conditional dependencies and independencies in a data distribution and the causal process that generates the data. This close correspondence is exploited by causal discovery algorithms to infer causality from observational non-experimental data. For details, readers can read refs. [4, 11] of the present chapter.

a backward-looking model is built to infer the causal processes that generated the data and then this model is used in a forward-looking way to predict events about contemplated actions or observed events. Ideally, the model is then refined based on information from prediction errors such that it is continually improved based on more accurate accounts of the causal processes that produce the data.

There is a growing literature to support the formal use of causal reasoning within medicine to improve predictive accuracy for disease-related events and to avoid biases in causal inference that can occur when causal reasoning is not employed [8–10]. Counter-intuitively, one of the most important barriers to progress in most medical fields is the near- exclusive reliance on the results from experimental studies for accepted causal knowledge. For many practical and ethical reasons experiments cannot be conducted with human subjects to understand causal processes for many forms of disease. Even in medical fields where experiments are more practical, they can rarely be conducted in a way that can capture the conditional dependencies for disease related events, particularly the scale of data and possible interactions unlocked by the Big Data information revolution. This information is contained within observational data sets, and inferences on causation from correlational observational data, *when not conducted with appropriate discovery procedures*, are notoriously prone to error and bias, particularly in mistaking the direction of cause versus effect relations, mistaking confounded relationships for true causal ones, and estimating poorly the quantitative cause-effect relationship. As described previously, there are powerful informatics tools to support rigorous causal inference with observational data and robust such methods have been previously described [4, 11–13].

Next, I describe how these challenges and opportunities manifest in the field of psychiatry.

Evolution of Conceptualization and Classification of Psychiatric Disorders and the Importance of Causal PPM

The field of psychiatry is illustrative because its causal knowledgebase for the etiology of psychiatric disorders is particularly underdeveloped compared to other medical fields. There are several reasons for this underdevelopment including, (1) the difficulty of conducting human experiments related to psychiatric disorders, (2) the likely complex etiology of many of these disorders, and (3) uncertainty about psychiatric phenotypes given that traditional psychiatric disease classification is not explicitly based on causation. The resulting limitations on knowledge of causation translates to great difficulty with evaluating alternative theories of diseases and a poor track record in predicting disease-related events (e.g., outcomes and responses to treatments). These challenges have been magnified considerably by the amount of information now available related to genetic, molecular, and neurologic processes. Although the problem of causality may be more significant in psychiatry compared to other medical fields, these same problems manifest in varying degrees in all medical fields. Thus the ideas presented through discussion of the challenges in the conceptualization and classification of psychiatric disorders for PPM are relevant for many other non-psychiatric disorders, particularly those with complex etiologies.

The landscape in psychiatry is now shifting with increasing calls for greater integration of causal understanding within the conceptualization of psychiatric disorders and the corresponding classification and diagnostic approaches. These changes most clearly manifest in controversies over the conventional diagnostic system used in psychiatry: the American Psychiatric Association's Diagnostic and Statistical Manual of Mental Disorders (DSM) [14] versus the more recent approach endorsed by the National Institute of Mental Health's Research Domain Criterion [15, 16].

In 1980, the field of psychiatry made a deliberate turn *away* from causation within its classification system when the DSM III was released [17]. One of the drivers of this change was that previous versions of DSM had tied diagnostic categories to presumed causal factors, with poor empirical evidence of causation. Such diagnostic categories were not only poorly supported by evidence, they were also applied inconsistently because psychiatrists did not agree on underlying causal processes that determined previous classification approaches. With DSM III, the diagnostic process became entirely descriptive. This system was based on observable groupings of symptoms that had defined functional relevance and were agreed upon by psychiatric experts. This led to a considerable increase in consistency of diagnosis but an abandonment of the usual function of medical diagnosis to point to specific underlying pathological processes. This rationale was defended in an influential editorial written by Gerald Klerman, former director of the federal *Alcohol, Drug Abuse and Mental Health Administration*, shortly after DSM III's release:

> …these [DSM III] criteria are based on manifest descriptive psychopathology rather than on presumed etiology…This reliance on descriptive rather than etiologic criteria does not represent an abandonment of the ideal of modern scientific medicine that classification and diagnosis should be by causation. Rather, it represents a strategic mode of dealing with the frustrating reality that, for most of the disorders we currently treat, there is only limited evidence for their etiologies. There are competing hypotheses and theories that involve various mixtures of biological, social, developmental, and intrapsychic causation, but for most disorders the evidence is insufficient and inconclusive [18].

An important implication of the field's turn from causality in diagnosis and classification is that causal discovery in the field was impeded. A disease is usually understood to be the phenotypic expression of underlying causal processes. If such a phenotypic expression is widely accepted as normal clinical practice, unconstrained by plausible causal processes, then the scientific pursuit of the causes of its expression is de-incentivized and weakened. In 1994 and 2013, the DSM IV and DSM 5 were launched, respectively, both with the same non-etiologic, non-causal approach contained in DSM III in part because the state of causal knowledge in the field had still not advanced sufficiently to help define psychiatric classification [14, 19].

Fortunately, crisis can reveal opportunity and the NIMH Research Domain Criterion (RDoC) initiative was launched to help establish an empirically-based diagnostic system that is integrally related to causal knowledge. Importantly, such a system integrates the diversity of possible causal processes that can help define PPM within psychiatry and has recently been conceptualized to be highly consistent with the causal inferential processes described previously. Although the RDoC initiative is only a decade old and its utility for the purposes described remains to be established, its central organizing ideas may have great utility for other medical fields seeking to leverage the information now available for PPM.

The NIMH Research Domain Criterion and the Bayesian Integrative Framework for Computational Psychiatry

NIMH's RDoC initiative was launched, in part, to address the problems described previously by locating causality within pathological brain circuits (and their upstream and downstream pathways). Recently, NIMH director Joshua Gordon has written about using RDoC for causal discovery-related Bayesian causal inference [20]. Briefly, RDoC represents a framework to categorize psychopathologic categories within five 'transdiagnostic' domains corresponding to variables selected for analysis. In this way, the RDoC framework can be useful for theory building because the variables discovered within the resulting causal models would be defined (as relevant) within the five transdiagnostic RDoC domains of: Negative Valence Systems, Positive Valence Systems, Cognitive Systems, Social Processes, Arousal and Regulatory Systems, and within specific units of analysis (genes, molecules, cells, circuits, physiology, behavior, self-report). These units of analysis are centered within brain circuits and corresponding upstream (e.g., genes, molecules, cells) and downstream (e.g., physiology, behavior, signs and symptoms) causal processes from these brain circuitry pathologies. At their downstream end, these are expressed in the signs and symptoms that are used for diagnoses and classification [15, 16]. Thus, the RDoC framework enables the inclusion of causal processes—and the dependencies between them—for creating models of psychiatric disorders that can be used to predict psychiatric disorder-related events.

Within the past few years, RDoC has been seen as a way to enable the formal integration of classification and causal inference within a causal reasoning approach, in order to support PPM within the field. This has been proposed as a Bayesian Integrative Framework at the influential Ernst Strüngmann Forum (ESF) on *Computational Psychiatry*. Details about this framework are available in the book documenting the ESF proceedings [21] by ESF organizers, Drs David Redish and Joshua Gordon, Director of the National Institute of Mental Health, and in a recently published article by Friston, Redish and Gordon entitled *Computational Nosology and Precision Psychiatry* [22]. In these articles, and others [23], this *Framework* has also been proposed as a promising means of applying Research Domain Criterion (RDoC) concepts to understanding underlying mechanisms of psychiatric disorders.

This *Bayesian Integrative Framework* is appealing for PPM because it offers a formalized—and empirically testable—approach to research related to prediction, causal inference, and prevention in psychiatry. This *Framework* starts with the notion that diagnostic categories in psychiatry are not the causes of psychopathology; they are the observable and measurable consequences of pathophysiologic and psychopathologic processes. Friston, Redish and Gordon highlight the importance of this notion within the consensus reached at the ESF, as follows:

> Although rather obvious in hindsight, this came as something of a revelation, largely because it exposed the missing link between the putative causes of psychiatric illness (e.g., genetic predisposition, environmental stressors, or iatrogenic outcomes) and the consequences, as observed by clinicians (e.g., symptoms, signs, and crucially, diagnostic outcome) (pg. 3) [22].

With such a perspective on psychiatric nosology, a formalized approach to prediction and causal discovery becomes necessary.

A *Bayesian Integrative Framework* calls for the building of a generative causal model[2] from psychiatric data. Such a generative model can estimate consequences from causes. For purposes of constructing the model the consequences are what are directly observed (e.g., symptoms, diagnoses, psychometric and biomarker measurement). The causes are identified from prior knowledge based on the literature (e.g., trauma exposure, losses, intervention exposure, genetic variation). These known causes, in turn, cause underlying (and latent) pathophysiologic states (e.g., a brain state, a neuroendocrine state), which then cause underlying psychopathologic states (e.g., cognitive, emotional, behavioral). These latent pathophysiologic and psychopathologic states then cause the measured symptoms, signs and diagnostic consequences available for observation. The causal discovery methods previously outlined can readily discover causal relationships between measured variables and indicate presence and properties of latent variables (states). Once such a model is built, it is then possible to conduct prognostication and estimate the effect of a potential intervention [11–13].

Next, I will describe application of this causal Framework to my own area of research: the prediction of deleterious outcomes (e.g., psychosocial dysfunction, Posttraumatic Stress Disorder (PTSD), aggression, self-destructive behavior) in children who experience traumatic events and the development of preventative interventions for children at risk. We know that between 15% and 40% of traumatized children will acquire such deleterious outcomes as PTSD [24–26]. In this area, ongoing research questions include what factors contribute to risk and what contributes to resilience? And which of these factors are remediable and will reduce a child's risk should an intervention be applied to the identified risk factor or causal process? Cumulatively, the research literature has not been sufficiently informative for predicting risk, and so computational methods that enable answers to these questions

---

[2] Editors' note: informally a *generative* model essentially captures the distributions of variables in some process of interest whereas a *discriminant* model aims to separate entities (for classification or prediction) without capturing the underlying process. A causal generative model furthermore represents causal relationships in the data generative process.

are extremely important [27]. These answers clearly relate to PPM because they can potentially offer specific risk profiles for an individual traumatized child and the identification of specific preventative interventions according to the nature of the risk. This research is ongoing but I include a description of it in this chapter to provide an example of how such a framework can be used to guide research for PPM of complex disorders, such as psychiatric disorders.

Of note, among psychiatric disorders, PTSD is one of the only ones that include etiology (a traumatic event) in its definition. Notwithstanding this fact, the great diversity of individual responses to traumatic events indicate that PTSD has a far more complex etiology than simply exposure to trauma and that PTSD may not fully capture the phenotype of human pathologic responses to traumatic events. That is why my research has studied a broad range of pathologic responses to trauma in children.

Applying a Causal Integrative Framework[3] for PPM for Child PTSD

Our application of a causal Integrative Framework led to the creation of a hypothesized model of causal processes and conditional dependencies for a traumatized child acquiring traumatic stress following trauma exposure, and is illustrated in Fig. 13.1. The framework integrates information from the Pre-traumatic, Peri-traumatic, and Post-traumatic Periods (the three columns in Fig. 13.1). Each of the columns indicates the Bayesian model building process described above and each of the models will be sequentially updated with new information from the next period (a Pre-trauma model is updated with information from the Peri-traumatic period, a combined Pre and Peri-traumatic model is updated with information from the Post- traumatic period). The Bayesian process shown in each column generates models by inferring latent Psychopathologic and Pathophysiologic causal states from measured evidence of signs, symptoms, diagnoses, and other outcomes. The gray arrows in Fig. 13.1 represent this causal inferential process. Once this generative model is built through such a causal inferential process, it is then used to predict signs, symptoms, diagnoses, and prognostic trajectories using new subject data pertinent to these causal processes defined within the generative model (the black arrows in Fig. 13.1). Data collected from later periods (e.g., Post-traumatic period) is used to refine models that made such prognostic predictions (e.g., Gray arrow from Post to Peri-trauma period). The process illustrated in Fig. 13.1 begins with defining putative causes. There is, however, a limitation in the field about the quality of available prior knowledge on causal factors for traumatic stress outcomes.

---

[3] The Integrative Framework applied emphasizes causality and prediction and can be instantiated either as a Bayesian model or as a Frequentist one depending on the suitability to the data and study or clinical goals at hand to a Bayesian or Frequentist framework. With this clarification in mind we will emphasize more the causal aspect in the remainder of the chapter.

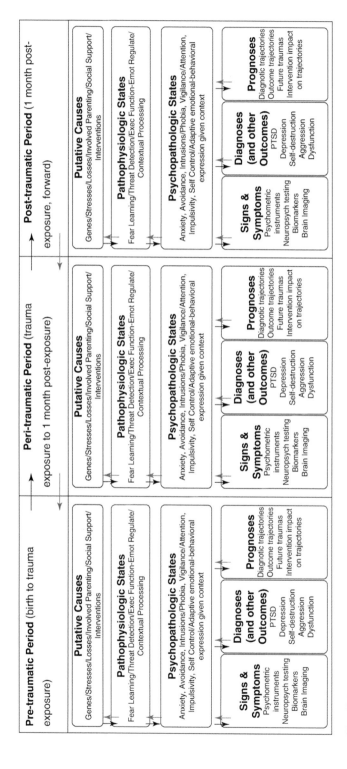

Fig. 13.1 A Causal Integrative Framework for Child PTSD (adapted from [21, 22])

Nevertheless, we cautiously choose variables in this category of putative causes to represent environmental stressors and traumas—or closely associated environmental variables—such as loss or parental neglect. We also include gene variations that have been associated with traumatic stress in several well-designed studies. In identifying plausible pathophysiologic and psychopathologic states associated with child PTSD outcomes, we are guided by recent influential theories on the pathophysiology of PTSD and its clinical application proposed by Liberzon and Abelson [28], Liberzon [29], and by Shalev et al. [30], respectively.

These reports are important because they give a strong account of the various pathophysiologic systems underlying traumatic stress and how dysfunction of these systems can be expressed in psychopathologic states. These articles identify similar systems involving: (1) Fear Learning (FL), (2) Threat Detection (TD), (3) Executive Function & Emotional Regulation (ExF-ER), and (4) Contextual Processing (CxP). Dysfunction of each of these systems have a well described brain circuitry, are associated with specific genomic, molecular, neuroendocrine, and physiologic relations, and are expressed in patterns of behavior, emotion, and cognition that would define specific psychopathologic states.

These specific patterns are summarized in Fig. 13.1 under the boxes on "Psychopathological States". Dysfunction in FL, for example, would be observed through such behavioral and emotional expressions as avoidance and persistent anxiety. Dysfunction in TD would be observed through a child's preferential attention to threatening stimuli, hypervigilance to the possibility of threat, and exaggerated responses when threat is introduced. Dysfunction in ExF-ER would be observed in problems with attention, working memory, planning, and impulsivity. Dysfunction in CxP would be observed in difficulties appraising the present demands of the environment, such that thoughts, emotions, behaviors would be expressed, that do not correspond to these present demands (e.g., mis-appraising safety and responding, instead, to threat).

There is a strong empirical literature supporting the importance of these systems for child PTSD, including the developmental manifestations of these systems and the influence on these systems from disordered developmental processes including influences from the child's social environment [31–36]. Indicators of pathophysiological and psychopathological states representing dysfunction in these four systems—and their developmental and social environmental influences—are captured in data collected from children and families using psychometric instruments, neuropsychological testing, and biomarker measurement. Such measured variables can be categorized according to these defined domains and according to the time period in which they were measured (Pre-trauma, Peri-trauma, Post-trauma). Such categorization includes symptom and diagnostic profiles and prognostic trajectories across time.

We are currently in the process of studying the application of a causal Integrative Framework in this way, and so it is important to not over interpret these ideas. They do, however, provide a powerful approach to bringing PPM to the problem of child traumatic stress and to other psychiatric and non-psychiatric problems and disorders. Our previous work demonstrated that causal discovery methods can successfully be applied to understand the etiology of PTSD and to build models that accurately predicted PTSD, supporting the promise of the ideas described in this chapter [37, 38].

How RDoC/Integrative Framework Enables PPM for Traumatized Children

As described previously, the goal in establishing PPM for any disease concerns building a model of the disease that will use all relevant information available, to accurately predict disease-related events (e.g., disease onset, prognosis, critical incidents, intervention response) for a specific patient. There are a number of disease-related events following childhood trauma that are known to be extremely important for a child's health and development. These include PTSD, aggressive behavior, self-destructive behavior, school performance difficulties, and difficulties in social relationships. The empirical literature indicates poor predictive performance for these outcomes from existing models related to children's response to traumatic events. Models developed from methods that are not able to provide knowledge on the causal process will both have limitations in predictive accuracy and in informing disease classification that would support prediction.

The advantage of using a causal Integrative Framework to support PPM is that, if successful, it would build accurate and reliable generative models from data on large numbers of traumatized children for a set of deleterious outcomes observed in the data. These models could point to meaningful ways to categorize traumatized children for given outcomes based on the conditional dependencies between identified causal processes for predicting specific outcomes. These models can then be used to classify a traumatized child based on information available about the child, in the service of predicting disease-related events of concern (e.g., PTSD, aggressive behavior, self-destructive behavior, school performance difficulties, and difficulties in social relationships). In the example given in the previous section, we may find that symptoms and signs associated with Fear Learning, Threat Detection, Executive Function & Emotional Regulation, and Contextual Processing are centrally important in a generative model of deleterious outcomes following trauma and, as hypothesized, signal different underlying pathophysiologic processes. It may also be found that these pathophysiological processes serve to influence different outcomes (e.g., processes related to fear learning produce anxiety related outcomes and processes related to Executive Function/Emotional Regulation produce more aggressive outcomes). Accordingly, the research that produced such a generative model would have strongly contributed to PPM for traumatized children by leading to the classification of a child, based on their personalized information that would accurately predict meaningful disease-related events.

This framework has been applied to other psychiatric disorders such as Psychosis and Obsessive-Compulsive Disorder [22]. To learn more about this framework and its applications in psychiatry, interested readers should consult the proceedings of the Ernst Strüngmann Forum (ESF) on *Computational Psychiatry* that is found in the book *Computational Psychiatry: New Perspectives on Mental Illness* [21], as previously noted. In particular, the Bayesian Integrative Framework is proposed and detailed in the chapter in this book entitled, "A Novel Framework for Improving Psychiatric Diagnostic Nosology" by Flagel and colleagues [39].

Application of a Causal Integrative Framework to Support PPM in Other Medical Fields

This chapter focused on redefining disease and the process of disease classification to support PPM, in an area of medicine—psychiatry—in which the current process of disease classification is problematic. As described, the focus on psychiatry is informative because its known problems have spawned a great amount of attention into how to address barriers to progress, that might enable PPM in psychiatry. The ideas that have been generated have application beyond the borders of psychiatry. Many medical disorders have complex etiologies and the respective medical field's knowledge base on causation of these disorders is curtailed by the limitations of experimental research. These problems become manifest in limitations in prediction of disease-related events as applied to individual patients. For such disorders, a causal Integrative Framework may be particularly helpful in the same way that it has been proposed for psychiatric disorders.

Using appropriate data sets containing well characterized patient symptoms and signs, and information on a diverse set of plausible causal processes for these symptoms and signs (based on theory in the field), causal discovery methods can be used to construct a generative model of disorder, including the optimal way of classifying patients to entail accurate prediction of disease-related events. This model can then be used to classify patients, based on available information about them, in such a way that the probability of relevant disease-related events can be used to guide their care. Such models can also be used to consider intervention alternatives based on the change in likelihood of disease-related events should a given intervention be applied. In most medical fields these ideas are still theoretical, but the main concepts underlying this approach has been proven, the methods to support this work are available, and the potential of redefining specific diseases for a robust PPM is now on the horizon.

References

1. Ashley EA. The precision medicine initiative. A new national effort. JAMA. 2015;313(21):2119–20. https://doi.org/10.1001/jama.2015.3595.
2. Moscatelli M, Manconi A, Pessina M, Fellegara G, Rampoldi S, Milanesi L, Casasco A, Gnocchi M. An infrastructure for precision medicine through analysis of big data. BMC Bioinformatics. 2018;19(S10):257–67. https://doi.org/10.1186/s12859-018-2300-5.

3. Chen R, Snyder M. Promise of personalized omics to precision medicine. WIREs Syst Biol Med. 2013;5:73–82. https://doi.org/10.1002/wsbm.1198.
4. Pearl J. Causality: models, reasoning, and inference. Cambridge: Cambridge University Press; 2009.
5. Friston K. The free-energy principle: a unified brain theory? Nat Rev Neurosci. 2010;11:127–38.
6. Hohwy J. The predictive mind. Oxford: Oxford University Press; 2013.
7. Kuhn TS. The structure of scientific revolutions. Chicago: University of Chicago Press; 1962.
8. Gill CJ, Sabin L, Schmid CH. Why clinicians are natural Bayesians. BMJ. 2005;330:1080.
9. Elstein AS. Heuristics and biases: selected errors in clinical reasoning. Acad Med. 1999;74(7):791–4. https://doi.org/10.1097/00001888-199907000-00012.
10. O'Connor GT, Sox HC. Bayesian reasoning in medicine: the contributions of Lee B. Lusted, MD. Med Decis Mak. 1991;11(2):107–11. https://doi.org/10.1177/0272989X9101100206.
11. Spirtes P, Glymour CN, Scheines R. Causation, prediction, and search, vol. xxi. 2nd ed. Cambridge, MA: MIT Press; 2000. p. 543.
12. Aliferis CF, Statnikov A, Tsamardinos I, Mani S, Koutsoukos XD. Local causal and Markov Blanket induction for causal discovery and feature selection for classification part I: algorithms and empirical evaluation. J Mach Learn Res. 2010;11:171–234.
13. Aliferis CF, Statnikov A, Tsamardinos I, Mani S, Koutsoukos XD. Local causal and Markov Blanket induction for causal discovery and feature selection for classification part II: analysis and extensions. J Mach Learn Res. 2010;11:235–84.
14. American Psychiatric Association. Diagnostic and statistical manual of mental disorders, vol. 5. Philadelphia: APA Press; 2013.
15. Insel TR. The NIMH research domain criteria (RDoC) project: precision medicine for psychiatry. Am J Psychiatry. 2014;171:395–7. https://doi.org/10.1176/appi.ajp.2014.14020138.
16. Morris SE, Cuthbert BN. Research domain criteria: cognitive systems, neural circuits, and dimensions of behavior. Dialogues Clin Neurosci. 2012;14(1):29–37.
17. American Psychiatric Association. Diagnostic and statistical manual of mental disorders-III. Philadelphia: APA Press; 1980.
18. Klerman GL. The advantages of DSM-III. Am J Psychiatry. 1984;141(4):539–53.
19. American Psychiatric Association. Diagnostic and statistical manual of mental disorders-IV. Philadelphia: APA Press; 1992.
20. Gordon J. RDoC: Outcome to Causes and Back. NIMH Directors Message, June 2017; 2017. https://www.nimh.nih.gov/about/director/messages/2017/rdoc-outcomes-to-causes-and-back.shtml.
21. Redish DA, Gordon JA, editors. Computational psychiatry: new perspectives on mental illness. Cambridge, MA: MIT Press; 2016.
22. Friston KJ, Redish AD, Gordon JA. Computational nosology and precision psychiatry. Comput Psychiatr. 2017;1:2–23. https://doi.org/10.1162/cpsy_a_00001.
23. Ferrante M, Redish AD, Oquendo MA, Averbeck BB, Kinnane ME, Gordon JA. Computational psychiatry: a report from the 2017 NIMH workshop on opportunities and challenges. Mol Psychiatry. 2019;24(4):479–83. https://doi.org/10.1038/s41380-018-0063-z.
24. Kilpatrick DG, Resnick HS, Milanak ME, Miller MW, Keyes KM, Friedman MJ. National estimates of exposure to traumatic events and PTSD prevalence using DSM-IV and DSM-5 criteria. J Trauma Stress. 2013;26:537–47. https://doi.org/10.1002/jts.21848.
25. Finkelhor D, Turner HA, Shattuck A, Hamby SL. Prevalence of childhood exposure to violence, crime, and abuse. JAMA Pediatr. 2015;169:746. https://doi.org/10.1001/jamapediatrics.2015.0676.
26. Fairbank J, Putnam F, Harris W. The prevalence and impact of child traumatic stress. In: Handbook of PTSD: science and practice. New York: Guilford Press; 2007. p. 229–51.
27. Trickey D, Siddaway AP, Meiser-Stedman R, Serpell L, Field AP. A meta-analysis of risk factors for post-traumatic stress disorder in children and adolescents. Clin Psychol Rev. 2012;32:122–38. https://doi.org/10.1016/j.cpr.2011.12.001.
28. Liberzon I, Abelson JL. Contextual processing and the neurobiology of post-traumatic stress disorder. Neuron. 2016;92:14–30. https://doi.org/10.1016/j.neuron.2016.09.039.

29. Liberzon I. Searching for intermediate phenotypes in posttraumatic stress disorder. Biol Psychiatry. 2018;83:797–9. https://doi.org/10.1016/j.biopsych.2017.06.005.
30. Shalev A, Liberzon I, Marmar C. Post-traumatic stress disorder. N Engl J Med. 2017;376(25):2459–69. https://doi.org/10.1056/nejmra1612499.
31. Teicher MH, Samson JA, Anderson CM, Ohashi K. The effects of childhood maltreatment on brain structure, function and connectivity. Nat Rev Neurosci. 2016;17(10):652–66. https://doi.org/10.1038/nrn.2016.111.
32. Wolf RC, Herringa RJ. Prefrontal-amygdala dysregulation to threat in pediatric posttraumatic stress disorder. Neuropsychopharmacology. 2016;41(3):822–31. https://doi.org/10.1038/npp.2015.209.
33. Crozier JC, Wang L, Huettel SA, De Bellis MD. Neural correlates of cognitive and affective processing in maltreated youth with posttraumatic stress symptoms: does gender matter? Dev Psychopathol. 2014;26(2):491–513. https://doi.org/10.1017/S095457941400008X.
34. Herringa RJ, Birn RM, Ruttle PL, Burghy CA, Stodola DE, Davidson RJ, Essex MJ. Childhood maltreatment is associated with altered fear circuitry and increased internalizing symptoms by late adolescence. Proc Natl Acad Sci U S A. 2013;110(47):19119–24. https://doi.org/10.1073/pnas.1310766110.
35. Hein TC, Monk CS. Research review: neural response to threat in children, adolescents, and adults after child maltreatment—a quantitative meta-analysis. J Child Psychol Psychiatry. 2017;58(3):222–30. https://doi.org/10.1111/jcpp.12651.
36. Herringa RJ. Trauma, PTSD, and the developing brain. Curr Psychiatry Rep. 2017;19(10):69. https://doi.org/10.1007/s11920-017-0825-3.
37. Saxe GN, Ma S, Ren J, Aliferis C. Machine learning methods to predict child posttraumatic stress: a proof of concept study. BMC Psychiatry. 2017;17(1):223. https://doi.org/10.1186/s12888-017-1384-1.
38. Saxe GN, Statnikov A, Fenyo D, Ren J, Li Z, Prasad M, Wall D, Bergman N, Briggs EC, Aliferis C. A complex systems approach to causal discovery in psychiatry. PLoS One. 2016;11(3):e0151174. https://doi.org/10.1371/journal.pone.0151174.
39. Flagel SB, Pine DS, Ahmari SE. A novel framework for improving psychiatric diagnostic nosology. In: Redish DA, Gordon JA, editors. Computational psychiatry: new perspectives on mental illness. Cambridge, MA: MIT Press; 2016. p. 169–200.

Chapter 14
Pragmatic Trials and New Informatics Methods to Supplement or Replace Phase IV Trials

Eneida Mendonca and Umberto Tachinardi

Introduction

A report developed by the U.S. Department of Health and Human Services in 2014 [1], identified that one of the main challenges to the process of developing new drugs are complex and expensive clinical drug trials. Given the necessity of clinical trials (CT) to approve a new drug, obstacles to trials result in fewer new drugs becoming available. The list of barriers is long and widespread and includes high costs (phase IV CT costs, in particular, are almost the same as the sum of the three preceding phases combined), lengthy processes, recruitment and retention issues; regulatory and administrative barriers, drug-sponsor imposed barriers, and the disconnect between clinical and academic worlds. The report suggests some solutions to the CT problems that include: the use of electronic health record (EHR) systems; simpler enrollment processes; and the wider use of mobile and electronic

E. Mendonca
Department of Biostatistics and Medical Informatics, School of Medicine and Public Health, Department of Industrial and Systems Engineering in the College of Engineering, Clinical/Health Informatics, UW Institute for Clinical and Translational Research, University of Wisconsin Madison, Madison, WI, USA
e-mail: emendonc@regenstrief.org

U. Tachinardi (✉)
Department of Biostatistics and Medical Informatics, School of Medicine and Public Health, University of Wisconsin-Madison, Madison, WI, USA

UW Institute for Clinical and Translational Research, University of Wisconsin-Madison, Madison, WI, USA

UW Health, University of Wisconsin-Madison, Madison, WI, USA
e-mail: utachina@iu.edu

© Springer Nature Switzerland AG 2020
T. Adam, C. Aliferis (eds.), *Personalized and Precision Medicine Informatics*, Health Informatics, https://doi.org/10.1007/978-3-030-18626-5_14

technologies. Informatics tools are replacing traditional processes with significant potential to overcome most of the problems listed above. Automation and reuse of data can reduce costs and time; new technologies (e.g., EHR systems, social media, mobile systems) are helping to improve recruitment and retention rates; and the use of EHRs also helps bridge the research and the clinical sides towards improved clinical trials.

It is clear that CT as previously defined, need to be dramatically improved to respond to the urgent need for more and better drugs [2]. It is even more critical that we improve how we use those drugs [3] and that we identify when we should not use them. That is the role of Phase IV. This chapter discusses enhancements to Phase IV along with new alternatives (that completely change the original definitions and may be seen as full replacements to Phase IVs).

A good example of the new "Phase IV" is the potential to improve drug repurposing. It is a fact that the drug development pipelines are not pumping out enough new drugs [4] to supply the growing need for more and better therapeutical options (This has been called "Eroom's Law", which is the literal and semantic reverse of Moore's Law). Drug repurposing is one of many solutions that can be used to alleviate this problem.

What Are Phase IV Trials, and Why Are They Needed?

Phase IV studies are developed to test the efficacy and safety of drugs *after* they are approved to be marketed by a designated regulatory authority (FDA in the United States). Both characteristics are critically important to the patients that depend on drugs that are efficacious and safe in the short and long term horizons. Randomized Clinical Trials (RCT), work well in efficacy determination, but drug safety assessment may require a different approach. The calculation of sample size is critical in establishing drug safety. Phase III studies usually enroll 1000 to 3000 patients who use the new drug. The probability of identifying a rare adverse event in this small population is low [5]. In fact, defining the right sample size is so critical that the European Medicines Agency (EMA) adopted well-defined guidelines for it: the post-authorization safety studies (PASS) [6]. PASS is designed to identify, characterize or quantify a safety hazard; confirm the safety profile of a medicine; and measure the effectiveness of risk-management measures [7] in healthcare.

While not specific to Phase IV drug safety testing, an interesting aspect of the EMA guidelines is the inclusion of non-interventional [8] alternatives. The *Guideline on good pharmacovigilance practices (GVP)* describes:

> ...non-interventional studies to include database research or review of records where all the events of interest have already happened (this may include case-control, cross-sectional, cohort or other study designs making secondary use of data). Non-interventional studies also include those involving primary data collection (e.g., prospective observational studies

and registries in which the data collected derive from routine clinical care), provided that the conditions set out above are met. In these studies, interviews, questionnaires, blood samples and patient follow-up may be performed as part of normal clinical practice.

Pragmatic Clinical Trials

The term pragmatic clinical trial (PCT) was coined nearly 50 years ago to distinguish between clinical trials that were explanatory in orientation (i.e., understanding whether a difference exists between treatments that are specified by strict definitions) and trials that were pragmatic in orientation (i.e., understanding whether a difference exists in treatment as applied in practice) [9]. PCT offers the potential to assess comparative effectiveness in broadly based patient populations receiving care in real-world clinical settings [10].

In August 2018, the website clinicaltrials.gov listed around 500 studies defined as "pragmatic clinical trials", 63 of those were labeled as Phase IV studies. As expected, the majority of those studies were funded at academic centers (total 40), but 18 of them were sponsored by industry. While small, when compared to almost 300,000 total studies in that database, those numbers seem to show a trend, since 60 of those 500 studies were not yet open to enrollment at the time of the query.

Whereas clinical trials are widely-accepted designs to establish the presence or absence of Rx efficacy as well as toxicity, they are often too rigid and with too short horizons. As a result, the efficacy and toxicity of approved drugs is not entirely known. Pragmatic trials take advantage of secondary use of EHR and other types of data (e.g., tumor registries and claims) to determine longer-term effects and personalized responses to treatments. Recent initiatives like PCORnet [11] are designed to share and exchange data across institutional boundaries to enable pragmatic trials by augmenting the sample size for all populations of interest.

The Role of EHR as a Phase IV Tool

Clinical Trials are designed to be highly controlled processes that define "how" and "what" data are collected and organized. Various mechanisms are usually in place to ensure data completeness and accuracy. Statistical methods are often used to analyze data, sometimes pre-analysis of data will require cleansing and or semantical harmonization (making sure all codes have one explicit and reproducible meaning).

Data in EHR systems are usually not at the same level of quality and standardization. For instance, both structured and unstructured data may be used for the same information. Therefore, mining data in EHR systems is a complex task. Nonetheless, the value of repurposing the wealth of EHR data available is high. This secondary use provides faster and cheaper ways to obtain data from patients. Different than "explanatory" trials that measure efficacy, "pragmatic clinical trials", designed to test "effectiveness" [12], match the goals of CT Phase IV.

EHR systems were primarily designed to support financial, clinical and administrative functions, while collecting data to support those processes. However, along their evolution, EHR databases became a valuable resource for other uses, such as quality and clinical research. Now virtually all data used in Phase IV studies (laboratory results, chief complaints, ER admissions, prescriptions) are being collected in modern EHR systems.

There are many strategies to assess drug safety, including active surveillance (pharmacovigilance), intensive monitoring schemes and registries. Active surveillance are continuous processes used to identify adverse events by tracking prospective findings for a group of patients that are using drugs of interest. Intensive monitoring is a system to collect data in specific areas of the healthcare system (e.g., ICUs, ERs). The selected sites may provide information, such as data from specific patient subgroups that would not be available in a passive spontaneous reporting system. Registries are systems that curate and organize data for specific populations, conditions or outcomes.

Is There a Difference Between Phase IV Clinical Trials and Drug Re-purposing?

Phase IV seeks to define if the drug is effective for the approved uses and if new adverse events develop in the long term that were not identified in the previous clinical phases (II and III). The combination of EHR data and PCT approaches can be used to either find new adverse effects; prove or disprove drug effectiveness for the approved uses; or identify new benefits of the drug that were not initially tested or approved, but are capable of yielding important benefits in areas where drugs do not exist or are still being tested [13].

Drug repurposing (or repositioning) is the process of expanding the use of currently available drugs to other indications than the approved ones. A well-known example is sildenafil (Viagra) which was initially developed to treat angina [14]. Many companies and academic centers are working in this area due to the reduced costs (when compared to brand new drugs) and the lack of new compounds past preclinical phases. The same process that results in drug repurposing can also be used for the prediction of adverse events of known or novel drugs [15].

In reality, in both Phase IV and drug repurposing, the challenge is quite similar: to establish the association of a drug with an outcome (positive or negative) and find out if that relationship is causal or not. If PCT is the chosen method, the technical approach for both should include a precise, computable and reproducible definition of markers (phenotypes) based on data that is already being collected.

Identifying and Acting on Adverse Drug Events (ADE)

Identifying adverse events is a critical step for any system aimed to provide data for conventional or pragmatic clinical trials. An analogy can be made with trigger tools designed to support Learning Health System models. Those are resources developed to help with a standardized identification of an adverse event (in this case any negative outcome determined by some healthcare action). The Institute for Healthcare Improvement Global Trigger Tool (GTT) has become one of the most widely used trigger tools for detecting harm in hospitalized patients [16].

A GTT "trigger" is a medical record-based "hint" (such as the use of the antidote naloxone) that "triggers" the search of the medical record to determine whether an adverse event (such as a clinical overdose of an opiate, as opposed to a therapeutic use in response to non-prescribed opiate use) might have occurred [17]. Similar triggers can be developed to track the use of individual or associate drugs, thus mimicking part of what Phase IVs are designed to do.

Once identified an ADE candidate needs to be processed to properly identify the cause of the problem (misuse, prescription error, drug adverse event), then appropriate action should follow: suspension/change of therapy, internal and external reporting (e.g., FDA, EMA).

Informatics Methods in Phase IV

The Food and Drug Administration (FDA) Adverse Event Reporting System (FAERS) is a database that contains adverse events reports, medication error reports, and product quality complaints resulting in adverse events that were submitted to the FDA [18]. FAERS adopts MedDRA (Medical Dictionary for Regulatory Activities), used in pharmacovigilance processes in the US, Europe and some eastern countries. MedDRA provides a single standardized international medical terminology which can be used for regulatory communication and evaluation of data pertaining to medicinal products for human use [19]. The database is a good resource for post marketing drug information, but investigators have shown that the resource is not sufficient because of challenges related to under-reporting [20, 21] and patterns of missing drug exposures [22, 23]. Data mining with effective analytical frameworks and large-scale medical data is a potentially powerful method to discover and monitor ADEs [24]. Pharmacovigilance studies have explored the examination of ADEs using a diverse number of data sources, including scientific literature, online publicly available databases, social media, and EHRs [20, 25].

Studies have also shown that just a small fraction of ADEs recorded in EHRs are reported to federal databases and authorities, making EHRs an important source of ADE information.

Existing observational studies have mainly relied on structured EHR data to obtain ADE information; however, ADEs are often buried in the EHR narratives and not recorded in structured data. A number of studies using EHRs have focused on using structured/coded information and drug ontologies [26, 27], showing somewhat limited results [24, 28, 29]. Furthermore, information contained in clinical notes are not likely to be presented in structured form in other parts of the record (e.g., signs, symptoms, severity of findings, disease progress).

Most studies that attempt to discover ADE information from narratives use a combination of natural language processing (NLP) methods and machine learning. Most recently, approaches integrating multi-faceted, heterogeneous data sources have become more common [25]. Two recent reviews of the literature on the use of NLP methods for pharmaco-vigilance and medication safety show a growing number of algorithms for automated detection of associations between medications and adverse events [20, 25].

Luo and colleagues [25] categorized the findings based on the characteristics of the NLP components and their complexity. Methods evaluated included basic keyword and trigger phrase search, algorithms exploring the syntactic and semantic patterns of drugs and adverse events, methods extending existing biomedical NLP systems and methods using existing or custom-built ontologies. The study also identified recent trends in EHR-based pharmacovigilance, such as the increased adoption of statistical analysis and machine learning, integration of temporal resolution, and the use of multiple data sources. Wong and colleagues [20] illustrated the fundamentals of NLP and discussed the application of these methods on medication safety in different data sources (e.g., EHRs, scientific literature, Internet-based data, and reporting systems). Both reviews demonstrate that it is important to consider the different approaches, as some of them are context and task-dependent. Combined approaches (hybrid) involving computational (statistical and machine learning) and linguistic methods may yield better results.

Despite the growing number of NLP, machine learning, and statistical methods for adverse event detection in EHR systems, several challenges remain. One example is the data fragmentation caused by movement of patients between multiple EHR systems. This is a big problem when longitudinality is required. Techniques designed to combine EHR data from multiple institutions while still protecting privacy are becoming increasingly available [30].

Data exchanges provide a powerful means to rapidly and significantly expand cohorts. Whether the data comes from research [31] or directly from EHR systems [32], the intent is to expand the cohorts faster than traditional methods. Larger cohorts increase the probability of identifying outliers (i.e. rare conditions), but also confirm key trends and patterns. Initiatives that make secondary use of data require additional measures to protect privacy and confidentiality. Several automated de-identification methods are available [33], helping promote safer data sharing.

Polypharmacy is the use of multiple medications [34], and one of the most understudied aspects of adverse event detection using EHR data. With the aging of the population and the increased number of chronic diseases, it is expected that a substantial percent of the population take more than one medication. In a national population-based study, Qato and collaborators found that 36% of older US adults were regularly using 5 or more medications or supplements and 15% were potentially at risk for a major drug-drug interaction [35]. Despite that, polypharmacy has not been the focus of the scientific community [25], with most studies assessing the adverse events based on a single drug. The "new Phase IV" paradigm presents a good opportunity to fix this problem, since EHR and pharmacy systems can more naturally identify associations of drugs, versus the specific targeted drugs monitored by traditional RCTs.

Data Integration and Analytical Tools

Phase IV studies (traditional or pragmatic) depend on collaboration from multiple sites. With EHR systems being added to the research protocols, data harmonization and integration becomes central to the process. Different sites may adopt different EHR systems, and even when the same EHR systems are used, the data may be represented in different ways at different levels of granularity.

Several initiatives have focused in data harmonization processes (i.e. use of Common Data Models). Others have focused on efforts on shared resources and community-wide tools to promote analytical solutions to the use of electronic health records.

Common data models standardize the representation of healthcare data from diverse sources in a consistent way. The goal is to facilitate the mapping of clinical observation to standard vocabularies and, consequently, improve how these data can be reused for research purposes and shared across institutions. This chapter does not intend to give a comprehensive view of common data models, but it is worth mentioning some examples.

PCORNet [11], the National Patient-Centered Clinical Research Network, is an initiative of the Patient-Centered Outcomes Research Institute (PCORI). The goal of PCORNet is to facilitate clinical research by facilitating the sharing of electronic health records across institutions. The PCORNet CDM [36] is a platform that enables rapid responses to research-related questions. The CDM is based on the FDA Sentinel Initiative Common Data Model [37]. It leverages the use of standard terminologies and coding systems such as ICD, SNOMED, CPT, and LOINC among others. PCORNet also provide a platform that allows simple creation, operation, and governance of distributed health data networks, called PopMedNet. PopMedNet allows for distributed querying, customizable workflows, and auditing and search capabilities, while enables the enforcement of varying governance policies.

The Observational Health Data Sciences and Informatics (OHDSI) [38, 39], an international collaborative initiative whose goal is to create and apply open-source data analytic solutions to a large network of health databases to improve human health and wellbeing. OHDSI was initially based on the Observational Medical Outcomes Partnership (OMOP) [40], which generated the OMOP CDM. In addition to EHR data, the OMOP CDM supports administrative claims data. ODSHI also provides tools for tools for data quality and characterization (ACHILLES), database exploration, standardized vocabulary browsing, cohort definition, and population-level analysis (ATLAS).

Another example is the Accrual to Clinical Trials (ACT) network, a federation of academic research institutions. The goals of this network are somewhat similar to the ones described above. ACT aims to facilitate cohort discovery by determining recruitment feasibility and patient identification. ACT uses the i2b2 tool's multi-site Shared Health Research Information Network (SHRINE), and the i2b2 CDM.

Despite these initiatives, data harmonization and data sharing are still major challenges in the design and implementation of Phase IV trials.

Data Challenges in Pragmatic Clinical Trials

Conventional Phase IV studies adopt several mechanisms to ensure that the data is complete, accurate and standardized. When EHR systems are used as the source, as opposed to traditional data collection tools like Case Report Forms (CRF), data quality becomes an important issue. There are informatics techniques that can help improve the quality: data harmonization, use of standard coding systems, data linkage and NLP are part of the informatics toolbox.

Data harmonization methods are used when the data comes from a variety of sources that originally used different definitions for the same concepts. The data harmonization process equalizes the granularity of the definition (e.g., reducing sex concepts to two genders M/F) at the coarsest common level of granularity. Standardized coding systems help data to be shared more easily. Examples of those coding standards include ICD, SNOMED, LOINC, RxNORM, and MedDRA. Data linkage is important when there are multiple sources containing part of the necessary data, a common identifier (usually name, date of birth or identity document number) is used as the link anchor. When a patient, for instance, has his or her data in multiple EHR systems those methods need to be used. NLP can produce codes out of unstructured data (i.e., plain text). The ability to extract codes from text can overcome some deficiencies like missing structured data (e.g., a behavioral condition) or confirm the accuracy of certain structured codes (e.g., an ICD code entered for billing).

Most EHR systems have the data available in two different databases. The first is the database used primarily by the system to support transactions using the user-interface in real-time, called the transactional database. The transactional database is optimized for performance, referential integrity and multiple users simultaneously editing the same information. Transactional databases are not good for analytics like machine learning, where intense querying occurs at very high frequencies. Consequently, EHR systems usually have a secondary database for analytics work. The Clinical Data Warehouses (CDW) are databases designed to respond to complex queries, and not to perform changes in the data (edits, insertions or deletions).

The CDW usually has a temporal lag with the transactional database, usually lagging around 24 h behind.

Those differences are important in designing a solution like a continuous Phase IV, where some processing can use past data, but others need to be computed in real-time. EHR systems are consolidators of data of several sub-systems (i.e., labs). Interfaces allow data to be transferred from the ancillary systems to the EHR. A popular interfacing standard is HL7 (Health Level Seven), where data is streamed from the source system (i.e., lab system) and received by the target system (i.e., EHR). Some solutions to track adverse events actually tap directly in that data stream to get the results faster (closer to realtime). Based on HL7, FHIR (Fast Healthcare Interoperability Resources) can also help applications (like adverse event detectors) request data from EHR systems quickly, process it and return an action (i.e., decision support) if applicable.

Linking Patient Data Across Multiple EHR Systems

There are two basic ways that EHR systems help with Phase IV trials: as a resource to the conventional Clinical Trials Management Systems (CTMS) or by replacing the CTMS with a pragmatic Phase IV solely using EHR systems data. The first model (Fig. 14.1—left box) assumes that a conventional Phase IV protocol will be in use, subjects will be enrolled given a defined criterion, subjects will consent and

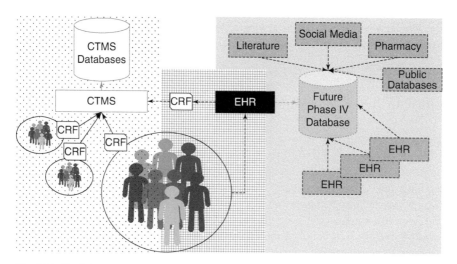

Fig. 14.1 Traditional Phase IV studies (left) use Clinical Trials Management Systems (CTMS) to manage participants, protocols and study teams; to be a source of record for study data and documents; and to produce reports. Those systems can be interfaced with EHR systems (checkered rectangle in the middle) reducing the need for human transcripts. The right box shows a hypothetical scheme where EHR systems and other data sources combined form a "future platform" for Phase IV studies (pragmatic approach)

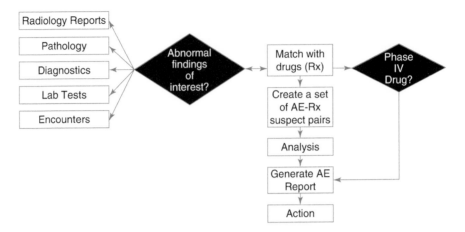

Fig. 14.2 EHR data can be used to identify triggers (potential AEs) out of different data sources: pathology reports, lab results, ICD codes, ER visits (encounters), radiology reports and others. If a pragmatic Phase IV study for a certain drug is in place, the ocurence of a finding of interest will trigger the generation of an AE report. If the system is being used as a pharmacovigilance tool, the pair EFI-Drug will be analyzed as a potential unpredicted AE

data will be collected using Case Report Forms (CRF). The EHR system of record for a given participant will be interfaced with the CTMS system, and the data will be transferred electronically from the EHR (Fig. 14.2).

A possible replacement to Phase IV as traditionally defined (Fig. 14.1—right box), this new platform would also connect to other data sources (e.g., publications, social media and pharmacy databases). The envisioned new Phase IV databases would be used for heavy analytics (i.e. machine learning).

Phase IV and Precision Medicine

The future of Phase IV CTs is one that relies heavily on data collected via the EHR. PCTs are one step forward, but the availability of both historical and real-time data enables a continuous and individualized Phase IV. The use of machine learning and AI can help "learn" the patterns of normality for a given person (or population) and detect changes or anomalies in that pattern. The same technologies can help differentiate the "good changes" (drug efficacy) from the "bad changes" (adverse events). Learning is always a more intense computational effort, but once the patterns are established, the detection of those occurrences can be performed in real-time using clinical decision support (CDS) tools. The detected changes (triggers) then become part of a registry of adverse events or positive outcomes, which in essence would be the basis of an endless Phase IV. The detected anomalies can also immediately become an actionable event (CDS) specific to one particular person (Fig. 14.3).

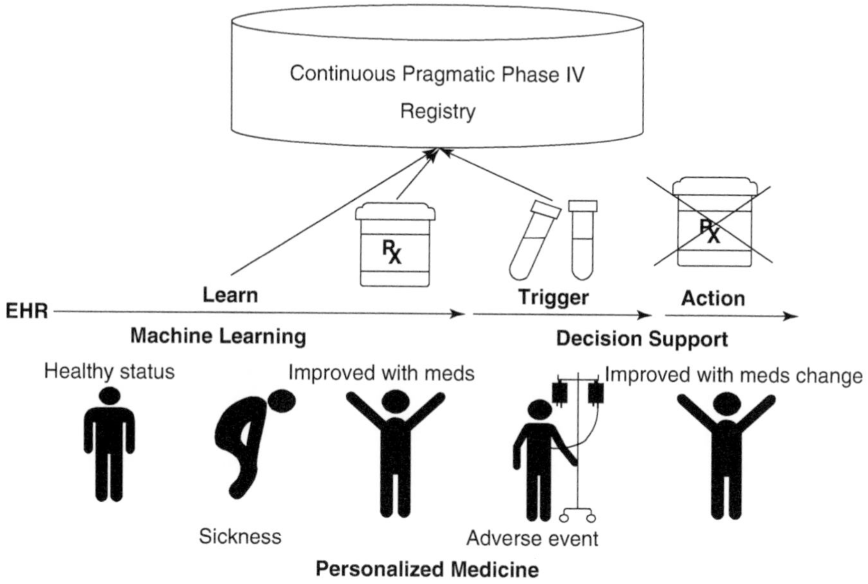

Fig. 14.3 The EHR system as a foundation to a continuous pragmatic Phase IV registry and a key tool in support of precision medicine. Using a person's EHR (or a large number of people's EHRs) as a training set, machine learning methods can define a "normal pattern" and identify when something does not fit the pattern. In this schematic example, the development of an adverse event after a new drug (to treat the sickness) was introduced. That trigger would define an action based on decision support logic implemented in the EHR system's clinical decision support system module. The detection, trigger, decision support sequence is typical of a personalized medicine approach. The finding for that individual, on the other hand, provides insights that, if repeated for other similar cases, can be used to produce generalizations like showing that the drug is not safe when this particular set of findings is present

Solutions like this one would definitely provide early signals in cases like the Vioxx (rofecoxib), given the amount of evidence that was available but not connected to make a compelling case towards a revision of the drug safety [41].

Final Remarks

The pressing and growing need for new more effective, safer and cheaper drugs is forcing the clinical trials industry toward radical innovation. Phase IV clinical trials, for instance, are transitioning from their original design into an agile and more efficient platform to track drug efficacy and adverse events. Those innovations also support more precise and targeted use of available drugs (i.e., precision medicine and re-purposing), an active way to improve efficacy and safety.

The ubiquity of EHR systems is a key factor driving this transformation. Not only are EHR systems helping improve data collection for traditional Phase IVs, but more importantly they are showing that a real-time, continuous, efficient solution can completely replace the old model. The current EHR systems still need to be improved in terms of data quality, use of standards, data sharing and data integration. Academic research institutions are developing solutions to overcome some of the current limitations of the EHR systems (e.g. developing standards for phenotyping, augmenting data with NLP and machine learning, integrating data with other sources and establishing data sharing networks). EHR vendors are adding new features (most of which developed by research groups) to new releases of their systems. But the backlog is enormous, and at the current rate of progress, it will take a long time to have all necessary advancements implemented in practice. Some of those changes may even require a complete reengineering of the current systems, since they were not designed to acquire and process bigger volumes of multi-dimensional data (as required in this case).

Certainly the "new Phase IV" will take advantage of more variety (more patients, more conditions, more findings), more data elements, and larger sample sizes for longer periods of time. Those new characteristics impose the need for novel tools and methods. In the current era of big data there are plenty of options for new computing (e.g., cloud computing) and analytics (e.g., deep learning) technologies to support those challenges.

Genomics data are slowly starting to be incorporated into EHR systems [42]. Since EHR systems were not designed to properly incorporate unstructured data like genomics, most institutions are adopting external solutions to provide that function. The addition of those new types of data can potentially transform how cohorts are defined for all clinical phases of clinical trials, including potentially the "N-of-1" model [43]. A "continuous EHR-based Phase IV" combined with a pharmacogenomics component can be truly transformational. The boundaries between the traditional CT phases would be less clear, and may even disappear.

References

1. Sertkaya A, Birkenbach A, Berlind A, Eyraud J. Examination of clinical trial costs and barriers for drug development. Washington, DC: US Department of Health and Human Services; 2014.
2. Bennani YL. Drug discovery in the next decade: innovation needed ASAP. Drug Discov Today [Internet]. 2011;16:779–92. https://www.sciencedirect.com/science/article/pii/S13596446110 01826?via%3Dihub.
3. Vallance P. Developing an open relationship with the drug industry. Lancet [Internet]. 2005;366:1062–4. https://www.sciencedirect.com/science/article/pii/S0140673605668353?vi a%3Dihub.
4. Scannell JW, Blanckley A, Boldon H, Warrington B. Diagnosing the decline in pharmaceutical R & D efficiency. Nat Rev Drug Discov [Internet]. 2012;11:191–200. http://www.ncbi.nlm. nih.gov/pubmed/22378269.
5. Cesana BM, Biganzoli EM. Phase IV Studies: some insights, clarifications, and issues. Curr Clin Pharmacol [Internet]. 2018;13:14–20. http://www.eurekaselect.com/161232/article.

6. Kiri VA. A pathway to improved prospective observational post-authorization safety studies. Drug Saf [Internet]. 2012;35:711–24. http://link.springer.com/10.1007/BF03261968.

7. Post-authorisation safety studies (PASS)|European Medicines Agency [Internet]. https://www.ema.europa.eu/human-regulatory/post-authorisation/pharmacovigilance/post-authorisation-safety-studies-pass. Cited 9 Sept 2018.

8. European Medicines Agency, Heads of Medicines Agencies. Guideline on good pharmaco-vigilance practices (GVP)Module VIII – Post-authorisation safety studies (Rev 3) [Internet]. 2017. https://www.ema.europa.eu/documents/scientific-guideline/guideline-good-pharmaco-vigilance-practices-gvp-module-viii-post-authorisation-safety-studies-rev-3_en.pdf.

9. Rosenthal GE. The role of pragmatic clinical trials in the evolution of learning health systems. Trans Am Clin Climatol Assoc [Internet]. 2014;125:204–16. discussion 217-8. http://www.ncbi.nlm.nih.gov/pubmed/25125735.

10. Oster G, Sullivan SD, Dalal MR, Kazemi MR, Rojeski M, Wysham CH, et al. Achieve control: a pragmatic clinical trial of insulin glargine 300 U/mL versus other basal insulins in insulin-naïve patients with type 2 diabetes. Postgrad Med [Internet]. 2016;128:731–9. http://www.ncbi.nlm.nih.gov/pubmed/27690710.

11. PCORnet The National Patient-Centered Clinical Research Network. PCORnet, the National Patient-Centered Clinical Research Network - PCORnet [Internet]. https://pcornet.org/.

12. Roland M, Torgerson DJ. What are pragmatic trials? BMJ [Internet]. 1998;316:285. http://www.ncbi.nlm.nih.gov/pubmed/9472515.

13. McCabe B, Liberante F, Mills KI. Repurposing medicinal compounds for blood can-cer treatment. Ann Hematol [Internet]. 2015;94:1267–76. http://www.ncbi.nlm.nih.gov/pubmed/26048243.

14. Hernandez JJ, Pryszlak M, Smith L, Yanchus C, Kurji N, Shahani VM, et al. Giving drugs a second chance: overcoming regulatory and financial hurdles in repurposing approved drugs as cancer therapeutics. Front Oncol [Internet]. 2017;7:273. http://www.ncbi.nlm.nih.gov/pubmed/29184849.

15. Deftereos SN, Andronis C, Friedla EJ, Persidis A, Persidis A. Drug repurposing and adverse event prediction using high-throughput literature analysis. Wiley Interdiscip Rev Syst Biol Med [Internet]. 2011;3:323–34. http://www.ncbi.nlm.nih.gov/pubmed/21416632.

16. AHRQ Agency for Healthcare Research & Quality. AHRQ Agency for Healthcare Research and Quality [Internet]. Rockville, MD: AHRQ Agency for Healthcare Research & Quality. https://www.ahrq.gov/.

17. Stockwell DC, Bisarya H, Classen DC, Kirkendall ES, Landrigan CP, Lemon V, et al. A trigger tool to detect harm in pediatric inpatient settings. Pediatr Int. 2015;135:1036–42. http://www.ncbi.nlm.nih.gov/pubmed/25986015.

18. Center for Drug Evaluation and Research- US Food and Drug Administration. Drug approvals and databases - FDA adverse event reporting system (FAERS) [Internet]. Silver Spring, MD: Center for Drug Evaluation and Research; 2017. https://www.fda.gov/drugs/informationon-drugs/ucm135151.htm.

19. MedDra Medical Dictionary for Regulatory Activities. Vision for MedDRA [Internet]. VA: McLean. https://www.meddra.org/about-meddra/vision.

20. Wong A, Plasek JM, Montecalvo SP, Zhou L. Natural language processing and its impli-cations for the future of medication safety: a narrative review of recent advances and chal-lenges. Pharmacother J Hum Pharmacol Drug Ther [Internet]. 2018;38:822–41. https://doi.org/10.1002/phar.2151.

21. Wang X, Hripcsak G, Markatou M, Friedman C. Active computerized pharmacovigilance using natural language processing, statistics, and electronic health records: a feasibility study. J Am Med Informatics Assoc [Internet]. 2009;16:328–37. https://doi.org/10.1197/jamia.M3028.

22. Munkhdalai T, Liu F, Yu H. Clinical relation extraction toward drug safety surveillance using electronic health record narratives: classical learning versus deep learning. JMIR Public Heal Surveill [Internet]. 2018;4:e29. http://www.ncbi.nlm.nih.gov/pubmed/29695376.

23. Begaud B, Moride Y, Tubert-Bitter P, Chaslerie A, Haramburu F. False-positives in spontaneous reporting: should we worry about them? Br J Clin Pharmacol [Internet]. 1994;38:401–4. http://www.ncbi.nlm.nih.gov/pubmed/7893579.

24. Zhan C, Roughead E, Liu L, Pratt N, Li J. A data-driven method to detect adverse drug events from prescription data. J Biomed Inform [Internet]. 2018;85:10–20. https://www.sciencedirect.com/science/article/pii/S1532046418301394?via%3Dihub.

25. Luo Y, Thompson WK, Herr TM, Zeng Z, Berendsen MA, Jonnalagadda SR, et al. Natural language processing for EHR-based pharmacovigilance: a structured review. Drug Saf [Internet]. 2017;40:1075–89. http://www.ncbi.nlm.nih.gov/pubmed/28643174.

26. Iqbal E, Mallah R, Rhodes D, Wu H, Romero A, Chang N, et al. ADEPt, a semantically-enriched pipeline for extracting adverse drug events from free-text electronic health records. PLoS One [Internet]. 2017;12:e0187121. https://doi.org/10.1371/journal.pone.0187121.

27. Combi C, Zorzi M, Pozzani G, Moretti U, Arzenton E. From narrative descriptions to MedDRA: automagically encoding adverse drug reactions. J Biomed Inform [Internet]. 2018;84:184–99. https://www.sciencedirect.com/science/article/pii/S1532046418301278?via%3Dihub.

28. Nadkarni PM. Drug safety surveillance using de-identified EMR and claims data: issues and challenges. J Am Med Informatics Assoc [Internet]. 2010;17:671–4. https://doi.org/10.1136/jamia.2010.008607.

29. Classen DC, Resar R, Griffin F, Federico F, Frankel T, Kimmel N, et al. 'Global trigger tool' shows that adverse events in hospitals may be ten times greater than previously measured. Health Aff [Internet]. 2011;30:581–9. https://doi.org/10.1377/hlthaff.2011.0190.

30. Kho AN, Cashy JP, Jackson KL, Pah AR, Goel S, Boehnke J, et al. Design and implementation of a privacy preserving electronic health record linkage tool in Chicago. J Am Med Informatics Assoc [Internet]. 2015;22:1072–80. https://doi.org/10.1093/jamia/ocv038.

31. Ohmann C, Banzi R, Canham S, Battaglia S, Matei M, Ariyo C, et al. Sharing and reuse of individual participant data from clinical trials: principles and recommendations. BMJ Open [Internet]. 2017;7:e018647. http://www.ncbi.nlm.nih.gov/pubmed/29247106.

32. Fleurence RL, Curtis LH, Califf RM, Platt R, Selby JV, Brown JS. Launching PCORnet, a national patient-centered clinical research network. J Am Med Informatics Assoc [Internet]. 2014;21:578–82. https://doi.org/10.1136/amiajnl-2014-002747.

33. Kayaalp M. Modes of de-identification. AMIA Annu Symp Proc [Internet]. 2017;2017:1044–50. http://www.ncbi.nlm.nih.gov/pubmed/29854172.

34. Masnoon N, Shakib S, Kalisch-Ellett L, Caughey GE. What is polypharmacy? A systematic review of definitions. BMC Geriatr [Internet]. 2017;17:230. http://bmcgeriatr.biomedcentral.com/articles/10.1186/s12877-017-0621-2.

35. Qato DM, Wilder J, Schumm LP, Gillet V, Alexander GC. Changes in prescription and over-the-counter medication and dietary supplement use among older adults in the United States, 2005 vs 2011. JAMA Intern Med [Internet]. 2016;176:473–82. http://www.ncbi.nlm.nih.gov/pubmed/26998708.

36. PCORnet The National Patient-Centered Clinical Research Network. PCORnet Common Data Model (CDM) - PCORnet [Internet]. 2018. https://pcornet.org/pcornet-common-data-model/.

37. Sentinel Coordinating Center. Sentinel Initiative [Internet]. 2018. https://www.sentinelinitiative.org/.

38. OHDSI Observational Health Data Sciences and Informatics. OHDSI – Observational Health Data Sciences and Informatics [Internet]. 2018. https://www.ohdsi.org/.

39. Hripcsak G, Duke JD, Shah NH, Reich CG, Huser V, Schuemie MJ, et al. Observational health data sciences and informatics (OHDSI): opportunities for observational researchers. Stud Health Technol Inform. 2015;216:574.

40. Overhage JM, Ryan PB, Reich CG, Hartzema AG, Stang PE. Validation of a common data model for active safety surveillance research. J Am Med Inform Assoc [Internet]. 2012;19:54–60. http://www.ncbi.nlm.nih.gov/pubmed/22037893.

41. Krumholz HM, Ross JS, Presler AH, Egilman DS. What have we learnt from Vioxx? BMJ [Internet]. 2007;334:120–3. http://www.ncbi.nlm.nih.gov/pubmed/17235089.

42. Ohno-Machado L, Kim J, Gabriel RA, Kuo GM, Hogarth MA. Genomics and electronic health record systems. Hum Mol Genet [Internet]. 2018;27:R48–55. https://academic.oup.com/hmg/article/27/R1/R48/4975618.

43. Silvestris N, Ciliberto G, De Paoli P, Apolone G, Lavitrano ML, Pierotti MA, et al. Liquid dynamic medicine and N-of-1 clinical trials: a change of perspective in oncology research. J Exp Clin Cancer Res [Internet]. 2017;36:128. http://jeccr.biomedcentral.com/articles/10.1186/s13046-017-0598-x.

Chapter 15
Precision Trials Informatics

Eric Polley and Yingdong Zhao

Precision Medicine Clinical Trial Designs

Precision medicine has been described as attempting to find the right drug, at the right dose, and the right time [1]. The precision medicine paradigm has also major implications for drug development and clinical trials. The advancement of precision medicine in oncology has motivated novel clinical trial study designs. The US Food and Drug Administration (FDA) provided a guidance letter on these study designs [2]. The various trial designs can be distinguished in their method of integration of clinical and biomarker data to determine eligibility and trial arm assignment. Figure 15.1 provides a visual guide for the common precision medicine clinical trial designs.

The first design is the *Basket study design*. A basket study in oncology is designed so that the eligibility is based on the presence of a biomarker and then patients are grouped into "baskets" (i.e., groups) based on their subtype of disease. The subtypes are usually based on the location of the primary tumor (e.g. lung, brain, colon). The primary analysis is pooled across all the subtypes, but individual subtype effects may also be estimated with sufficient sample sizes.

The complement of the basket trial is the *Umbrella trial design*. In an umbrella trial, patients with a common subtype (e.g. lung cancer) are screened for multiple biomarkers and are then assigned to different independent sub-studies based on the biomarker results.

E. Polley (✉)
Division of Biomedical Statistics and Informatics, Department of Health Sciences Research, Mayo Clinic, Rochester, MN, USA
e-mail: Polley.Eric@mayo.edu

Y. Zhao
Computational and Systems Biology Branch, Biometric Research Program, Division of Cancer Treatment and Diagnosis, NCI, Bethesda, MD, USA
e-mail: zhaoy@ctep.nci.nih.gov

© Springer Nature Switzerland AG 2020
T. Adam, C. Aliferis (eds.), *Personalized and Precision Medicine Informatics*, Health Informatics, https://doi.org/10.1007/978-3-030-18626-5_15

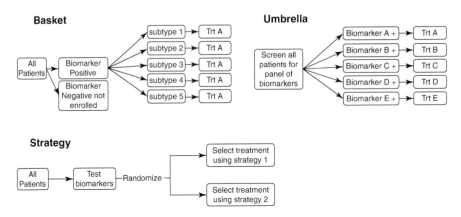

Fig. 15.1 Common precision medicine clinical trial designs

A third study design is a *Platform study*, which combines the features of an Umbrella study with a Basket study. Patients from a variety of subtypes are tested for a panel of biomarkers. An example of a Platform study is the NCI-MATCH clinical trial.

The fourth study design is a *Strategy study*. A strategy study differs from the usual clinical trial in that by design it is not testing for the effect of a treatment or drug. A strategy clinical trial randomizes patients to a specific treatment selection strategy and compares the efficacy of the selection strategies. For example, one strategy could utilize genomic mutation assay results in the selection of a drug and be compared with a strategy that follows current standard of care for drug selection for patients with advanced cancer.

An in-depth review of the statistical designs and considerations for oncology precision medicine clinical trials can be found in Renfro and Sargent [3] and Simon and Polley [4].

The NCI-MPACT Study

The NCI-MPACT study was one of the first precision medicine clinical trials in oncology [5]. It was designed by the National Cancer Institute (NCI) to test the hypothesis of whether selecting a treatment based on molecular alterations in the tumor versus not using the information improved response rates in patients with advanced cancer. Patients with advanced solid tumors who had exhausted standard treatments were enrolled and underwent a study-specific biopsy of their tumor. The tumor sample underwent DNA sequencing using a targeted panel of 20 genes to evaluate over 380 unique actionable variants. The results of the molecular characterization of the tumors combined with clinical information formed the basis for a predefined treatment selection strategy utilizing the information. The study was designed as a strategy clinical trial with patients and clinicians blinded to the treatment selection strategy. Figure 15.2 shows the NCI-MPACT study design.

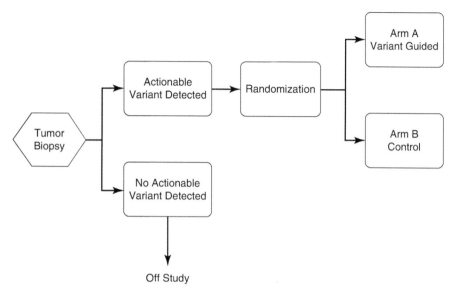

Fig. 15.2 NCI-MPACT study design

GeneMed Precision Clinical Trial Management System (CTMS)

The GeneMed [6] informatics system was developed to facilitate the implementation of the NCI-MPACT clinical trial. Precision Clinical trials are logistically and operationally complex, requiring a new tumor biopsy that is rapidly shipped to a Clinical Laboratory Improvement Amendments (CLIA)-accredited molecular characterization laboratory for application of an analytically validated sequencing assay, development of a computational pipeline for detecting genomic variants, annotation of the variants to determine the actionable mutations, real time evaluation of the clinical and laboratory results for determination of eligibility, complex informed consent and randomization procedures, and reporting of the sequencing results in the medical record.

An informatics system is required for such clinical trials to enable the translation of clinical grade sequencing data into clinically meaningful information in a short timeframe. The informatics system also serves as a communication hub linking the sequencing lab, the study oversight team, and the clinic team. In addition to the upstream bioinformatics pipeline for raw data processing and sequence alignment, the system must have the ability to quickly annotate the sequencing data, predict the functional impact of somatic mutations, and match the detected mutations to the pre-specific genomic changes in tumors found in previous studies (i.e., the actionable mutations of interest). The informatics hub should translate the mutation data from a sequencing result into a concise and easy-to-read actionable report for the study oversight team in a timely manner. Potential clinical trial participants are often waiting for the sequencing results to determine their eligibility on the clinical trial; therefore, the system needs to be as efficient as possible to avoid delays in patient treatment. The biopsy and evaluation of the somatic mutations in the DNA can take a few days for the assay results and must occur before the team submits the mutation summary to the informatics system, which then assigns patients to different arms based on their detected mutations. The informatics system also collects and stores patient data, including response data for prior therapies, which are required to evaluate eligibility of each treatment in the study and assist the treatment selection team and the clinic team in the development of a treatment plan. Finally, the system is required to make both sequencing data and clinical response data available to biostatisticians who are able to evaluate whether there is any improvement in the clinical outcomes of the study.

GeneMed System Design

Informatics systems for clinical trials are designed around study teams with unique roles and responsibilities on the study. The study teams often require specific access and control within the clinical trial system. For a precision medicine trial, we define, in addition to the CTMS and Bioinformatics, the following four study teams:

- Clinical Team: Includes physicians, research nurses, and study coordinators
- Lab Team: Includes members of the clinical laboratory involved in the molecular characterization of biospecimens
- Treatment Review Team: Often referred to as a Tumor Board in oncology
- Biostatistics Team: Includes statisticians and data managers

Each team had specific roles defined in the study protocol or study operational manuals and components which can be programmed into the informatics system. For the NCI-MPACT study, we defined workflows for how the teams interacted within GeneMed. A design goal for GeneMed was to reduce delays in communication between the study teams. This is necessary because potential study participants are waiting for test results to determine if they are eligible for the clinical trial.

GeneMed Workflow

A schema summarizing the roles and workflows is shown in Fig. 15.3.

1. From a study participant perspective, the workflow starts when they are recruited to the study and provide informed consent.
2. A study coordinator from the clinical team will register the participant in the GeneMed system and collect baseline clinical data.
3. When a participant is registered in the system, a unique study ID is generated and assigned.

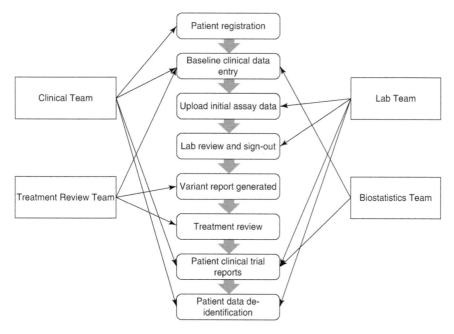

Fig. 15.3 NCI-MPACT workflow implemented in GeneMed system

4. The baseline clinical data is used to evaluate study eligibility and will be combined with the molecular characterization data to guide the treatment review team.

5. The participant will be scheduled for a tumor biopsy or other biospecimen collection appointment as required for the molecular characterization assay.

6. The biospecimen will be shipped to the lab team for analysis. GeneMed incorporates basic sample tracking capabilities, but doesn't replace a laboratory LIMS system.

7. When the initial results from the molecular characterization assay are generated, they are uploaded to GeneMed and associated with the study ID generated at the registration phase. These initial results are automatically reviewed for basic quality controls and annotated for study protocol specific rules.

8. A report is generated within GeneMed that allows the lab team to review the initial assay results with the additional quality and study specific annotations. The review is done entirely within GeneMed and allows the approved results to be exported and incorporated into the final lab results report.

9. When the assay results are approved and signed out, the study protocol specific rules are applied to the results combined with the clinical data collected at registration.

10. If the participant does not meet the study protocol eligibility, a notification is sent to the clinical team and physician with this information.

11. If the participant appears to be eligible for the clinical trial, a notification is sent to the treatment review team informing them to log into GeneMed for this participant.

12. The treatment review team will evaluate if the study protocol eligibility rules have been correctly applied and the precision medicine guided treatments have been assigned appropriately. The review team can either override the eligibility or treatment assignments or approve the report.

13. When a report is accepted, the system will run the adaptive randomization to assign the participant to either the arm A where treatment is based on the mutations identified in the tumor or arm B where a treatment is selected based on the complementary set of treatments not matched to the mutation identified in the tumor.

14. Following the randomization, a notification with the treatment assignment is sent to the clinical team, but blinded to whether the assignment came from arm A or arm B.

15. Participants know which treatment they are receiving on the clinical trial, but do not know if they are receiving the treatment as a variant guided or control arm assignment. The lab assay report is only accessible to the lab team on GeneMed while the participant is still active in the study to maintain the randomization blinding, but will be available to the participant when their participation is completed.

16. As participants are enrolled on the study and assigned to treatment arms, an accrual report is updated within GeneMed. The biostatistics team are able to access GeneMed with an accrual dashboard containing real time data on the number of participants registered and undergoing biopsies, the number of participants eligible and randomized along with the frequency of identified variants and treatment assignments. Since many variants may be rare, it is important to monitor the rates to maintain the feasibility of identifying enough individuals with specific treatment matched variants to complete accrual within the study period.

17. While the participant is active on the clinical trial treatment, outcome data on the response to treatment is collected by the clinical team and recorded in GeneMed. The outcome data in GeneMed is used by the biostatistics team for interim monitoring reports and designed per-protocol evaluations of treatment response rates. The final clinical trial analysis can also be done in GeneMed mapping the randomization assignments with the treatment responses.

18. A workflow was developed to de-identify the clinical information and subsequent additional genomic assays conducted using the tumor biospecimens when a participant goes off-study.

19. All data and lab material are moved to a research component and relabeled with new study IDs delinked for the participant's clinical records from the study. The de-identified data are used for additional studies of novel biomarkers and drug development.

Bioinformatics

A common component for all precision medicine clinical trials is molecular characterization of a biospecimen. In oncology, a sample of the tumor is collected for analysis. Tumor deoxyribonucleic acid (DNA) or ribonucleic acid (RNA) is extracted from the sample and the nucleic acids undergo high throughput sequencing to identify somatic alterations in the patient's tumor. Advances in sequencing technology allow for the sequencing of millions of short nucleic acid fragments within a timeframe necessary for a screening assay, with an ideal turnaround time from collection of the sample to return of results of less than a week.

Extensions: OpenGeneMed

The GeneMed system was designed for the NCI-MPACT clinical trial, but was subsequently generalized as a standalone application with additional flexibility as the OpenGeneMed system [7]. The OpenGeneMed system allows the user to develop an informatics system for a precision medicine clinical trial that adapts to their protocol specific rules. The user roles and workflows build upon the GeneMed concepts, with the addition of an IT team to manage the system design and modification to align with a new study protocol. The system is provided as a customizable virtual machine and user access the system via a web browser similar to the GeneMed system.

References

1. Salgado R, Moore H, Martens JWM, Lively T, Malik S, Mcdermott U, et al. Societal challenges of precision medicine: bringing order to chaos on behalf of the IBCD-faculty. Eur J Cancer. 2017;84:325–34. https://ac-els-cdn-com.kuleuven.ezproxy.kuleuven.be/S0959804917311486/1-s2.0-S0959804917311486-main.pdf?_tid=51419b46-8fd3-4835-bb76-2de50e387c87&acdnat=1524130410_d4b2eabe31b3628a238944d08d8cb499.
2. CDER, CBER. Master protocols: efficient clinical trial design strategies to expedite development of oncology drugs and biologics (Draft) [Internet]. Guidance. 2018. https://www.fda.gov/Drugs/GuidanceComplianceRegulatoryInformation/Guidances/default.htm.
3. Renfro LA, Sargent DJ. Statistical controversies in clinical research: basket trials, umbrella trials, and other master protocols: a review and examples. Ann Oncol. 2017;28:34–43.
4. Simon R, Polley E. Clinical trials for precision oncology using next-generation sequencing. Per Med. 2013;10:485–95.
5. Do K, O'Sullivan Coyne G, Chen AP. An overview of the NCI precision medicine trials-NCI MATCH and MPACT. Chin Clin Oncol. 2015;4:31. http://www.ncbi.nlm.nih.gov/pubmed/26408298.

6. Zhao Y, Polley EC, Li MC, Lih CJ, Palmisano A, Sims DJ, et al. Genemed: an informatics hub for the coordination of next-generation sequencing studies that support precision oncology clinical trials. Cancer Inform. 2015;14:45–55.

7. Palmisano A, Zhao Y, Li MC, Polley EC, Simon RM. OpenGeneMed: a portable, flexible and customizable informatics hub for the coordination of next-generation sequencing studies in support of precision medicine trials. Brief Bioinform. 2017;18:723–34.

Chapter 16
Informatics for a Precision Learning Healthcare System

Marc S. Williams

Introduction

If the nineteenth century was the Industrial Age and the twentieth century was the Atomic Age, it is possible that the twenty-first century will be remembered as the Age of Precision Medicine. While this may seem presumptuous given that we have yet to experience a fifth of the century, the dramatic breakthroughs in genomics, informatics, and other enabling technologies culminating in the announcement by President Obama at the 2015 State of the Union address that called for investment in a large-scale precision medicine initiative, All of Us [1, 2], would seem to make this assertion plausible.

Medicine as currently practiced is empiric and dependent on how much knowledge and experience the individual provider has, leading to care that has high variability and sub-optimal outcomes. Christensen et al. refer to this as 'intuitive medicine' defined as "care for conditions that can be diagnosed only by their symptoms and only treated with therapies whose efficacy is uncertain [3]." The same authors define precision medicine as "The provision of care for diseases that can be precisely diagnosed, whose causes are understood, and which consequently can be treated with rules-based therapies that are predictably effective." While some conflate genomic medicine with precision medicine, genomics is a subset of information used to inform precision care in conjunction with other information. The concept that best captures what is needed to attain precision medicine at the level of the individual was first stated in 1987 by Pauker and Kassirer [4].

> Personalized medicine is the practice of clinical decision-making such that the decisions made **maximize the outcomes that the patient most cares about and minimizes those that the patient fears the most**, on the basis of **as much knowledge about the individual's state as is available**.

M. S. Williams (✉)
Genomic Medicine Institute, Geisinger Health, Danville, PA, USA
e-mail: mswilliams1@geisinger.edu

© Springer Nature Switzerland AG 2020
T. Adam, C. Aliferis (eds.), *Personalized and Precision Medicine Informatics*, Health Informatics, https://doi.org/10.1007/978-3-030-18626-5_16

There are three key points captured by this definition. First is the focus on the outcomes of care. Second is the central role of the patient in defining what outcomes, positive or negative, are most important. Third, the words "genetic" or "genomic" do not appear only "…as much knowledge about the individual's state as is available." There are no assumptions that genetic or genomic information is superior to other information. The discussion of precision medicine has been dominated by new technologies, with less attention paid to the critical role of the patient to define the desired outcomes of care from their perspective. Precision health encompasses precision medicine but extends it beyond the identification and treatment of disease, to emphasize the role of genomics and other technologies in prevention and health maintenance.

The healthcare system as currently realized is ill-equipped to deliver precision health at the individual level. In 2007, the National Academy of Medicine (formerly the Institute of Medicine) published the first workshop summary defining the Learning Healthcare System [5], as "science, informatics, incentives, and culture are aligned for continuous improvement and innovation, with best practices seamlessly embedded in the delivery process and new knowledge captured as an integral by-product of the delivery experience." This approach contains the components needed to synthesize complex and disparate information and present this information to the clinician and patient at the time of clinical decision-making in a reliable and reproducible fashion.

Precision medicine and health are emerging in clinical practice, mostly in the setting of clinical research. Anticipating the emergence of genomics into practice and in recognition of the challenges identified by prior efforts, in 2015 the National Academy of Medicine published a workshop summary describing Genomics-Enabled Learning Health Care Systems [6]. While much of the focus was on the electronic health record (EHR) and data management, on page 19 Friedman notes, "A health care system in which an infrastructure supports complete learning cycles that encompass both the analysis of data to produce results and the use of those results to develop changes in clinical practices is a system that will allow for optimal learning."

This chapter describes the implementation of a large-scale population precision health initiative in a rural, integrated healthcare delivery system using the principles of a learning healthcare system. The primary focus will be on the informatics challenges and opportunities related to the implementation, within the larger context of the precision health project. The chapter begins with a description of the implementation setting. This is followed by a detailed description of the precision health research program which is divided into four discrete sections (Fig. 16.1): Consenting and sample collection; Sequence interpretation, confirmation, and reporting; Reporting results to participants and family; Measuring outcomes attributable to reporting. Each section will present clinical problems and research issues, a depiction and description of the processes involved in that section, relevant standards and technologies supporting the process, and other contextual factors that can impact the process. To conclude the chapter, a description of the migration of the precision health research program into a clinical program will be provided.

Fig. 16.1 Overview of the four essential components of a precision health program. While the depiction is linear, the Learning Healthcare model means that information from all components feeds back to program leadership and is used to continuously improve the program

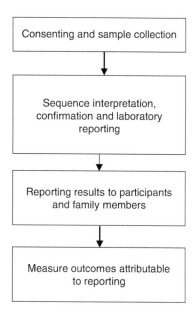

Setting

Geisinger is a rural, integrated healthcare delivery system in central Pennsylvania and southern New Jersey serving approximately 4.2 million residents. About one-third of Geisinger's patients are insured by the provider-owned Geisinger Health Plan (GHP). This creates a "sweet spot" which allows Geisinger to test innovations in care delivery first with those patients with GHP health insurance, before rolling out the innovations to the entire Geisinger patient community. Research has been a key element of Geisinger's mission since its beginnings. The theme of the Research Strategic Plan is Personalized Healthcare Research with an emphasis on developing and testing innovative approaches that will enable us to identify the unique differences between patients—genetic, environmental, or social—so that each patient receives the 'right care at the right time in the right way' to increase quality and improve outcomes.

Enabling Factors

The *Genomic Medicine Institute* (GMI) was launched in 2007 as a focal point for genomics research. In January 2012, the Institute's mission was expanded to include translational and clinical genomics. To fulfill the mission, the GMI is actively engaged with clinical care departments, clinical innovation, informatics and the broader research enterprise. The GMI has the primary responsibility for leading the implementation of the MyCode® Community Health Initiative.

The *MyCode® Community Health Initiative* (MyCode) began in 2007 [7]. This initiative is a precision health project enrolling Geisinger patients of all ages from across the system. It includes a system-wide biobank designed to store blood and other samples for research use by Geisinger and Geisinger collaborators. MyCode participants have a median of 12 years of EHR data coupled with data from whole exome sequences, high density genotyping chips, and HLA typing. This is made possible through a collaboration with Regeneron Pharmaceuticals and the Regeneron Genomic Center, which generates the research sequences for the participants. While the primary purpose of the genomic data is to support discovery research, Geisinger has full and unrestricted use of the data for clinical care. MyCode participants are enrolled under a broad, opt-in research consent that supports research, but also allows recontact of participants, and return of results that are deemed medically actionable including placing results in the EHR. This provides the opportunity to benefit participants, something that was valued by Geisinger patients in the extensive community consultation used to design and continuously improve the program. The initiative is governed by the Geisinger Institutional Review Board and the MyCode Governing Board, with input from several advisory boards, including participant, youth, and clinician advisory boards; a genomic council consisting of all genetic providers in the system, and an external ethics advisory board. This ongoing commitment to seek input from the Geisinger community is key to maintaining trust and provides opportunities to adapt the initiative to the changing needs of the community. As of April 2019, over 230,000 Geisinger patients have been consented for participation and nearly 93,000 have completed exome sequencing. Results have been reported to more than 1000 patients across a variety of genes and conditions [8, 9].

At the outset of the program, the Clinical Genomic team identified 76 actionable genes associated with 27 different conditions eligible for return [10], including the 56 genes identified as reportable by the American College of Medical Genetics and Genomics (ACMG) [11]. This was recently updated to 80 genes associated with 29 conditions, inclusive of the ACMG secondary findings policy revision [12]. Approximately 3.5% of participants have a variant eligible for return [13]. The Geisinger gene list is revised annually at a minimum. Changes to the list necessitate reanalysis of all the previous sequences which has been added to the pre-return of result process. The reanalysis also allows incorporation of new knowledge about variant pathogenicity.

Clinical care re-engineering and quality improvement: Geisinger has over 10 years of experience creating evidence-based care pathways to reduce unexplained clinical variation resulting in high quality care at a lower cost, optimizing value to the patient, health system, and payer [14]. The pathways are implemented with the full support of the EHR system and associated data sources coupled with dashboards and other metrics to track outcomes and identify process failures. Patient engagement is essential to the success of this approach and supports the need for patient context if precision health is to be successful. This approach demonstrates that linking several improvement concepts (evidence-based guidelines, data feedback, reliability science, patient-centered care) in a single design model can effectively reduce unwarranted variation in care delivery to reduce cost and optimize outcomes from the perspective of the patient.

Creation of a learning healthcare system: Geisinger has committed to transform to a learning healthcare system. To this end, working groups consisting of leaders from the delivery system, research, and the health plan are meeting to identify current assets and gaps that need to be filled to attain this system goal. A 1-year timeline has been set to accomplish four phases needed to support development of an LHS.

- Phase 1: (a) Survey Geisinger to identify 'pockets of goodness' and local learning health care initiatives to develop evaluation criteria, and (b) Develop a knowledge management system to represent these existing efforts.
- Phase 2: Create linkages between these existing efforts to enhance collaboration and replication.
- Phase 3: Develop an enabling core of providers to lead development of the Geisinger learning healthcare system by developing additional local learning healthcare initiatives that will enhance knowledge and dissemination of best practices.
- Phase 4: Use the information from phases 1–3 to develop conceptual and business models for a LHS core that will lead system-wide efforts to implement a system-wide learning healthcare system culture.

It is the goal of the GMI to implement genomic medicine as a local learning healthcare initiative.

Realizing the Precision Health Learning Healthcare System

Implementing the Precision Health learning healthcare system is complex and requires multi-disciplinary expertise coupled with a communication strategy that crosses traditional institutional boundaries. At its foundation is a robust information system that utilizes data derived from the EHR but extends data collection beyond the EHR to capture critical data that are not part of the EHR ecosystem. This includes collecting data from outside Geisinger, as the variants identified by the research sequencing must be confirmed in a clinical laboratory before being used for patient care. As noted in the NAM report on the Genomic Learning Healthcare System workshop, communication of genomic data between different systems is not standardized, necessitating creation of customized workflows to ensure data are available for care and tracking. It is important for the reader to understand that the processes discussed below are dependent on a robust informatics infrastructure. The overall workflow of the Precision Health learning healthcare system can be divided into Consenting and sample collection; Sequence interpretation, confirmation, and laboratory reporting; Reporting results to participants and family; and Measuring outcomes attributable to reporting (Fig. 16.1), each of which are discussed in detail.

Implementing Precision Health

Consenting and Sample Collection

The workflow for these activities is outlined in Fig. 16.2.

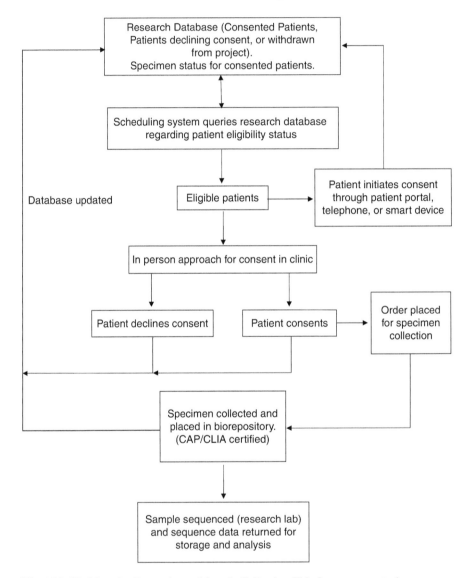

Fig. 16.2 Workflow for Consenting and Sample Collection. This figure represents the necessary communication between research and clinical systems needed to optimize recruitment and sample collection while minimizing burden on the patient. Most of the interfaces to support this workflow have been purpose-built for this process

MyCode is a clinical research program. In consultation with patients and other stakeholders, the decision was made to use an opt-in consenting process. Given the desire to develop a large cohort very quickly, a multi-pronged approach to consent was developed. In addition to traditional in person consenting, IRB approval was obtained to consent for participation through the tethered patient portal associated with the Geisinger EHR (MyGeisinger), by telephone, and using smart devices. In response to patient feedback, the consent form itself is 2 pages. An accompanying educational brochure provides additional information about the program, including links to online resources and contact numbers. This approach has allowed consenting of 800–1200 patients per week from virtually any location within the Geisinger service area (Central Pennsylvania and Southern New Jersey). Most consents are obtained by MyCode consenters located in clinics across the system. The strongest predictor of participation in MyCode is the number of clinic visits a patient has, which explains in part why the MyCode cohort is older and more female than the Geisinger population as a whole.

To minimize the burden on participants, the decision was made to align sample collection with routine laboratory blood draws, rather than requiring a separate research blood draw. Once consented, a standing laboratory order is entered for the participant such that whenever the participant presents for a blood draw, they are reminded that they are in MyCode and are asked if they are willing to provide a specimen. This approach has several advantages including reminders to the participant that they are in the program, opportunities to decide if they wish to provide a specimen or continue in the program, and replenishment of sample in the biorepository reducing the challenge of sample depletion faced by many biorepositories. One drawback is that some participants do not have routine laboratory work, meaning that while they are consented to participate in the program, there is no specimen available for sequencing, such as pediatric patients. To address this issue, saliva kits are now being mailed to interested consented participants who have no scheduled laboratory work, and likewise saliva is being collected from pediatric patients.

A clear message that emerged from the community engagement efforts was that patients did not want to be repeatedly approached about consent for the MyCode project. If they had consented to participate, they wanted the consenters to know that, so they wouldn't be approached to consent again. If they opted not to participate, they wanted that decision to be respected so that they wouldn't be disturbed going forward when they presented for medical care. There are also implications for where to place consenters in clinics to maximize the number of patients approached for consent. After a period of time, clinics with consenters achieve saturation, meaning that the number of patients in the clinic that have consented to (or declined) participation begins to plateau. All of these issues informed an informatics strategy.

Traditionally, a list of research participants is maintained by the research team. This is the case with MyCode. However, it was recognized that if this list could be dynamically linked to the scheduling system, this could be used to address the challenges outlined above. Geisinger informaticists developed an interface between the MyCode participant database and the scheduling system such that any patient scheduled to come in for an outpatient visit is identified as being consented as a participant, a patient who had declined participation, previously approached for consent, but still considering, or not previously approached. The consenter located in the clinic can review the clinic schedule and identify those patients who have not been previously approached for participation allowing them to approach those patients before or after their appointment. In some clinics with strong provider advocacy, this information is shared with the provider who can choose to discuss MyCode as part of the encounter. Clinics that use this proactive approach involving providers have the highest consent rates for the program. The second use of this interface is to track the number of patients eligible for participation in MyCode that are not yet consented. As the number of eligible patients in a given clinic plateaus, consenters can be moved to other clinics with more eligible patients. This improves the efficiency of the consenter. Using this approach, consenters average 10–20 consents per day, supporting the rapid accrual needed to support the goals of the program.

A second issue involving consent is versioning. The MyCode program has evolved over its 11 years of existence from a traditional biorepository operating under more traditional research principles where return of research results is not expected, to the current community health initiative where medically significant results are actively sought and reported to participants and their providers. As such, depending on when the participant enrolled in the program, they may be on a different consent. An additional complication has been the assimilation of biospecimens into MyCode that are derived from studies that operated under project-specific consents. While these are no longer in use for future Geisinger research, the specifics of the consent for a participant in one of these projects that has not enrolled in MyCode must be understood. Analysis of the consent forms has allowed development of a database where each participant's consent is represented, allowing segregation of certain consented participants from participation in projects for which their version of consent is not appropriate.

Once consent is obtained, collection of a blood specimen for DNA extraction and storage is critical for the project. For this step, the standard order function in the EHR is used. A standard order was created for MyCode that details the amount of blood and the type of tubes used for collection. The order is associated with a project physician and a research billing code so that the participant is not charged for contributing samples for the project. The order is represented in the vendor EHR as a standing order, such that additional specimens can be collected as the participant receives care in the system. No customization to the vendor ordering system is needed to support specimen collection. This has been implemented in two different EHR systems within Geisinger.

Specimen handling also leverages existing procedures. All specimen collections are performed in clinical phlebotomy sites that are under the laboratory's College of American Pathology/Clinical Laboratory Improvement Amendment (CAP/CLIA) certification. To avoid having to create a separate specimen tracking system, the decision was made to bring the biorepository under the laboratory's CAP/CLIA certification. This not only takes advantage of pre-existing technology and workflow but has benefits for the clinical confirmation step that will be described later. The biorepository also uses vendor provided specimen annotation software that supports characterization of the specimen with project-defined attributes and associates the relevant consent with the specimen.

Implementation Challenges

While the specimen collection process was able to use existing information systems, the consenting process required development of several custom systems to support the workflow in order to create interfaces to share data between the research database and the software used for scheduling patients in near real-time to support the consenting workflow.

Despite extensive effort in the development and implementation of the consenting and specimen collection process, problems were encountered that necessitated modification of the program to achieve optimal performance. The structure of a learning healthcare system that includes robust process monitoring and response to process failures supports rapid iterative project improvement. As an example, the consent versioning issue was identified when participants contacted to receive a result contacted the program stating that they had not consented for such a return. Result return was immediately suspended until all consents had been reviewed and a system put in place to ensure results are only returned to those who are appropriately consented. A second issue is identifying individuals who have died since enrolling in the project. Since death can occur at any point in the process, the participant's status must be checked at multiple times during this process and as part of results reporting.

Monitoring also identified a process failure in the specimen collection process. It is well known that upgrading a system in a complex network of systems can have unintended consequences. After an upgrade to the laboratory information system, it was noticed that there was a decline in specimen collection for the project. Investigation revealed that the upgrade had affected the standing order process. Once identified, a new order set was implemented and specimen collection resumed. Real-time monitoring of processes is essential to identify and fix the process failures that will inevitably arise.

A challenge that was not encountered in this aspect of the project involved clinician workflow. Consultation with providers and clinic staff allowed the consenting and specimen collection process to proceed independent of the clinical workflow. The support of providers and staff for the project itself, and for a process that did not disrupt the clinic workflow allowed rapid and effective implementation.

Sequence Interpretation and Confirmation

Bioinformatics Analysis and Variant Annotation

The high-level process of taking the research sequence and transforming it for use in clinical care is depicted in Fig. 16.3a. The key aspect of this process is the bioinformatics analysis of the sequence data to identify high confidence expected pathogenic variants that can be returned to participants. It is important to remember that the MyCode participants are not selected for the presence of any disease or condition. Therefore, the interpretation must consider the low prior probability of an individual having any one of the conditions of interest for the project. This necessitates conservative variant calling protocols to minimize the return of false positive results. This is a challenging paradigm for clinical labs for which most testing is based on a clinical

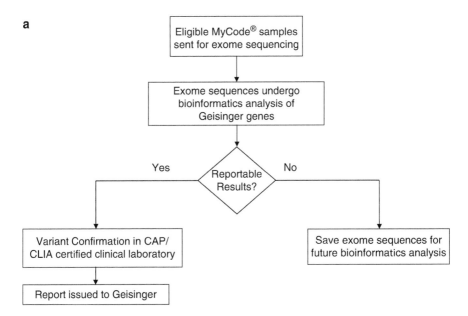

Fig. 16.3 (**a**) Sequencing, Data Analysis and Confirmation Workflow (idealized). This flow diagram represents the ideal process for sequence analysis, confirmatory sequencing, and laboratory reporting. (**b**) Sequencing, Data Analysis and Confirmation Workflow (mapped). This flow diagram represents the actual process with one laboratory to achieve the objectives of sequence analysis, confirmatory sequencing, and laboratory reporting. Information systems must be assessed for their ability to support the various processes. This includes assessment of the interactions between systems such as the EHR and laboratory information systems, both local and at the referral laboratory. The box identifies a process that was used initially, but has now been transitioned to the internal workflow, reflecting the dynamic nature of the process. This workflow is specific to one referral laboratory. The analysis must be performed for each laboratory contracted to perform confirmatory sequencing (currently a total of four—the Geisinger molecular laboratory and three external referral labs). Lack of standard interfaces and standards for genomic data representation limit the ability to develop standard interfaces that are reusable

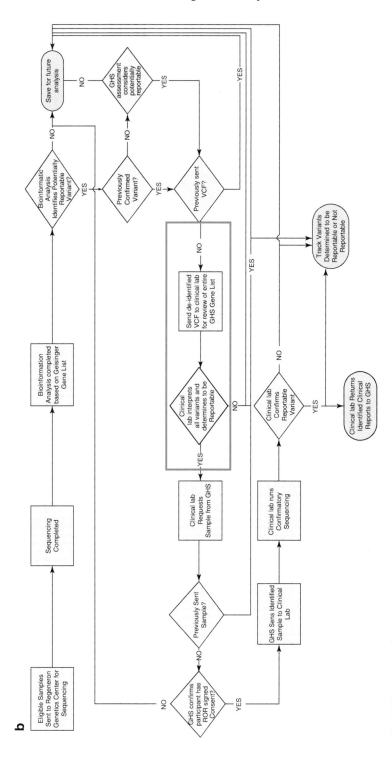

Fig. 16.3 (continued)

indication, implying a higher prior probability to inform interpretation. Recognizing this challenge, Geisinger has invested in developing a robust variant annotation infrastructure combining conservative variant calling algorithms with an additional layer of manual interpretation involving biomedical informaticists, variant scientists and clinicians. Variants that are annotated as pathogenic or likely pathogenic by this process are further evaluated through the process of clinical confirmation.

When the relatively straight forward high-level process is mapped to a real-world implementation it becomes much more complex, as shown in Fig. 16.3b. This figure details the process as it was initially developed with the first clinical laboratory at the initiation of the process. It included an independent review of all the variant call files (VCF) generated by the research laboratory (indicated by the box). This was necessary at the outset of the project, as the internal variant calling pipeline was just being developed and there was concern that the internal pipeline might over- or under-call variant pathogenicity.

A second review by an experienced clinical laboratory using an established clinical pipeline increased confidence in the selection of the variants to send for clinical confirmation. As the internal pipeline was enhanced and additional experienced personnel were added to the annotation team, a comparison of concordance of the internal pipeline with the laboratory pipeline was undertaken. This analysis identified a very low rate of discordance. A further review of the discordant variants determined that these were not of high clinical significance. As a result, the external review of VCF files was discontinued, reducing the cost and complexity of variant annotation.

Clinical Confirmation and Laboratory Reporting

The nature of the research collaboration with our pharmaceutical partner means that the exome sequencing is not performed in a CAP/CLIA certified laboratory, so they must be confirmed in a CAP/CLIA certified laboratory before they can be returned to a participant. As noted above, the biospecimens are collected and maintained in a CAP/CLIA compliant environment, obviating the need to collect another specimen from the participant, which removes a barrier and reduces burden on the participant. In addition to testing the specimen to see if the variant confirms using an orthogonal sequencing approach, the laboratory performs an annotation of the variant to independently validate the Geisinger annotation.

Only those variants that are confirmed by clinical sequencing and categorized as pathogenic or likely pathogenic by both the internal and external processes are eligible for return to the participant.

The clinical confirmation process leverages existing clinical genetic testing processes. An order for variant specific testing is entered in the EHR order system with a research physician of record, so as not to add work to clinical staff. With one exception, the clinical confirmation is done by external referral laboratories. Project staff worked with the Geisinger referral laboratory to develop a standard process for sending out the specimens with the test order to the referral laboratory. This included using billing codes that routed charges for the order and testing to the MyCode project for reimbursement under a research code. Beyond adding some new codes, no modifications to existing information systems were required.

If the variant is confirmed by the clinical laboratory, a report is issued to Geisinger. This uses the standard reporting process. Unfortunately, the 'state of the art' for genetic test reporting in EHRs at this time is transmission of the report as a text, or portable document format file, which is placed in the EHR as a scanned image [15]. This means that the information contained in the report is not represented as structured data, thus cannot be used to support clinical decision support to aid patient and provider decision-making. Reports must be compliant with CLIA reporting requirements (42 CFR §493.1291) and there are recommendations from professional societies about the organization of the report [16, 17], however, at present, there are no recommendations or requirements that the genetic information contained in such a report be represented as structured data. A full discussion of the issues is beyond the scope of this chapter, but interested readers are referred to this paper for more information, and emerging approaches [18]. As genetics and genomics is increasingly utilized in clinical practice it is anticipated that vendor-provided EHRs and laboratory information systems will add the capability to represent these results as structured data. In addition, to issue the laboratory report, as part of the laboratory's contract with Geisinger, the variant with annotation is deposited into the Clinical Variant Resource (ClinVar) [19] to promote data sharing and enhance information availability for clinical variant annotation efforts.

Implementation Challenges

Most of the challenges in this step are ones experienced by most groups looking to use genomic sequence in a clinical or clinical research setting. Variant annotation pipelines are being continuously improved but still require significant manual curation effort. One unique aspect of our program that impacts the annotation pipeline is the screening paradigm. Most variant calling pipelines have been designed for interpretation in the context of clinical signs and symptoms that suggest a genetic disease. In this setting, the pipeline needs to emphasize sensitivity such that variants that are potentially disease causing are not automatically filtered, including so-called variants of uncertain significance. In some settings, such as rare undiagnosed complex disease (e.g., the Undiagnosed Diseases Network) [20, 21], there may be a discovery component that expands annotation to variants in genes that do not currently have an established gene-disease association. However, for MyCode, the emphasis of the variant annotation pipeline is on specificity, that is on only reporting variants for which there is strong evidence of causality. This first requires a definitive gene-disease association followed by an understanding of the variants that are damaging and associated with the disease.

Several sources are used to establish the pathogenicity of variants. ClinVar, which has been mentioned previously, is a very important resource, as it not only has one of the largest collections of variants with assertions of pathogenicity, but it also includes a rating system for the evidence associated with the variant. If a variant is identified in a MyCode participant that is represented in ClinVar with a three star assertion of pathogenicity, there is high confidence that it is associated with the condition of interest, while if it has zero or one star, the interpretation must be more circumspect and more clinical contextual factors including personal or family history of disease must be included in the review. The information associated with genes and variants is constantly changing and updating these sources for the project is critical. A recent example was the publication by Hosseini et al. [22] that comprehensively reviewed gene-disease assertions for Brugada syndrome. After a critical review, only one of the 21 genes asserted to cause Brugada syndrome actually had definitive evidence supporting gene-disease causality. Several of the other genes had been included on the Geisinger list for reporting and are now being assessed for potential removal. The same issue exists at the variant level even for some relatively well-characterized variants. Manrai et al. [23] demonstrated the impact of lack of race and ethnic diversity in variant databases in the context of hypertrophic cardiomyopathy. At present the updating is heavily dependent on manual processes, a problem compounded by the proliferation of relevant databases [24]. A number of approaches to automate this process are emerging, particularly in commercially available products and services. While these lower the time required to identify relevant resources, they are not robust enough to be used autonomously.

Another problem is the high rate of novel variants in disease-associated genes found when sequencing a population. While the vast majority of these likely represent benign variation, identifying the suspected pathogenic variants from the rest is important. For genes where the mechanism of disease is loss of function, this is somewhat more straightforward. In-silico variant predictors perform well to identify loss of function variants. If these occur early in the sequence, then it is likely the gene product would be subject to nonsense mediated decay leading to haploinsufficiency, and probably disease. Diseases where the mechanism is a gain of function, or a dominant negative interaction are more difficult to parse when a novel missense variant is encountered. In-silico prediction of the pathogenicity of missense variants relies on assessments of the likelihood that a given variant would damage the resulting protein combined with the conservation of the variant evolutionarily, the assumption being that the more conserved the reference nucleotide is, the more likely a variant is deleterious. Another issue is the nature of the gene itself. Genes code for a variety of different protein products, so a predictor that works well for a gene that codes for a structural protein such as collagen, may perform very poorly when applied to a gene that codes for an ion channel [25]. Many predictors have been used alone and in combination to assist in variant annotation. While there is some value to using this information as part of the variant interpretation process, over reliance on in-silico predictors is problematic as reflected in professional guidelines for variant interpretation [26].

An additional benefit of a large-scale sequencing project associated with longitudinal health records is the opportunity to incorporate clinical information from participants to aid in the annotation of novel variants. In addition, the stable population in MyCode means that many families have relatives also participating in the project. This allows the construction of virtual pedigrees based on the genomic degree of relatedness coupled with inferences about the nature of the relationship based on demographic information. In at least two instances, a novel presumed pathogenic variant was identified in multiple family members participating in MyCode, allowing a disease segregation analysis which provided additional evidence for the pathogenicity of the variant.

Informatics challenges associated with the lack of structured data for genes and variants in laboratory reports was discussed above and will be discussed more in the following section.

Reporting Results to Participants and Family

The process for the reporting of results to participants is shown in Fig. 16.4.

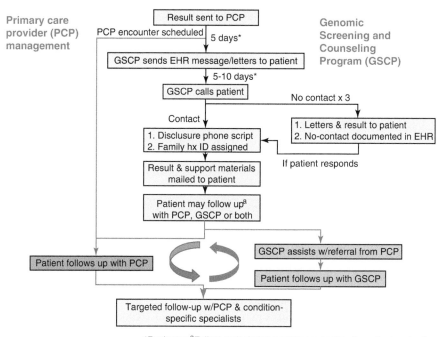

*Business; ªFollow-up includes genetic counseling & medical evaluation

Fig. 16.4 Reporting results to patients. This figure depicts the results reporting workflow which involves coordination between the Genetic Screening and Counseling Program (GSCP) and the clinical system as represented by the participant's primary care physician (PCP). GSCP uses communication channels in the Geisinger healthcare informatics ecosystem to coordinate care with Geisinger PCPs and specialists. A physician advisory council provides input on the preferred communication strategies which are implemented. Approximately 40% of PCPs are not employed by Geisinger and have less integration of information systems. The GSCP uses existing communication strategies the institution has developed to coordinate care with external PCPs, so no new infrastructure was required to support care for participants. A multimodal approach to participant contact reflects the rural nature of the system where internet connectivity is variable, leading to more reliance on telephone and mail contact. Smart devices are supported, so as penetration of these devices increases, strategies that utilize device capability will be expanded. The use of a certified letter for participants that cannot be contacted directly allows the GSCP to close the loop for reporting results

The process was informed by extensive consultation with participants and providers. One key feature is notification of the providers prior to patients in order to allow the provider time to access materials relevant to conditions with which they may not be familiar. This includes mini-CME courses for each condition available online through the system's goals site which is used for mandatory compliance training. The Genetic Screening and Counseling Program (GSCP) consisting of geneticists, genetic counselors, and support staff is on call for consultation at the request of clinicians. After 5 days, results are released to the EHR where they are available for participants through the patient portal tethered to the EHR. It is essential to close the loop with the participant who receives a result. This is done through a combination of letters and phone calls by the GSCP. Participants that cannot be reached are sent a certified letter with the result, information to help them understand the implications for their healthcare, information for family members and contact information for the GSCP. About half the participants have a primary care physician outside the Geisinger system. The team uses existing communication channels developed by the system for non-Geisinger providers to return results for these participants. Consultation is available for Geisinger and non-Geisinger providers.

Participants are given the choice to follow-up with their primary care provider, or to have a visit with a member of the GSCP. Since this result is being returned as part of a research program, the initial return of results visit is provided without charge to the participant. Subsequent follow-up transitions into usual clinical care. Specialty referral is also offered. A network of specialists with expertise in the conditions relevant to the genomic result has been identified and works closely with the GSCP to ensure guideline-based care is offered to the participant.

The existing EHR with its tethered patient portal is used to support the results reporting. No additional functionality was necessary to support the process. The implementation of the International Classification of Disease, Tenth Revision, Clinical Modification (ICD10) has greatly enhanced the ability to precisely code diseases and related processes. This is of importance to the project, as the identification of a pathogenic variant is not equivalent to having a diagnosis of a disease [27]. Prior versions of ICD did not provide the ability to represent the presence of a variant that confers risk for disease. However, ICD10 includes a range of codes for genetic carrier and genetic susceptibility to disease (Z14–Z15). When a pathogenic variant is returned to a participant, in addition to the scanned laboratory report in the EHR, an appropriate Z code that describes the patient's genetic variant status is added to the problem list with explanatory text entered as a comment associated with the problem. This is a structured data element that supports searching by gene, a function to support outcomes research that will be described in the subsequent section. This also supports knowledge representation which will be discussed in the Implementation Challenges in this section.

Communication of genomic results to at risk relatives to support cascade testing enhances the value of the program. This is supported by collecting family history information from the participant and providing copies of information for all at risk relatives to the participant for distribution. The GSCP is available to support relatives that want to consider testing. This process is manual and is supported by a purpose-built database that is separate from the EHR. The current functionality for family history in the system's EHR is insufficient to represent family history at the detail needed to support the cascade testing program. Geisinger has invested in standalone family history tools that have the necessary functionality and developed interfaces to allow these tools to be used within the EHR environment. This has been quite successful but represents a local solution that is not generalizable without extensive expertise and customization.

Implementation Challenges

Given the limitations of the laboratory-issued genomic test report, an additional innovation to support the return of results was to design and implement paired patient and provider genome test reports and make these available through an application that interfaces with the EHR [28, 29]. In a prospective study, the reports were found to improve communication between patients and providers and increased patient empowerment and satisfaction [30]. These reports were designed based on input from patients and providers and contain information deemed important for interpreting genomic results from each of the stakeholder groups. The format is standardized and the content for each of the patient-facing reports is assessed for readability and comprehension. Links to additional resources are embedded in the report and allow navigation from the EHR. Paper versions of the report can be sent for participants without access to reliable internet—a significant issue in our service area. The reports were implemented using an existing local application, COMPASS, that interacts with the EHR through a standard application programming interface (API). This API is also compatible with emerging standards such as Fast Healthcare Interoperable Resources (FHIR) including more advanced initiatives including SMART on FHIR and SMART genomics. The use of standard APIs facilitates the generalizability of this approach, particularly as EHR standards are requiring the availability of APIs as part of EHR certification. Details of the informatics strategy to create and deploy Genome COMPASS are published [31].

As noted above, the nature of the Geisinger patient population is such that multiple generations of family are cared for by the system. This makes Geisinger an ideal place to study how information systems can be used to support cascade testing of family members following identification of a genetic variant in a family member. Unfortunately, family history collection and representation in the EHR is not adequate at the present time [32]. An additional function that would support cascade testing would be the association of individual health records under an overarching family record. This was relatively straightforward with paper records, but has proven challenging with EHR systems, even for a seemingly simple use case of associating a child with its parents. There are some early efforts, mostly to support payer and public health programs [33], but these have yet to be implemented in vendor provided systems. While newer versions of these systems will provide enhanced capabilities to represent family history to support risk assessment for an individual patient, more advanced functionality remains aspirational.

Studies have consistently shown that health care providers are not adequately trained to deal with genomic information, and self-report low confidence in their ability to use this information to care for patients [34]. Providing information and support at the point of care to assist providers in the care of their patients is essential if the anticipated benefits of precision health are to be realized. Clinical decision support (CDS) in the form of ready access to knowledge resources in the clinical workflow (Passive) and computerized algorithms triggered by clinical information coupled with genomic information that guide care through alerts, reminders, and care pathways (Active) is an essential component of the precision health informatics ecosystem. There is an extensive literature on both passive and active CDS, a review of which is beyond the scope of this chapter but is covered extensively in the Institute of Medicine workshop summary, Genomics-Enabled Learning Health Care Systems: Gathering and Using Genomic Information to Improve Patient Care and Research [6].

At Geisinger, we are exploring native functionality in our EHR to support CDS. Active CDS in the form of best practice advisories (BPAs) are available to guide care in several places in the EHR. We have implemented BPAs in a set of use cases related to pharmacogenomic-guided therapy. As more pharmacogenomic information on our participants becomes available, this will be expanded. These are informed by evidence-based guidelines available from the Clinical Pharmacogenetics Implementation Consortium (CPIC) [35]. To promote generalizability and facilitate implementation, the CPIC guidelines are unusual, and possibly unique, in that the guidelines are designed with computability in mind. Input from the CPIC informatics working group ensures that the guidelines are adequately explicit. Narrative descriptions of the guideline (an L1 CDS artifact) and a decision tree (an L2 CDS artifact) are created and published with the guidelines. As more pharmacogenomic information on our participants becomes available, this will be expanded. We deposit L1 and L2 artifacts in a publicly available database of clinical decision support algorithms, CDSKB [36], which was created and is supported with funding from the National Human Genome Research Institute through the electronic Medical Records and Genomics (eMERGE) and Implementing Genomics in Practice (IGNITE) networks. One barrier at present is that the pharmacogenomic variants are not able to be stored as structured data in the EHR, meaning that they must be manually converted into structured data elements that can be placed in the EHR such that they can appropriate trigger the relevant BPA. It is anticipated that EHR upgrades will support storing genomic variants as structured data to support passive and active CDS.

The genomic test reports described above are one modality being used to provide knowledge at the point of care. As more clinically relevant knowledge about genomics becomes available, it is imperative that these knowledge repositories can be accessed by clinicians through the EHR. The challenge is how to facilitate provider access to the information within the clinical workflow in a time frame compatible with the limited visit length. Extensive research on this problem has been conducted. A promising approach is to use a tool such as an infobutton. Infobuttons are context-sensitive links embedded within an EHR or other information system, which allow easy retrieval of relevant information. The author in concert with investigators within eMERGE and the NIH-funded Clinical Genome Resource (ClinGen) [37] have investigated how online genomic knowledge repositories can be configured to support infobutton queries. The ClinGen repository represents an active test bed for this technology given its stated mission is "…dedicated to building an authoritative central resource that defines the clinical relevance of genes and variants for use in precision medicine and research." A summary of this work has been published [38–40]. A technical problem encountered locally was that while the EHR system has infobutton functionality, it was not active within the production EHR environment, so could not be used to provide information to clinicians at the point of care. Infobuttons will be activated with the next system upgrade (fall 2018). This upgrade will also add the functionality to represent genomic information as structured data, which will support context-specific information retrieval, once the native infobuttons are configured. This will also support deployment of active CDS to support care for the prioritized conditions in our precision health initiative.

Measuring Outcomes Attributable to Reporting

Precision health is an exciting idea that conceptually promises to transform the way medicine is practiced. To achieve the goal of precision health in the context of a learning healthcare system, it is necessary to 'close the loop' to determine the impact of the return of results to the participant and to the system. The healthcare system can no longer afford to add new interventions that don't provide value to the patient or system. This means that an essential component of a precision health program is to define and measure the outcomes attributable to the interventions. Outcomes of relevance to healthcare stakeholders are diverse (Table 16.1).

Capturing the outcomes requires a variety of approaches. For participants that receive their care from Geisinger, the process, intermediate and health outcomes can be captured from the EHR. Health outcomes may take years to measure, even decades when considering the impact of screening for familial hypercholesterolemia in the pediatric population. The stability of the Geisinger population with little in and out migration provides an ideal opportunity to measure the long-term impact of a genomic medicine-informed precision health program. Capturing outcomes data for participants not cared for at Geisinger is more difficult but can be addressed in three ways. Some of these participants are covered by Geisinger Health Plan, meaning that claims data can be used to measure some of the outcomes (mostly process). Secondly, Geisinger leads the Keystone Health Information Exchange which allows information from participating healthcare organizations to be collected for care coordination and, more recently research. Finally, participants are contacted by the GSCP on a periodic basis after the return of results. This provides an additional opportunity to collect information on process outcomes, and potentially intermediate and health outcomes if the participants provide access to medical records. Contact is also critical to obtain information about whether the measured outcome

Table 16.1 Outcomes for precision health implementation

Outcome type	Description	Precision health example
Process	These measures are the specific steps in a process that lead—either positively or negatively—to a particular health outcome	Lipid profile performed after return of a pathogenic variant in *LDLR* a gene associated with familial hypercholesterolemia
Intermediate	A biomarker associated—either positively or negatively—to a particular health outcome	An LDL cholesterol level at or below the target level of 100 mg/dl in response to interventions recommended based on presences of a pathogenic variant in *LDLR*
Health	Change in the health of an individual, group of people, or population which is attributable to an intervention or series of interventions	Decrease in myocardial infarction, or cardiac revascularization procedures in response to interventions recommended based on presences of a pathogenic variant in *LDLR*
Cost	Standard costs associated with the interventions and health states experienced by the patient. Can also include costs associated with patient reported outcomes from self-reported health state and life disruption	Cost of sequencing Cost of return of result infrastructure Direct costs of care related to return of results Utilization
Patient-reported	Report of the status of a patient's health condition, knowledge, or service outcomes that comes directly from the patient, without interpretation of the patient's response	Satisfaction with service Engagement with self-care Knowledge about gene and disease Access to recommended care Self-assessed well being
System-defined	Outcomes that are of relevance to the system as whole. In addition to those listed above, other outcomes could include, patient experience, employee benefits, resource utilization, visibility, and market differentiation	Visibility related to precision health program Sequencing program as a service differentiator to health care purchasers (payer, employer) Sequencing offered to employees as a benefit

can be confidently attributed to the return of result. As an example, if a participant has a mammogram after the return of a pathogenic variant in the *BRCA1* gene it could be due to the result being returned, or because it was performed as part of routine preventive care. Accurate attribution is essential to determine the true value of the precision health program. Cost outcomes can be determined by applying standard costing to the clinical data obtained above.

Follow-up phone calls to the participants also supports the collection of patient-reported outcomes. This can be done using standard tools but also requires the development of validated patient-reported outcomes relevant to precision health, as these currently do not exist. Geisinger has active research in this area alone, and in collaboration with networks like eMERGE.

These outcomes can be used to populate economic models to examine the cost-effectiveness of the intervention and identify which data elements have the most impact on cost-effectiveness. This can prioritize the collection of the most critical data elements, while saving resources by not collecting outcomes that have little impact. Geisinger is currently funded with two other institutions to develop economic models to study the cost-effectiveness of population sequencing.

Informatics Challenges

For the health-related outcomes, while the information is frequently available in the transactional data derived from the EHR, laboratory and radiology information systems, and claims data from the provider-owned health plan, the retrieval of this information requires significant effort. This requires an inventory of what outcomes data is generated routinely from clinical care, assessment of whether these data are in a structured format that can be retrieved, mapping the relevant data elements to facilitate retrieval, and a critical evaluation of the data to determine its quality and completeness. As is frequently the case in healthcare, some of the outcomes information is not structured but resides in unformatted text blobs. Utilization of text-mining and natural language processing may be necessary to provide a more complete representation of outcomes. For any given participant, there will be variability of the available data and the location of that data, depending on their healthcare utilization patterns. Retrieval strategies must account for this variability and be able to flag missing data that may need to be acquired using manual methods.

Michael Porter, in his landmark article "What is Value in Healthcare?" [41] introduced the outcome measures hierarchy. In discussing the hierarchy, he notes that health outcomes must be evaluated *from the perspective of the patient.* In the last 10 years, patient-reported outcomes have been increasingly prominent in healthcare. To support collection of these measures, the United States Department of Health and Human Services through the National Institutes of Health funded the development of the Patient-Reported Outcomes Measurement Information System (PROMIS®) [42]. PROMIS® is a publicly available set of person-centered measures that evaluates and monitors physical, mental, and social health in adults and children. Over 300 measures are currently available. A review of the measures identifies some that would be of use in the context of precision medicine, but none that account for unique issues associated with genetics and genomics. Also, these measures have been primarily developed to support research, so, while they are applicable to clinical care, the ability of current health information systems to collect and store these measures is limited.

Outcomes specific to business require data from systems that are outside of the EHR and other health information systems. Claims data generated by payers is segregated by law from other health related data and can only be merged under specified conditions to support business operations or research. Health systems that do not have a payer associated with the system (which is the case for most systems in the United States) will have very limited access to claims data at the individual patient level. An additional issue is that many provider systems are limited to inpatient or outpatient services, such that data on utilization is difficult to aggregate.

Outcomes at the system level requires a business intelligence approach that aggregates and synthesizes data from a variety of disparate sources. While health information systems contribute some data (primarily related to cost and utilization), they are insufficient, in and of themselves, to generate system outcomes.

The Future: Precision Health in the Clinic

Almost all the projects that would be considered under the general heading of precision health have been launched either as pilots or in the context of clinical research. As such, there has not been a strong need for clinically deployed health information systems to accommodate the components needed to support precision health. This has not prevented experts in the field from assessing the weaknesses of current systems and identifying desirable features that will be needed to support genomic medicine—a key component of precision health. Masys et al. [43] and Welch et al. [44] reported on desiderata for integrating genomic information into the EHR and CDS respectively. In 2014, the National Human Genome Research Institute convened Genomic Medicine Workshop VII (GM7), **Genomic Clinical Decision Support: Developing Solutions for Clinical and Research Implementation** co-chaired by the author and Blackford Middleton [45]. The objectives for GM7 were to convene key thought leaders in genomic implementation and application of clinical decision support to compare current state with ideal state of genomic clinical decision support (GCDS) to define gaps and strategies to close the gaps; identify and engage US and international health IT initiatives that would support recommended strategies; and, define a prioritized research agenda for GCDS. The meeting was organized around five key questions:

1. Is clinical decision support an essential element in the successful implementation of genomic medicine?

   (a) Does GCDS differ significantly from decision support used for other purposes? If yes, what are the key differences?
   (b) What is the ideal state of GCDS?
   (c) How can the impact of GCDS be defined and measured?

2. What are data issues that impact GCDS?
3. How do we manage knowledge for GCDS?
4. What are implementation issues surrounding GCDS?
5. What are areas that should be prioritized for the research agenda for GCDS?

While the focus of the meeting was CDS, many of the key questions involve broader aspects related to informatics support of precision health. A major product of the meeting was a survey of the attendees.

A pre-meeting survey asked attendees to rank the 14 desiderata against two metrics: the importance of the element to achieve the ideal state of GCDS and the ability current information systems had to support the element. These results are summarized in Table 16.2.

Table 16.2 Desiderata for Genomic Medicine and Genomic Clinical Decision Support

Desiderata (1–7 Masys [44]; 8–14 Welch [45])	Importance of the element to achieve the ideal state of GCDS (mean score)	Technical ability of current information systems to support (mean score)
1. Maintain separation of primary molecular observations from the clinical interpretations of those data	2	3.6
2. Support lossless data compression from primary molecular observations to clinically manageable subsets	2.4	4.4
3. Maintain linkage of molecular observations to the laboratory methods used to generate them	1.6	2.9
4. Support compact representation of clinically actionable subsets for optimal performance	1.6	3.2
5. Simultaneously support human-viewable formats and machine-readable formats in order to facilitate implementation of decision support rules	1.4	3.8
6. Anticipate fundamental changes in the understanding of human molecular variation	1.9	4.2
7. Support both individual clinical care and discovery science	1.4	3.5
8. CDS knowledge must have the potential to incorporate multiple genes and clinical information	1.2	3.5
9. Keep CDS knowledge separate from variant classification	3.0	4.1
10. CDS knowledge must have the capacity to support multiple EHR platforms with various data representations with minimal modification	1.6	4.4
11. Support a large number of gene variants while simplifying the CDS knowledge to the extent possible	1.8	3.7
12. Leverage current and developing CDS and genomics standards	1.7	4.1
13. Support a CDS knowledge base deployed at and developed by multiple independent organizations	1.6	4.1
14. Access and transmit only the genomic information necessary for CDS	3.0	3.9

This table lists the 14 desiderata of Masys and Welch. These were presented to the attendees of the NHGRI-sponsored Genomic Medicine VII meeting, Genomic Clinical Decision Support: Developing Solutions for Clinical and Research Implementation. The survey asked two questions for each of the desiderata, Respondents answered on a 5-point Likert scale: (1) Strongly Agree, (2) Agree, (3) Neither Agree nor Disagree, (4) Disagree, (5) Strongly disagree. The survey was sent to 33 meeting attendees and 25 completed the survey for a response rate of 75%

Table 16.3 Importance of components to support Genomic Clinical Decision Support

Question	Essential	Desirable	No opinion
Always updateable	25	2	1
Provides guidance for all target users	17	10	1
Explains all of its actions and recommendations	15	12	1
Monitors process or outcome measures and tracks uptake of decision support advice by clinicians	14	13	1
Tracks decision support events and provides basis for correlating subsequent clinical course with guidance provided	14	12	2
Has recognition logic for conditions of interest as represented in EHR systems (both genotype and phenotype)	16	8	4
Sensitive to different users' health and genomics literacy and numeracy	12	14	2
Builds a shareable knowledge repository for GCDS artifacts (rule/alerts, algorithms, etc.)	12	14	2
Stores content that can be (re)purposed for different types of users	9	16	3
Contributes to local continuous process improvement to a shared national learning healthcare system	7	17	4
Generates de-identified outcomes data to be transferred and stored in a public library to inform a national learning healthcare system	5	19	4
Adaptively learns what each user knows with use over time	3	18	7
Improves quality and consistency by autonomous individual entities	7	9	12

This table presents the results of a post-meeting survey. Thirteen items were identified from the meeting discussion as being relevant components for genomic clinical decision support. Respondents were asked to select a response from three choices for each of the components: (1) Essential, (2) Desirable, but not essential, (3) No opinion. Twenty-eight meeting attendees returned surveys for a response rate of over 50%. The table is ordered from most essential to least essential

Attendees overwhelmingly agreed that 12 of the 14 desiderata were important to achieve the ideal state. In contrast, most disagreed that current systems are technically capable of supporting the ideal state. A synthesis of the meeting identified 13 components needed to achieve the ideal state of GCDS. A post-meeting survey was distributed to attendees that asked which of these components are essential as opposed to desirable, with an option for no opinion. Results are presented in Table 16.3.

Even though the meeting took place in 2014, the state of information systems has not appreciably changed based on the response of attendees of the 2018 American College of Medical Informatics Meeting (data not shown). Nonetheless, this represents a valuable road map to support the implementation of precision health in the clinic.

In 2018, Geisinger announced it was launching a program to provide exome sequencing as part of clinical care [46]. Moving this from the research to the clinical setting accelerates the strategy to create a health information ecosystem that can support precision health. Anticipated upgrades to the vendor EHR will provide additional capabilities to support genomic information as structured data lowering barriers to the presentation of relevant information to patients and providers at the point of care. Active clinical decision support best practice advisories have already been created and tested to support the return of pharmacogenomic information which will occur shortly after the system upgrade. Geisinger investigators, in conjunction with other investigators in the eMERGE network are developing clinical decision support artifacts that instantiate care guidelines developed by professional organizations, such as the American College of Medical Genetics and Genomics, in a computable format that can be deployed in the EHR to promote evidence-based care. Storage of the exome sequence in an ancillary system [47] that interfaces with the EHR is under development. This will support the use of the sequence as needed over the course of clinical care for the individual. Prior work has identified the 'known unknowns' that need to be addressed through collaboration between research and clinical informaticists. Undoubtedly, 'unknown unknowns' will arise as the program is implemented; however, the framework of the learning healthcare system powered by the tools of implementation science allows for rapid identification of these unknowns to allow iterative modifications and improvements to achieve a robust genomically-informed precision health program.

Conclusion

Chambers et al., recognize the convergence of implementation science, precision medicine, and the learning healthcare system [48]. They note two major themes of this convergence: (1) clinical research is not complete prior to implementation and (2) research and practice can coexist. The authors go on to state, "Although precision medicine remains a story to be written, implementation science can substantially add value to learning health care systems, and in turn, the evolutionary nature of precision medicine can reshape current thinking about and approaches to research-practice translation." To this one must surely append the critical need for data and intelligent systems to transform the data into clinical intelligence, for which informatics plays a key role. This is central to Geisinger's vision to realize the value of implementing precision health as reflected in a quotation by JoAnne Wade, then Executive Vice President in charge of Strategic Program Development for Geisinger, in an article describing the value proposition for Geisinger's investment in genomic medicine [49], "In the midst of such change, opportunity to innovate new systems of care and payment models to improve the value of healthcare for patients, providers, payers, and employers requires reframing traditional means of integrating research within a clinical setting to add to the value proposition of improving patient outcomes and reducing the total cost of care."

References

1. The White House. The precision medicine initiative [Internet]. [Cited 2018 Aug 28]. https://obamawhitehouse.archives.gov/precision-medicine.
2. Collins FS, Varmus H. A new initiative on precision medicine. N Engl J Med. 2015;372:793–5. http://www.nejm.org/doi/10.1056/NEJMp1500523.
3. Christensen CM, Grossman JH, Hwang J. The innovator's prescription: a disruptive solution for health care. New York: McGraw-Hill; 2009.
4. Pauker SG, Kassirer JP. Decision analysis. N Engl J Med. 1987;316:250–8. http://www.nejm.org/doi/abs/10.1056/NEJM198701293160505.
5. Institute of Medicine. In: Olsen L, Aisner D, McGinnis JM, editors. The learning healthcare system: workshop summary. Washington, DC: National Academies Press; 2007. https://www.ncbi.nlm.nih.gov/books/NBK53494/.
6. Institute of Medicine. Genomics-enabled learning health care systems gathering and using genomic information to improve patient care and research: workshop summary. Washington, DC: National Academies Press; 2015. http://www.nap.edu/catalog/21707.
7. Carey DJ, Fetterolf SN, Davis FD, Faucett WA, Kirchner HL, Mirshahi U, et al. The Geisinger MyCode community health initiative: an electronic health record-linked biobank for precision medicine research. Genet Med. 2016;18:906–13. [cited 2018 Aug 28]. http://www.ncbi.nlm.nih.gov/pubmed/26866580.
8. Geisinger Health. MyCode results reported [Internet]. 2019 [cited 2019 Apr 1]. p. 1–3. https://www.geisinger.org/MyCode-results.
9. Geisinger Health. MyCode conditions [Internet]. 2019 [cited 2019 Apr 1]. https://www.geisinger.org/precision-health/mycode/mycode-conditions.
10. Geisinger Health. Geisinger Health system list of clinically actionable genes for the mycode community health initiative [Internet]. 2016 [cited 2018 Aug 28]. https://www.geisinger.org/-/media/OneGeisinger/pdfs/ghs/research/departments-and-centers/genomic-medicine-institute/PDFs/clinically-actionable-genes.ashx?la=en.
11. Green RC, Berg JS, Grody WW, Kalia SS, Korf BR, Martin CL, et al. ACMG recommendations for reporting of incidental findings in clinical exome and genome sequencing. Genet Med. 2013;15:565–74. http://www.nature.com/articles/gim201373.
12. Kalia SS, Adelman K, Bale SJ, Chung WK, Eng C, Evans JP, et al. Recommendations for reporting of secondary findings in clinical exome and genome sequencing, 2016 update (ACMG SF v2.0): a policy statement of the American College of Medical Genetics and Genomics. Genet Med. 2017;19:249–55. http://www.ncbi.nlm.nih.gov/pubmed/27854360.
13. Dewey FE, Murray MF, Overton JD, Habegger L, Leader JB, Fetterolf SN, et al. Distribution and clinical impact of functional variants in 50,726 whole-exome sequences from the DiscovEHR study. Science. 2016;354:aaf6814. http://www.ncbi.nlm.nih.gov/pubmed/28008009.
14. Paulus RA. ProvenCare: Geisinger's model for care transformation through innovative clinical initiatives and value creation. Am Heal Drug Benefits. 2009;2:122–7. http://www.ncbi.nlm.nih.gov/pubmed/25126281.
15. Tarczy-Hornoch P, Amendola L, Aronson SJ, Garraway L, Gray S, Grundmeier RW, et al. A survey of informatics approaches to whole-exome and whole-genome clinical reporting in the electronic health record. Genet Med. 2013;15:824–32. http://www.ncbi.nlm.nih.gov/pubmed/24071794.
16. Gulley ML, Braziel RM, Halling KC, Hsi ED, Kant JA, Nikiforova MN, et al. Clinical laboratory reports in molecular pathology. Arch Pathol Lab Med. 2007;131:852–63. http://www.ncbi.nlm.nih.gov/pubmed/17550311.
17. Chen B, Gagnon M, Shahangian S, Anderson NL, Howerton DA, Boone DJ, Centers for Disease Control and Prevention (CDC). Good laboratory practices for molecular genetic testing for heritable diseases and conditions. MMWR Recomm Rep. 2009;58(RR-6):1–37.

18. Dorschner MO, Amendola LM, Shirts BH, Kiedrowski L, Salama J, Gordon AS, et al. Refining the structure and content of clinical genomic reports. Am J Med Genet C: Semin Med Genet. 2014;166:85–92. http://www.ncbi.nlm.nih.gov/pubmed/24616401.

19. National Center for Biotechnology Information—U.S. National Library of Medicine. ClinVar [Internet]. [Cited 2018 Aug 28]. https://www.ncbi.nlm.nih.gov/clinvar/.

20. The Undiagnosed Diseases Network. UDN Undiagnosed Diseases Network [Internet]. 2017 [cited 2018 Aug 28]. https://undiagnosed.hms.harvard.edu/.

21. Ramoni RB, Mulvihill JJ, Adams DR, Allard P, Ashley EA, Bernstein JA, et al. The undiagnosed diseases network: accelerating discovery about health and disease. Am J Hum Genet. 2017;100:185–92. http://www.ncbi.nlm.nih.gov/pubmed/28157539.

22. Hosseini SM, Kim R, Udupa S, Costain G, Jobling R, Liston E, et al. Reappraisal of reported genes for sudden arrhythmic death: evidence-based evaluation of gene validity for Brugada syndrome. Circulation. 2018;138:1195–205. [cited 2018 Aug 28]. https://www.ahajournals.org/doi/10.1161/CIRCULATIONAHA.118.035070.

23. Manrai AK, Funke BH, Rehm HL, Olesen MS, Maron BA, Szolovits P, et al. Genetic misdiagnoses and the potential for health disparities. N Engl J Med. 2016;375:655–65. http://www.nejm.org/doi/10.1056/NEJMsa1507092.

24. Lathe WC, Williams JM, Mangan ME, Karolchik D. Genomic data resources: challenges and promises. Nat Educ. 2008;1:2. https://www.nature.com/scitable/topicpage/genomic-data-resources-challenges-and-promises-743721.

25. Crockett DK, Lyon E, Williams MS, Narus SP, Facelli JC, Mitchell JA. Utility of gene-specific algorithms for predicting pathogenicity of uncertain gene variants. J Am Med Inform Assoc. 2012;19:207–11. http://www.ncbi.nlm.nih.gov/pubmed/22037892.

26. Richards S, Aziz N, Bale S, Bick D, Das S, Gastier-Foster J, et al. Standards and guidelines for the interpretation of sequence variants: a joint consensus recommendation of the American College of Medical Genetics and Genomics and the Association for Molecular Pathology. Genet Med. 2015;17:405–23. http://www.ncbi.nlm.nih.gov/pubmed/25741868.

27. Murray MF. Your DNA is not your diagnosis: getting diagnoses right following secondary genomic findings. Genet Med. 2016;18:765–7. http://www.nature.com/articles/gim2015134.

28. Stuckey H, Williams JL, Fan AL, Rahm AK, Green J, Feldman L, et al. Enhancing genomic laboratory reports from the patients' view: a qualitative analysis. Am J Med Genet A. 2015;167A:2238–43. http://www.ncbi.nlm.nih.gov/pubmed/26086630.

29. Williams JL, Rahm AK, Stuckey H, Green J, Feldman L, Zallen DT, et al. Enhancing genomic laboratory reports: a qualitative analysis of provider review. Am J Med Genet A. 2016;170:1134–41. http://www.ncbi.nlm.nih.gov/pubmed/26842872.

30. Williams JL, Rahm AK, Zallen DT, Stuckey H, Fultz K, Fan AL, et al. Impact of a patient-facing enhanced genomic results report to improve understanding, engagement, and communication. J Genet Couns. 2018;27:358–69. http://link.springer.com/10.1007/s10897-017-0176-6.

31. Williams MS, Kern MS, Lerch VR, Billet J, Williams JL, Moore GJ. Implementation of a patient-facing genomic test report in the electronic health record using a web-application interface. BMC Med Inform Decis Mak. 2018;18:32. https://bmcmedinformdecismak.biomedcentral.com/articles/10.1186/s12911-018-0614-x.

32. Polubriaginof F, Tatonetti NP, Vawdrey DK. An assessment of family history information captured in an electronic health record. AMIA Annu Symp Proc. 2015;2015:2035–42. http://www.ncbi.nlm.nih.gov/pubmed/26958303.

33. Angier H, Gold R, Crawford C, O'Malley JP, Tillotson CJ, Marino M, et al. Linkage methods for connecting children with parents in electronic health record and state public health insurance data. Matern Child Health J. 2014;18:2025–33. http://www.ncbi.nlm.nih.gov/pubmed/24562505.

34. Mikat-Stevens NA, Larson IA, Tarini BA. Primary-care providers' perceived barriers to integration of genetics services: a systematic review of the literature. Genet Med. 2015;17:169–76. http://www.ncbi.nlm.nih.gov/pubmed/25210938.

35. Clinical Pharmacogenetics Implementation Consortium (CPIC®). Guidelines [Internet]. 2018 [cited 2018 Aug 28]. https://cpicpgx.org/guidelines/.
36. Clinical Decision Support Knowledgebase (CDS_KB). About [Internet]. [Cited 2018 Aug 28]. https://cdskb.org/about/.
37. ClinGen Clinical Genome Resource. ClinGen clinical genome resource [Internet]. [Cited 2018 Aug 28]. https://www.clinicalgenome.org/.
38. Heale B, Overby C, Del Fiol G, Rubinstein W, Maglott D, Nelson T, et al. Integrating genomic resources with electronic health records using the HL7 infobutton standard. Appl Clin Inform. 2016;7:817–31. http://www.ncbi.nlm.nih.gov/pubmed/27579472.
39. Overby CL, Rasmussen LV, Hartzler A, Connolly JJ, Peterson JF, Hedberg RE, et al. A template for authoring and adapting genomic medicine content in the eMERGE infobutton project. AMIA Annu Symp Proc. 2014;2014:944–53. http://www.ncbi.nlm.nih.gov/pubmed/25954402.
40. Crump JK, Del Fiol G, Williams MS, Freimuth RR. Prototype of a standards-based EHR and genetic test reporting tool coupled with HL7-compliant infobuttons. AMIA Jt Summits Transl Sci Proc. 2018;2017:330–9. http://www.ncbi.nlm.nih.gov/pubmed/29888091.
41. Porter ME. What is value in health care? N Engl J Med. 2010;363:2477–81. http://www.nejm.org/doi/abs/10.1056/NEJMp1011024.
42. HealthMeasures. PROMIS [Internet]. 2018 [cited 2018 Aug 28]. http://www.healthmeasures.net/explore-measurement-systems/promis.
43. Masys DR, Jarvik GP, Abernethy NF, Anderson NR, Papanicolaou GJ, Paltoo DN, et al. Technical desiderata for the integration of genomic data into electronic health records. J Biomed Inform. 2012;45:419–22. http://www.ncbi.nlm.nih.gov/pubmed/22223081.
44. Welch BM, Eilbeck K, Del FG, Meyer LJ, Kawamoto K. Technical desiderata for the integration of genomic data with clinical decision support. J Biomed Inform. 2014;51:3–7. http://www.ncbi.nlm.nih.gov/pubmed/24931434.
45. National Human Genome Research Institute (NHGRI). Genomic Medicine Centers Meeting VII: genomic clinical decision support—developing solutions for clinical and research implementation [Internet]. 2017 [cited 2018 Aug 28]. https://www.genome.gov/27558904/genomic-medicine-centers-meeting-vii/.
46. DNA sequencing to become part of Geisinger's routine clinical care [Internet]. 2018 [cited 2018 Aug 28]. [Less than one page]. https://www.geisinger.org/about-geisinger/news-and-media/news-releases/2018/05/07/12/18/dna-sequencing-to-become-part-of-geisingers-routine-clinical-care.
47. Starren J, Williams MS, Bottinger EP. Crossing the omic chasm. JAMA. 2013;309:1237. [cited 2018 Aug 28]. http://jama.jamanetwork.com/article.aspx?doi=10.1001/jama.2013.1579.
48. Chambers DA, Feero WG, Khoury MJ. Convergence of implementation science, precision medicine, and the learning health care system. JAMA. 2016;315:1941. http://jama.jamanetwork.com/article.aspx?doi=10.1001/jama.2016.3867.
49. Wade JE, Ledbetter DH, Williams MS. Implementation of genomic medicine in a health care delivery system: a value proposition? Am J Med Genet C: Semin Med Genet. 2014;166:112–6. http://www.ncbi.nlm.nih.gov/pubmed/24619641.

Part IV
Integrative Informatics for PPM

Chapter 17
The Genomic Medical Record and Omic Ancillary Systems

Luke V. Rasmussen, Timothy M. Herr, Casey Overby Taylor, Abdulrahman M. Jahhaf, Therese A. Nelson, and Justin B. Starren

Background

With growth in the number of genetic tests that are available to providers and patients [1], an increasing amount of data is becoming available for integration into the clinical workflow. Germline tests can aid in diagnosing rare diseases, assessing

L. V. Rasmussen · T. M. Herr · A. M. Jahhaf
Division of Health and Biomedical Informatics, Department of Preventive Medicine, Feinberg School of Medicine, Northwestern University, Chicago, IL, USA
e-mail: luke.rasmussen@northwestern.edu; tim.herr@northwestern.edu; abdulrahman.jahhaf@northwestern.edu

C. O. Taylor
Division of General Internal Medicine, School of Medicine, Johns Hopkins University, Baltimore, MD, USA

Division of Health Sciences Informatics, Johns Hopkins University, Baltimore, MD, USA
e-mail: overby-taylor@jhu.edu

T. A. Nelson
Socio-Technical Innovation, Northwestern University Clinical and Translational Sciences, Northwestern University, Chicago, IL, USA
e-mail: therese.nelson@northwestern.edu

J. B. Starren (✉)
Division of Health and Biomedical Informatics, Department of Preventive Medicine, Feinberg School of Medicine, Northwestern University, Chicago, IL, USA

Northwestern University Clinical and Translational Science Institute (NUCATS), Northwestern University, Chicago, IL, USA

Center for Data Science and Informatics (CDSI), Northwestern University, Chicago, IL, USA
e-mail: Justin.starren@northwestern.edu

© Springer Nature Switzerland AG 2020
T. Adam, C. Aliferis (eds.), *Personalized and Precision Medicine Informatics*, Health Informatics, https://doi.org/10.1007/978-3-030-18626-5_17

253

Table 17.1 Facets of omic data

Facet	Description	Examples
Omic type	The type of omic data to be used and integrated	Genomic, proteomic, metabolomic, epigenomic, expression profile
Cell source	The source of the cells from which the omic data is derived	Germline vs. somatic
Biological cell type	The specific type of cell (if isolated) for analysis	E.g., macrophage, neurons
Result source	Where the omic data is coming from (where it was interpreted)	Internal laboratory, external laboratory
Clinical significance	The degree of potential impact on clinical care (depending on levels of evidence)	Pathogenic, likely pathogenic, variant of uncertain significance, likely benign, benign

disease risk, or targeting appropriate medications and doses. In addition, somatic variants can be used to guide cancer treatment. As proteomics and metabolomics see increased use, and as even more types of "omics" are translated from research settings into clinical care, providers and patients have access to rich new sources of data to guide care pathways.

Medical centers and providers ordering omic tests can find multiple avenues by which to acquire results. Some institutions have the ability to perform omic testing in-house. In this case, the laboratory workflow is often tightly integrated with the clinical workflow, and health information technology (HIT) systems are more likely to share information. External, commercial laboratories also provide a large number of genetic and genomic tests. Depending on the capabilities of the laboratory, the results may be sent back as a scanned fax or a PDF that is imported into the electronic health record (EHR), running the risk of the results getting lost in the "Miscellaneous" section of the EHR.

As our understanding of omics increases, questions arise as to how omic results should be interpreted, and how that interpretation may change with new evidence. Evidence may also come with a level of disagreement. For example, the ClinVar database [2], which provides variant interpretations reported by laboratories, has conflicting reports of pathogenicity for the same variants [3]. Likewise, healthcare systems, and even individual providers, may differ in how they choose to interpret or act on recommendations, which can make the integration and use of omic data specific to an institution.

The heterogeneity of omic data (see Table 17.1) makes data management an interesting informatics challenge. It is especially important to better acquire, manage and integrate omic data within the clinical and EHR workflow. Otherwise, already burdened clinicians can be faced with a deluge of additional data to wade through when trying to make clinical decisions.

Omic Data as Clinical Data

EHRs today are primarily centered around encounters with patients, and record a history of what healthcare providers observe and assess (e.g., vitals and diagnoses), as well as what they provide for the patient (e.g., medication or laboratory orders, procedures performed). This information is confirmed and documented each time the provider sees the patient, in order to track changes over time. Relatively speaking, the amount of storage needed for most types of clinical data is small, although total storage grows as more patients have more observations recorded over a long period of time. We contrast this with genomic data, which can require large amounts (several hundred gigabytes) of storage for a single whole exome sequencing result, but is usually a one-time assessment for germline results.

Another difference between omic data and conventional clinical data is that providers do not collect conventional data that they do not need or intend to use. However, our understanding of omic data is constantly evolving. At present we are able to sequence an entire genome, but do not yet fully understand how to interpret it. Because of this, omic data management needs to consider data that is currently actionable for a provider, while retaining the remaining data for when additional knowledge can turn it into action.

EHRs try to encourage the storage and presentation of data in a structured format, so that clinical data normally has a set "home" within an EHR, with separate places for medications, diagnoses, problem lists and laboratory lists. A survey of several academic medical centers revealed that the location of documentation about genetic information in the EHR can depend on which laboratory is performing the testing, how the laboratory interfaces with the EHR, the ordering clinician's department, and the source tissue [4]. Furthermore, genetic results were found to be stored in multiple locations of the EHR, and often in multiple modalities (e.g., a discrete result, mentioned in a clinical note, or stored as a document image). This complicates healthcare providers' ability to access available genetic results.

Interpretation of Results

One challenging aspect of omic data is that our understanding of it is changing more rapidly than other types of clinical data. For example, guidelines for the management of high blood pressure were recently updated for the first time in 14 years [5]. In contrast, the American College of Medical Genetics and Genomics revised actionability guidelines for genes after just 4 years of additional research [6, 7]. As genomics is an active area of study, it is perhaps not surprising that its rate of change is different. However, this rapid rate of change is challenging for HIT systems that are built around omic data.

Rethinking Omic Data in the EHR

Given these issues, we must determine the optimal strategy for storing, analyzing and using omic data in clinical workflows. One model proposed is to treat omic data the same way we treat radiology images [8]. Both data types have higher storage requirements than typical clinical data, both require specialized processing and interpretation (with tools to support this process), and both most commonly provide a synthesized result of the original data to the EHR (linking back to the original data). For radiology, a picture archiving and communication system (PACS) addresses these needs, coupled with specialized viewers provided by imaging device manufacturers to aid in review for diagnostic purposes. Similarly, an omic ancillary system (OAS) may serve these purposes for omic data [8]. An OAS allows storage for large files containing results, as well as specialized tools and processing pipelines to aid in their interpretation. This is also similar to laboratory systems that reference laboratories use to manage interpreting results and releasing reports, with the notable exception that such a system allows a healthcare organization to receive and manage the omic data itself—not just an interpretation report.

Masys et al. [9] presented a list of seven desiderata for integrating omic data into the EHR, which may be addressed by OASs and eventually omic enabled EHRs (OE-EHRs) [10]. Table 17.2 shows these relationships, which are described in more detail in the following sections.

Table 17.2 Desiderata for integrating omic data into the EHR [9], and how the proposed omic ancillary system (OAS) meets the desiderata

EHR integration desideratum	How met by omic ancillary system (OAS)
1. Maintain separation of primary molecular observations from the clinical interpretations of those data	Molecular data are preserved within the OAS and are converted to an actionable clinical interpretation that is transmitted to the EHR.
2. Support lossless data compression from primary molecular observations to clinically manageable subsets	As a storage location for molecular observations, the OAS ensures these data are not discarded.
3. Maintain linkage of molecular observations to the laboratory methods used to generate them	Methodology from laboratories providing omic data should be provided, which is then retained as a link to the underlying data.
4. Support compact representation of clinically actionable subsets for optimal performance	Specialized processing may be done within an OAS to convert the molecular observations to an actionable interpretation that is then made available within the OE-EHR.
5. Simultaneously support human-viewable formats and machine-readable formats in order to facilitate implementation of decision support rules	The OAS provides a user-friendly viewer of data, in addition to supporting and providing computable representations of the data that can be used for interpretation and decision support.
6. Anticipate fundamental changes in the understanding of human molecular variation	Translating the molecular observations into an actionable interpretation, as opposed to just having an interpretation, allows a health system to react to changes in the understanding of omic data.
7. Support both individual clinical care and discovery science	By providing a home for the molecular observations, the OAS makes these data accessible for discovery science as well as clinical care.

Informatics Challenges

As we will describe in the following sections, much work has been done to propose and implement both the OAS and OE-EHR [8–12]. However, the optimal solution is not yet known. Many opportunities exist to expand our understanding in the following areas:

- **Data and Knowledge Management**—the section "Translating Omic Data into Clinical Action" describes how omic data management and knowledge management may be done with an OAS, as well as how omic data can be optimized for action in the healthcare setting.
- **Display of Information**—it is necessary to determine the optimal location within the EHR to show the results of genetic tests and their interpretation. For example, if a patient has a variant that predisposes them to be a poor metabolizer of a certain drug, where should that be shown so that it is intuitive (a provider readily knows where to look for genetic results), appropriately linked to decision support, and does not get lost in (or cause) additional noise? This is explored further in the section "Integrating Omic Data into User Workflows."
- **Implementation**—much of the work reported to date has been within large academic medical centers and healthcare systems, which have led research and disseminated the understanding of OASs and OE-EHR development. As the field matures, a deeper understanding is needed of how to commoditize OASs and OE-EHRs, and how they may be more routinely integrated into workflows at practices of all sizes. This is also covered within the section "Integrating Omic Data into User Workflows."
- **Standards**—the section "Data Standards and Technologies" describes the past and current state of standards for storing and transmitting omic data, as well as terminologies for representing the concepts. However, these standards have not been exhaustively evaluated to date.
- **Ethical Concerns**—because knowledge of genomic results can impact a person for life, and may also have bearing on family members, genetic information for precision medicine must be treated with care. In the section "Ethical, Legal & Social Issues", we look at how ethical considerations for this data should be factored into the design and use of an OAS and OE-EHR.
- **Health Economics**—to integrate omic data effectively into the clinical workflow, additional investment is needed in technology and personnel. In the section "Cost Considerations", we explore considerations for organizations to weigh costs against potential benefits.

Translating Omic Data into Clinical Action

The Challenges of Omic Data

Though our understanding of genomics and other omic data is constantly improving, these are still relatively novel data types that few clinicians [13], and few HIT systems [14], are adequately prepared to handle. A complete human genome has approximately 3 billion base pairs—an overwhelming amount of data for even the most astute of healthcare providers to process. Even just the 1% of the genome that encodes for proteins (the whole exome), is a cumbersome 30 million base pairs. Add in additional omic data types, such as proteomic, metabolomic, and tumor sequencing, and it becomes clear that omic data presents unique challenges when compared to traditional clinical lab testing.

Moreover, the problem is not merely one of data management—it is also a knowledge problem. Distilling useful knowledge out of 3 billion base pairs is difficult enough, but because of the young nature of the clinical genomics field, our knowledge of the clinical impact of omic data is constantly evolving. When new interpretations of genetic variants are being published on a seemingly daily basis, it is unreasonable to expect busy clinicians to fully understand the clinical effects of all of the latest research.

If we are to unlock the full potential of omic-based PPM medicine and provide improved care, we must have a method for managing vast amounts of omic data and extracting useful knowledge. Here, we present a conceptual model and roadmap for this process [15].

A Conceptual Model

The core process for integrating omic data into the clinical setting is to filter clinical action from raw data. Consider a funnel shape, as in Fig. 17.1 [15]. Vast amounts of raw omic data start at the top, where the funnel is wide. As the data filter down the layers of the funnel, they are successively distilled and simplified into something that can be acted upon.

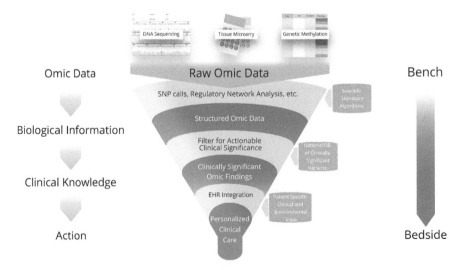

Fig. 17.1 Omic Funnel (based on Herr et al., J Path Info 2015 [15])

The four major steps of this model—*Omic Data*, *Biological Information*, *Clinical Knowledge*, and *Action*—run parallel to translational medicine's popular "bench to bedside" paradigm. Applying a filter to each level of the funnel leads to a narrower, but more actionable, state.

Omic Data to Biological Information

Raw omic data (genomic, proteomic, metabolomic, etc.) sit at the top of the funnel. For the purposes of this explanation, we will focus on genomic data. Genomic data might be unprocessed alignment data from next-generation sequencing (NGS) platforms, containing DNA segments represented as a sequence of A, C, G, and T, along with read-quality metadata. Common file formats at this level include Sequence Alignment Map (SAM) [16] and BAM (the binary equivalent of a SAM text file), though other formats, such as FASTA and FASTQ are also possible.

At the *Omic Data* stage, we have a complete picture of a patient's genome, but we have little to no understanding of its meaning. Here, our biological understanding of the structure of the human genome can provide context and give us a better picture of what is unique about the patient. By applying this scientific understanding (for instance, by comparing the patient's sequence to the human reference genome), we can take the step from *Omic Data* into *Biological Information*.

The biological understanding needed to make the translation from *Omic Data* into *Biological Information* is the domain of bioinformaticians and geneticists. These scientists perform their research and publish in the scientific literature, then their findings are integrated into standard genome interpretation pipelines.

Biological Information to Clinical Knowledge

Biological Information constitutes the second layer of the "Omic Funnel" and consists of refined, but still relatively raw, omic data. In our genomics example, this layer contains information about the unique biological structure of the patient, as compared to the human reference genome. This includes information about what specific genetic variations are present and where, such as single nucleotide polymorphisms (SNP), copy-number variations, rearrangements, insertions, and deletions. Common file formats at this level include Variant Call Format (VCF) [17] and BCF (the binary equivalent of a VCF text file). SNPs may be encoded as a Reference SNP Cluster ID (or "rs#") [18] and gene variants may be encoded in star allele nomenclature.

At the *Biological Information* stage, we understand what genetic variations a patient has, and where those variations exist in his or her genome, but we have little understanding of how those variations are relevant to the patient's health. Here, our understanding of the clinical implications of certain genetic variants can provide context and help us diagnose, treat, and prevent disease. By applying this clinical context, we can take the step from *Biological Information* into *Clinical Knowledge*.

The clinical understanding needed to make the translation from *Biological Information* to *Clinical Knowledge* is the domain of medical informaticists and clinical researchers, and requires significant coordination in the research and clinical communities. Scientific studies, such as Genome Wide Association Studies (GWAS), can identify genes of clinical interest. Bench and clinical studies can then confirm those associations and help determine how specific genes and gene variants affect health outcomes. Significant informatics effort is also required to centralize and standardize that knowledge for consumption by HIT applications. Efforts such as the ClinVar [2] database and the Clinical Pharmacogenetics Implementation Consortium (CPIC) [19] are examples of the sort of databases and curation that are required at this level.

Clinical Knowledge to Action

Clinical Knowledge is the third level of the Omic Funnel, and is generally the first point at which most clinicians will be able to interpret and assimilate omic-related data. This layer contains not only information about how a patient's genotype varies, but also knowledge about how those variations may affect his or her health. This may also include recommendations for how to best treat a patient with those specific variations. There are currently no true standards for encoding knowledge at this level, though CPIC has proposed a limited set of consensus pharmacogenetic terms. Clinical genetic knowledge and recommendations may exist in journal articles, on public websites such as PharmGKB, or as logic coded into HIT systems.

At the *Clinical Knowledge* stage, we have a useful understanding of the patient's genetics, as well as how to interpret and apply that knowledge to clinical care, but we have limited ability to actually effect change in physician behavior. Most clinicians are still not well educated on genomics and are generally unaware of the omic resources that are available to help them in their decision-making process. Here, we must have tools that easily integrate clinically relevant omic knowledge with patient-specific omic, clinical, and environmental data in the user's existing workflow (i.e., in the EHR). By seamlessly combining knowledge and data, we can provide clinicians with recommendations that are relevant, timely, and easily digested. With well-presented recommendations, clinicians can make more informed actions and provide truly personalized, precise medical care.

The tools required to make the transition from *Clinical Knowledge* to *Action* are largely the domain of health and biomedical informaticists and the makers of HIT systems. Health and biomedical informaticists must study knowledge presentation and workflow integration and create effective tools for disseminating omic-based recommendations. Ideal presentation models will require socio-technical research and the application of implementation science. When effective models are discovered, makers of HIT systems, such as EHR vendors, must provide the technical framework for displaying and streamlining clinical recommendations. This will allow the healthcare system to truly realize the benefits of an omic-enabled EHR.

Action

The final layer, *Action*, is the point at which the clinician provides precision (or personalized) care, tailored to the specific needs of the individual patient. This is not to say that current clinical practices are not personalized, but rather, that incorporation of omic data can even further refine and individualize care to make it more effective and further improve outcomes. Tools such as clinical decision support (e.g., pharmacogenetic alerts at the time of medication order entry) or distilled, individualized reference materials (e.g., infobuttons [20] on a patient's EHR chart) can aid in the delivery of precision care.

Though *Action* is the final layer of the "Omic Funnel", it is not a final destination. Instead, it can be considered part of a feedback loop that enables further research to expand our *Clinical Knowledge* and refine *Action*-inducing omic-based tools. By recording and observing the actions users take in response to these tools, we can improve upon them and discover better and better ways to care for patients.

Practical Applications of Omic Data

Though we provided some practical examples in the above description of our conceptual model, it is worth a closer look at how to achieve real-world applications of omic data. We start by asking what, exactly, we want to do with omic data (again, with a focus on genetics and genomics).

To answer that question, keep in mind that physicians are not the only people that may have a need for this data. Genetic counselors, nurses, pharmacists, researchers, and patients are all potential consumers of genetic and genomic data, and each will have their own needs. Potential applications of genomic data include clinical decision support (CDS), problem list integration, searchable genetic results, automated reinterpretation of results, patient communication, and genetic research.

These are all uses that will be driven by health IT applications, especially EHRs. In order to support such uses of genetic data, EHRs must be able to store and present the relevant data. As we established earlier, most health IT applications are not designed to handle the unique challenges of omic data, due to its size and rapidly evolving nature. This is where OASs play a critical role. As Fig. 17.2 depicts, an OAS can provide many of the necessary intermediate steps described in the Omic Funnel and translate raw omic data into clinically relevant knowledge, which can then be presented to end-users and acted upon [8].

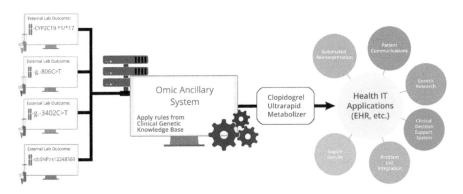

Fig. 17.2 Translating omic data into action

In real-world implementations, this generally means that an OAS will work in concert with a commercial EHR and a laboratory information system (either in-house or third-party). Laboratories complete their testing and return omic results to the ordering organization, with a format and interpretation that is generally specific to that lab. The OAS stores those results, translates them into one or more standardized "computed observations" that represent clinically relevant knowledge suitable for patient care, and then sends those observations to the EHR via an electronic interface (e.g., HL7). The EHR can then employ that information in any useful way—for example, by driving CDS or updating problem lists. The benefit of the "computed observation" is that it allows complex, rich omic data to be synthesized as a single actionable concept, while retaining links to the original data. This allows users of the computed observation to be able to dive down to the molecular measurements (if present in the OAS) to aid in interpretation, if needed.

To illustrate this chain of events, consider an example where a patient has a genetic test performed and the laboratory reports that he has the CYP2C19 *2/*3 genotype. At first glance, without additional context, this is not a particularly meaningful statement. With the aid of an OAS, this result could be translated to a more actionable computed observation "Clopidogrel Poor Metabolizer." This value could be stored in the patient's record as a discrete laboratory result, genetic test result, or problem list entry. If a physician tries to prescribe clopidogrel to the patient, CDS could then use that knowledge to drive alerts and display a recommended alternate medication to the clinician. This is in contrast to workflows that are common today, where genetic test results are commonly returned as textual reports, PDFs, or even non-computable document scans that require extensive human interpretation.

Figure 17.3 provides a model for how an OAS may fit into an existing HIT ecosystem, with multiple options for data flow. As an ancillary system, it lives alongside applications such as EHRs [8]. Ultimately, existing HIT applications will provide the framework necessary for displaying clinically relevant knowledge, while the OAS is responsible for supplying, maintaining, and updating omic knowledge. For example, commercially available EHRs may include a framework for displaying

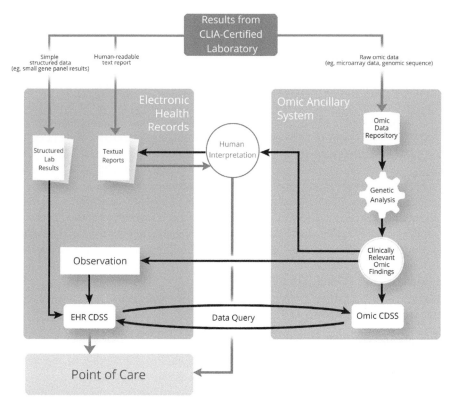

Fig. 17.3   Information flows for an omic ancillary system (based on Starren et al., JAMA 2013 [8])

pop-up alerts during order entry, but the OAS would supply the data that drives the underlying logic of those alerts. In the future, EHR vendors may even supply pre-built alerts that expect knowledge in a standardized format that can be provided by an OAS.

Integrating Omic Data into User Workflows

Though omic ancillary systems can serve many functions, perhaps their most important role is in facilitating the presentation of clinically relevant omic knowledge to healthcare providers. Although presentations will vary, there are general principles that will be true for most implementations. Specifically, this knowledge should be presented to the user in a way that seamlessly integrates with their existing workflow, provides timely and relevant advice, and is properly tailored to context and to the specific details of the patient in question. Here, we detail two CDS strategies that can help accomplish these goals: active and passive CDS.

Active Clinical Decision Support

Active CDS can take on many forms, though the classic example is of a pop-up alert advising a clinician of a recommended course of action. Existing applications warn physicians of potential adverse effects of medications (either due to interactions with other medications or to a recorded allergy), or remind physicians to conduct recommended best practice care such as vaccinations or routine mammograms.

Critics of this form of CDS often point out problems with alert fatigue [21], but well-designed alerts have the potential to be an important vector for the dissemination of clinical omic knowledge. As previously discussed, omic knowledge is constantly evolving and most clinicians are not well trained in fields like genetics and genomics. Active CDS can serve to fill this gap and provide users with timely and informative guidance on how to correctly apply omic knowledge to patient care. In fact, a number of healthcare organizations have begun to integrate omic knowledge into their workflows through the use of CDS [22–25]. Such efforts are largely in their nascent stages but hold significant promise. Organizations such as the Clinical Pharmacogenetics Implementation Consortium (CPIC) provide genetically guided dosing recommendations based on current scientific knowledge, and these recommendations are written so as to facilitate encoding into the programming logic of active CDS.

Omically-driven CDS must be designed with both technical and socio-technical considerations in mind, and while some basic standards are starting to emerge in the literature, best practices are still an open question. Figure 17.3 (see previous section) depicts one area where a consensus still does not exist around a technical aspect. That figure shows two possible locations for CDS logic. In one option, it can live in the EHR and be informed by data already stored in the EHR. Alternatively, the CDS logic can live in the OAS and be queried in real time by the EHR in order to calculate the proper recommendation. Real-world implementations have leaned towards the former option, though exploration into the latter still exists.

Passive Clinical Decision Support

The use of passive decision support can also provide a way to meet the information needs of providers. Specifically, infobuttons—context-sensitive links embedded in an EHR or patient portal [20]—can encode information about the patient and the current step of the clinical workflow to provide more targeted guidance. For example, an infobutton may contain not only the specific variant interpretation (e.g., VKORC1 results in relation to prescribing warfarin), but may also provide age, gender, race and ethnicity. These additional pieces of context about the patient may allow an information resource to provide more targeted, relevant information. Fortunately, several information resources exist specific to genomics and genetics that offer levels of support for infobuttons [26]. Given this, embedding infobuttons within an OAS or EHR may offer the support providers need to more widely adopt and apply omic data.

There are numerous socio-technical questions yet to be answered about the proper design of any omically-driven CDS, such as the best time in the user's workflow to display recommendations, whether active/interruptive alerts are more effective compared to passive alerts that clinicians would check at their own discretion, and precisely how to phrase recommendations and how much information to provide the user in an alert. All of these questions must balance the need to educate users on proper omic-driven care with the danger of overwhelming them with information. In short, recommendations must be timely, useful, and relevant, without being an additional burden on valuable clinician time and cognitive resources. These can best be answered through the use of implementation science and socio-technical design concepts.

Implementation Science Considerations

Omic knowledge is still quite new to most clinicians, so the design and implementation of software depending on it requires particular care. The implementation science field has a number of models that represent the processes involved in software implementation, evaluation, and acceptance. Examples of IT-adoption models include Technology Acceptance Model (TAM) [27], Task, Technology, Fit Model (TTF) [28], and the Fit between Individuals, Task, and Technology (FITT) Framework [29]. At the core of each of these models is the concept that users and technology must work together to achieve a goal. Technology must be both useful and usable in order for individuals to accept it [30].

However, it is often difficult to build software that is simultaneously useful and usable. Socio-technical design attempts to address this issue by incorporating human factors into software design [31, 32]. There is no single, canonical "socio-technical design cycle," but Koberg and Bagnall present a useful starting model [33]. Though their seven-step general design and problem-solving model is not specific to technology, it is clearly applicable to software design. It is defined as follows:

1. **Accept**: Stating initial intentions; accepting the problem as a challenge; allowing the problem to become the generator of process; self-motivation
2. **Analyze**: Becoming familiar with the insides and outsides of the problem; discovering what the "world of the problem" contains
3. **Define**: Determining the main issues of the problem; conceptualizing and clarifying aims, ends, and goals of problem resolution
4. **Ideate**: Identifying all possible ways of realizing the goals
5. **Select**: Comparing the destination with the possible ways of getting there; determining the best match or matches
6. **Implement**: Giving form to the selected "best ways;" "realizing" intentions
7. **Evaluate**: Reviewing the journey to determine the degree of success and its overall value

Most omic-based software tools currently in place can be considered first-generation tools, as many are custom-built for research purposes. Though efforts to evaluate and refine such tools are underway, there are few commercial options for such products, and few comprehensive studies in the literature evaluating the current solutions.

Standards and Technologies

Many standards exist for omic data; however, in this section we will concentrate on those that are more relevant to OASs and OE-EHRs. We will consider three general categories: (1) standards related to the structure of the data (storage and transmission), (2) standards and guidelines related to the vocabularies, terminologies and nomenclatures that represent concepts within those structures, and (3) standards that allow expanded user interfaces for omic results.

Structural and Transmission Standards

One may consider omic data at any point, from molecular measurements to a final interpretation applied in a clinical setting. Although it is possible to store sequence and read alignment data within an OAS, we will first consider Variant Call Format (VCF) files (and its binary counterpart, BCF) [17, 34]. VCF files are structured to represent multiple types of genomic variations—SNPs, insertions, deletions, structural variants—in conjunction with annotations. Although VCF files can be several gigabytes in size for whole genome results, the use of compression along with indexing tools such as tabix [35] helps improve access and processing times of results when they are needed. OASs do not need to be built using relational databases, and this makes the VCF file an option for supplemental data storage. A number of freely available tools exist to aid with processing and subsetting VCFs [17], which can be incorporated into an OAS processing pipeline.

Standards are also required for transmission of data between laboratories and an OAS or OE-EHR. Several standards for system interoperability have been produced by Health Level Seven International (HL7). The HL7 v2.x series of standards is based on plain-text files with pre-defined field positions and delimiters. It has remained ubiquitous within the U.S. healthcare system, despite the introduction of newer standards. As omic data is typically transmitted from a laboratory, the HL7 observation result (ORU) message format is a good fit. This message includes two primary parts: the observation request (OBR) segment, which contains information regarding the requisition of the test, including the type of testing performed, and the observation (OBX) segment, which contains the actual observations (results) of the test. Recognizing that HL7 v2.x is still widely used, recent drafted guidance exists around the use of v2.x messages for returning clinical genomic results [36, 37]. These genomic implementation guides recommend conventions for coordinate systems (using one-based coordinates), and strand orientation (positive strand), as opposed to explicitly specifying these attributes within the message.

Following upon HL7 v2.x, HL7 produced an XML-based v3 set of standards, which utilizes XML to represent results. This format offers greater verbosity in the attributes that can be represented (improving semantic interoperability), but comes with increased complexity. Recognizing the challenges of incorporating genomic results into this new format, HL7 created an implementation guide for representing genetic test results as a Clinical Document Architecture (CDA) document [38]. The implementation guide provides specific templates (prescriptive structures with a unique object identifier [OID]) for multiple types of genetic and genomic test results, and has sections for different results, like genetic variation, cytogenetics and gene expression.

In the commercial space, the GeneInsight platform [39] also uses an XML format for representing and transmitting reports. As demonstrated within the electronic Medical Records and Genomics (eMERGE) network, this format (which has been made publicly available) allowed two different sequencing centers to transmit results to ten different institutions for use in a clinical setting [40]. The importance of this work is not just as a competing standard, but also in its role as a real-world format for representing sequencing results. These experiences have been used in turn to inform development of other standards. The developers of the GeneInsight XML format have been active contributors to standards development in HL7, and the additional experience gained from the formats used within the eMERGE network will allow additional contributions to another more recent standard—HL7's Fast Healthcare Interoperability Resources (FHIR) [41].

The FHIR standard provides a robust set of resource definitions for many types of healthcare data (clinical and operational). Recognizing the work that the Global Alliance for Genomics and Health (GA4GH) [42] has done in defining standards and application programming interfaces (APIs) for the transmission of genomic data for research purposes, FHIR focuses primarily on the clinical space (although, adoption does not need to be limited to research or clinical domains for any of these standards). As its name indicates, FHIR is built around the concept of "resources," which represent a specific entity (e.g., AllergyIntolerance, Condition, Procedure). FHIR also allows for the definition of profiles and extensions, which allow implementers to build upon existing resources as opposed to creating new ones. Within the omic space, FHIR Draft Standard for Trial Use 2 (DSTU2) defined genetic data within the context of Observation resources, further defined by a genetics profile [43]. More recent work within FHIR DSTU3 has introduced a new Sequence resource specifically to capture sequencing data, while expanding upon profiles on the Observation, DiagnosticReport and ProcedureRequest resources for additional omic use cases. Currently, the FHIR

Sequence resource supports amino acid, DNA and RNA sequences. It supports the inclusion of reference sequence data along with the observed sequence, making an observed resource self-contained when the information is included. Unlike the HL7 v2.x messages, which build upon assumed conventions, the Sequence resource allows the explicit representation of coordinate system and strand orientation. As FHIR also specifies how to structure requests for specific data over APIs as they are needed (as opposed to fully self-contained documents), it represents an attractive standard for integrating OASs and OE-EHRs for real-time data exchange.

Vocabularies, Terminologies and Nomenclatures

In many of the omic data representations previously described, Logical Observation Identifiers Names and Codes (LOINC®) are heavily used to represent results [44]. As a code system that represents both laboratory tests and the resulting clinical observations, LOINC® acts as a rich source for helping to standardize omic data. LOINC® includes test and result codes for variations at the chromosome, gene, and individual SNP level, and has adopted the Human Genome Organization Gene Nomenclature Committee's (HGNC) terminology for naming genes [45], as well as the Human Genome Variation Society's (HGVS) nomenclature for variations [46, 47], and the International System for Human Cytogenetic Nomenclature (ISCN) for cytogenetic tests [48].

Since the 1990s, star alleles for representing pharmacogenetic (PGx) reports have provided a convenient representation of findings [49]. For example, the CYP2C19 gene can provide predictive ability regarding metabolism of the drug clopidogrel. The wild-type (meaning, no variation was found) for this gene is represented as *1, with a homozygous finding represented as *1/*1. Variants are then assigned other numbers—a poor metabolizer with a homozygous variant could be *2/*2. Heterozygous findings are typically represented in ascending numerical order (e.g., *1/*3, *2/*3). These findings are then translated into a clinical interpretation—normal, poor, intermediate or ultra-rapid metabolizer. A limitation with the star allele nomenclature is that it is dependent upon the actual variants checked by a test. In the example of CYP2C19, if the variant associated with the *4 allele is not tested, the interpretation given for a patient may be incorrect. Realizing this, more recent recommendations have been made for PGx result nomenclature [50]. This includes the use of HGNC and HGVS nomenclature, reference sequences, and the identification of variants that can be detected by a laboratory test. To aid in interpretations both under the new nomenclature and under the legacy star allele representation, both representations might be provided simultaneously. It is important for an OAS, then, to consider the need to store multiple representations of the same findings as aliases, as laboratories adopt these new guidelines.

Standards for EHR User Interface Integration

Integration between an OAS and an EHR need not be limited to transmission of messages across interfaces. As OASs gain more traction, the question remains how best to integrate with current day EHRs to allow omic data to be readily accessible and interpretable by healthcare providers. One such standard that we will describe was developed for general clinical use, but has seen increasing adoption in the omic world. The Substitutable Medical Applications and Reusable Technologies (SMART) framework, built using the FHIR data model (referred to as SMART-on-FHIR) [51], allows third party developers to create novel and optimized displays for certain types of clinical data—including omic. The ability to extend existing EHRs with novel displays optimized for omic data has allowed developers and health systems to realize the promise of OE-EHRs [52, 53].

Ethical, Legal and Social Issues

As national programs such as the *All of Us* Research Program in the United States are collecting data, building infrastructure and establishing mechanisms to share data, several important ethical, legal and social challenges have come to light specifically around the broader collection, storage, and use of omic data. Two key considerations for the use of an omic-enabled EHR are the potential for genetic discrimination and the management of genomic results with uncertain clinical significance.

One important consideration is who should receive and use personal genomic information, with insurance companies and relatives being of particular relevance. In the United States, the *Genetic Information Nondiscrimination Act* (GINA) prohibits insurers from using genetic information in health insurance decisions, but there is no prevention against this practice in life insurance or long-term care insurance. As an example of family considerations, it is only recently that Meaningful Use Stage 2 required EHRs to capture family history as structured data for at least one first-degree relative [54]. It is not commonplace for a health system to have a direct link between a patient's record and a family member's record (making sharing of familial information, like genomics, possible).

In traditional research settings, the establishment of an omic-enabled EHR has the potential to bring new challenges as information with uncertain clinical significance could be presented to the healthcare provider based upon patient preferences or institutional policies for returning results. To date, programs such as the electronic Medical Records and Genomics (eMERGE) Network in the United States have simplified the challenge of returning uncertain information by differentiating return of results from patient care. While project findings are often fed back to participants at affiliated healthcare practices by their healthcare providers, it is made clear that the results are as part of a research study to which they consented and are not part of their patient care. Many questions and concerns raised by the Institutional Review Boards (IRBs) of eMERGE institutions were related to the consent process (e.g., balancing detail and readability), and communicating results (e.g., counseling, and mechanisms to answer questions) [55]. Challenges with implications for an omic-enabled EHR included differentiating actionable genes in adult and pediatric populations and providing options for participants to receive limited results or to withdraw from the study at a later stage. Within the EHR this requires capturing life-stage (adult vs. pediatric) and participant preferences.

Cost Considerations

Having discussed the benefits of an OAS, a consideration is if there are compelling reasons for a healthcare institution to take on the cost of storing additional omic data versus requesting new tests and just storing a laboratory report. We do not attempt to assess the entire economic impact of a precision medicine program, but specifically look at the storage and reuse of omic data.

To help quantify this, we will use the Renaissance Computing Institute's (RENCI's) proposed archival value criterion (AVC) [56]. The AVC is defined as:

$$AVC = \frac{P_{reuse} \times S'}{S} \tag{17.1}$$

where:

P_{reuse} = the estimated probability that the stored data will be reused
S' = the cost to re-generate the data
S = the total cost to curate and store the data

A higher AVC indicates that there is likely more value to archiving the data, and a lower AVC indicates that there may be more value in regenerating the data. Many considerations go into these factors, including the availability of the storage (fast or archival) and adjustments over time as sequencing costs and storage costs both change. We note that there are two considerations not explicitly accounted for in the AVC calculation, but that can be incorporated in the analysis. The first is the depreciation of the data. As improvements to sequencing technologies are made, we need to consider if we still want to use 5- or 10-year-old sequencing results or if we may have more reliable data from resequencing. The second consideration is the number of times the data is accessed, both for clinical and research purposes. If omic data is obtained once, and can be used clinically as well as for multiple research studies, the overall value of the data increases.

For considering costs, a 2016 study at Partners HealthCare estimated (after initial sequencing costs) their total internal cost to process and store a single genome is around $245 per year [57]. This includes an estimate of approximately $40–$55 for storage only, depending on if the genome is placed on secondary (archival) storage, or primary (fast) storage, respectively. Given that they are performing the whole analysis pipeline (including the storage of FASTA, BAM and VCF files at ~300 GB total per genome), these costs do not entirely reflect what an OAS would incur. A 2014 study estimated the total upstream costs to generate WGS data clinically were closer to $10,000 [58], although costs for WGS have decreased since then. Most recent estimates from NHGRI put the cost of a sequence at around $1500 for a research setting. We will then consider four price points for the cost of re-generating a sequence: $10,000 [58], $1500 [59], $250 and $100 (the latter two being ideal future cost). For storage, we will use four price points as well: $55, $40, $25 and $10. The first two are fast and archival storage from [57], respectively. The $25 and $10 play two roles in estimation—they can be seen as ideal future states as storage costs decrease, and also a reduced cost for less storage per sequence as higher estimates [57] reflect storage costs for FASTA, BAM and VCF files. For the OAS, we may just receive (or just choose to store) the VCF.

To simplify the discussion, we are assuming that the probability of reusing the data is guaranteed. Given the amount of omic research, it is highly likely that the data would be used at least for a research study. We show estimated AVC values for these different cost points in Fig. 17.4, where the size of the circle correlates to the AVC value.

The RENCI report recommends that with an AVC of 100 or higher, archival is an effective solution. Using this threshold, we can see points where it may be preferential to regenerate a sequence (especially as cost goes down) as opposed to storing it in an OAS. However, the AVC should be used purely as a guideline, as there are some considerations mentioned above not directly reflected in these calculations.

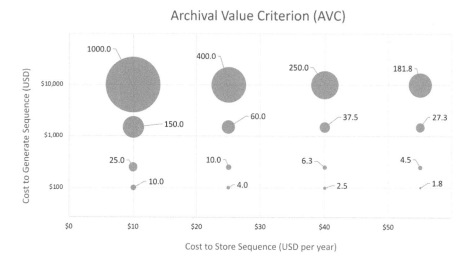

Fig. 17.4 Estimated Archival Value Criterion (AVC) calculations for several estimated costs to sequence and store omics data. The size of the circle represents the AVC, with a larger circle better justifying archiving the data

Conclusion

As we have described, the multiple facets of omics data make their integration into the EHR a different challenge than that of routinely collected clinical data. We present the concept of the omic ancillary system as a mechanism by which we can embrace the complexities of omic data in a special environment, similar to how radiological images are handled by PACS. As data moves through the four stages of the "Omic Funnel"—*Omic Data, Biological Information, Clinical Knowledge,* and *Action*—the OAS may be introduced at any stage, depending on the needs of the implementing institution. Ultimately, the goal of the omic-enabled EHR is to facilitate the *Action* stage within clinical workflows, including the use of both active and passive clinical decision support. These critical supports allow healthcare providers and patients to make better use of the increased volume of data that comes with precision medicine. While we note that much work that has been done in this area, we have also highlighted opportunities for ongoing and future research for health and biomedical informatics practitioners. This includes implementing and evaluating the systems and standards that support interoperability, weighing the cost and benefit tradeoffs inherent in managing omic data, and considering the ethical, legal, and social issues that come with genetic and genomic results.

Author Disclosures

Therese A. Nelson and Casey L. Overby Taylor have no relevant disclosures. Abdulrahman M. Jahhaf is the founder and CEO of GROA, a health information technology company. GROA is not directly related to the content of this chapter. Luke V. Rasmussen, Timothy M. Herr and Justin B. Starren are part of an initiative to commercialize an omics ancillary system developed at Northwestern University. The initiative did not fund or influence the content of this chapter, and no proprietary information is contained within. Timothy M. Herr and Justin B. Starren received research funding from AbbVie for an unrelated project.

References

1. Concert Genetics. The current landscape of genetic testing: market growth, reimbursement trends, challenges and opportunities [Internet]. http://www.concertgenetics.com/wp-content/uploads/2018/04/12_ConcertGenetics_CurrentLandscapeOfGeneticTesting2018.pdf.
2. Landrum MJ, Lee JM, Riley GR, Jang W, Rubinstein WS, Church DM, et al. ClinVar: public archive of relationships among sequence variation and human phenotype. Nucleic Acids Res. 2014;42:D980–5.
3. Yang S, Lincoln SE, Kobayashi Y, Nykamp K, Nussbaum RL, Topper S. Sources of discordance among germ-line variant classifications in ClinVar. Genet Med. 2017;19:1118–26.

4. Shirts BH, Salama JS, Aronson SJ, Chung WK, Gray SW, Hindorff LA, et al. CSER and eMERGE: current and potential state of the display of genetic information in the electronic health record. J Am Med Inf Assoc. 2015;22:1231–42.
5. Whelton PK, Carey RM, Aronow WS, Casey DE Jr, Collins KJ, Dennison Himmelfarb C, et al. 2017 ACC/AHA/AAPA/ABC/ACPM/AGS/APhA/ASH/ASPC/NMA/PCNA guideline for the prevention, detection, evaluation, and management of high blood pressure in adults: executive summary: a report of the American College of Cardiology/American Heart Association Task Force. Hypertension. 2018;71:1269–324.
6. Green RC, Berg JS, Grody WW, Kalia SS, Korf BR, Martin CL, et al. ACMG recommendations for reporting of incidental findings in clinical exome and genome sequencing. Genet Med. 2013;15:565–74. http://www.nature.com/articles/gim201373.
7. Kalia SS, Adelman K, Bale SJ, Chung WK, Eng C, Evans JP, et al. Recommendations for reporting of secondary findings in clinical exome and genome sequencing, 2016 update (ACMG SF v2.0): a policy statement of the American College of Medical Genetics and Genomics. Genet Med. 2017;19:249–55. http://www.ncbi.nlm.nih.gov/pubmed/27854360.
8. Starren J, Williams MS, Bottinger EP. Crossing the omic chasm: a time for omic ancillary systems. JAMA. 2013;309:1237–8.
9. Masys DR, Jarvik GP, Abernethy NF, Anderson NR, Papanicolaou GJ, Paltoo DN, et al. Technical desiderata for the integration of genomic data into electronic health records. J Biomed Inform. 2012;45:419–22. http://www.ncbi.nlm.nih.gov/pubmed/22223081.
10. Hoffman MA. The genome-enabled electronic medical record. J Biomed Inf. 2007;40:44–6.
11. Warner JL, Jain SK, Levy MA. Integrating cancer genomic data into electronic health records. Genome Med. 2016;8:113.
12. Jacob HJ, Abrams K, Bick DP, Brodie K, Dimmock DP, Farrell M, et al. Genomics in clinical practice: lessons from the front lines. Sci Transl Med. 2013;5:194cm5.
13. Korf BR, Berry AB, Limson M, Marian AJ, Murray MF, O'Rourke PP, et al. Framework for development of physician competencies in genomic medicine: report of the Competencies Working Group of the Inter-Society Coordinating Committee for Physician Education in Genomics. Genet Med. 2014;16:804–9.
14. Kho AN, Rasmussen LV, Connolly JJ, Peissig PL, Starren J, Hakonarson H, et al. Practical challenges in integrating genomic data into the electronic health record. Genet Med. 2013;15:772–8.
15. Herr TM, Bielinski SJ, Bottinger E, Brautbar A, Brilliant M, Chute CG, et al. A conceptual model for translating omic data into clinical action. J Pathol Inform. 2015;6:46. http://www.ncbi.nlm.nih.gov/pubmed/26430534.
16. Li H, Handsaker B, Wysoker A, Fennell T, Ruan J, Homer N, et al. The sequence alignment/map format and SAMtools. Bioinformatics. 2009;25:2078–9. https://www.ncbi.nlm.nih.gov/pubmed/19505943.
17. Danecek P, Auton A, Abecasis G, Albers CA, Banks E, DePristo MA, et al. The variant call format and VCFtools. Bioinformatics. 2011;27:2156–8.
18. Sherry ST, Ward MH, Kholodov M, Baker J, Phan L, Smigielski EM, et al. dbSNP: the NCBI database of genetic variation. Nucleic Acids Res. 2001;29:308–11. https://www.ncbi.nlm.nih.gov/pubmed/11125122.
19. Caudle KE, Klein TE, Hoffman JM, Muller DJ, Whirl-Carrillo M, Gong L, et al. Incorporation of pharmacogenomics into routine clinical practice: the Clinical Pharmacogenetics Implementation Consortium (CPIC) guideline development process. Curr Drug Metab. 2014;15:209–17. http://www.ncbi.nlm.nih.gov/pubmed/24479687.
20. Cimino JJ. Infobuttons: anticipatory passive decision support. In: AMIA Annual Symposium Proceedings. Washington, DC: American Medical Informatics Association; 2008. p. 1203–4.
21. Phansalkar S, van der Sijs H, Tucker AD, Desai AA, Bell DS, Teich JM, et al. Drug-drug interactions that should be non-interruptive in order to reduce alert fatigue in electronic health records. J Am Med Inform Assoc. 2013;20:489–93. https://www.ncbi.nlm.nih.gov/pubmed/23011124.

22. Rasmussen-Torvik LJ, Stallings SC, Gordon AS, Almoguera B, Basford MA, Bielinski SJ, et al. Design and anticipated outcomes of the eMERGE-PGx project: a multicenter pilot for preemptive pharmacogenomics in electronic health record systems. Clin Pharmacol Ther. 2014;96:482–9.

23. Dunnenberger HM, Crews KR, Hoffman JM, Caudle KE, Broeckel U, Howard SC, et al. Preemptive clinical pharmacogenetics implementation: current programs in five US medical centers. Annu Rev Pharmacol Toxicol. 2015;55:89–106. http://www.ncbi.nlm.nih.gov/pubmed/25292429.

24. Gottesman O, Scott SA, Ellis SB, Overby CL, Ludtke A, Hulot JS, et al. The CLIPMERGE PGx program: clinical implementation of personalized medicine through electronic health records and genomics-pharmacogenomics. Clin Pharmacol Ther. 2013;94:214–7. http://www.ncbi.nlm.nih.gov/pubmed/23588317.

25. Bell GC, Crews KR, Wilkinson MR, Haidar CE, Hicks JK, Baker DK, et al. Development and use of active clinical decision support for preemptive pharmacogenomics. J Am Med Inform Assoc. 2014;21:e93–9. http://www.ncbi.nlm.nih.gov/pubmed/23978487.

26. Heale B, Overby C, Del Fiol G, Rubinstein W, Maglott D, Nelson T, et al. Integrating genomic resources with electronic health records using the HL7 Infobutton standard. Appl Clin Inform. 2016;7:817–31. http://www.ncbi.nlm.nih.gov/pubmed/27579472.

27. Davis FD, Bagozzi RP, Warshaw PR. User acceptance of computer-technology—a comparison of 2 theoretical-models. Manag Sci. 1989;35:982–1003.

28. Goodhue DL, Thompson RL. Task-technology fit and individual-performance. MIS Q. 1995;19:213–36.

29. Ammenwerth E, Iller C, Mahler C. IT-adoption and the interaction of task, technology and individuals: a fit framework and a case study. BMC Med Inf Decis Mak. 2006;6:–3. http://www.ncbi.nlm.nih.gov/pubmed/16401336.

30. Davis FD. Perceived usefulness, perceived ease of use, and user acceptance of information technology. MIS Q. 1989;13:319–40.

31. O'Day VL, Bobrow DG, Shirley M. The social-technical design circle. In: Proc 1996 ACM conf comput support coop work. New York: ACM; 1996. p. 160–9.

32. Baxter G, Sommerville I. Socio-technical systems: from design methods to systems engineering. Interact Comput. 2011;23:4–17. http://iwc.oxfordjournals.org/content/23/1/4.full.pdf.

33. Koberg D, Bagnall J. The universal traveller: a soft-systems guide to creativity, problem-solving, and the process of reaching goals. Los Altos, CA: Kaufmann; 1976.

34. Samtools. The variant call format specification [Internet]. 2018. https://samtools.github.io/hts-specs/VCFv4.3.pdf.

35. Li H. Tabix: fast retrieval of sequence features from generic TAB-delimited files. Bioinformatics. 2011;27:718–9.

36. Health Level Seven International. HL7 version 2.5.1 implementation guide: Lab Results Interface (LRI), release 1, STU release 3—US Realm. 2017.

37. Health Level Seven International. HL7 version 2 implementation guide: clinical genomics; fully LOINC-qualified genetic variation model, release 2. 2013.

38. Health Level Seven International. HL7 implementation guide for CDA® release 2: Genetic Testing Report (GTR), DSTU release 1. 2013.

39. Aronson SJ, Clark EH, Babb LJ, Baxter S, Farwell LM, Funke BH, et al. The GeneInsight Suite: a platform to support laboratory and provider use of DNA-based genetic testing. Hum Mutat. 2011;32:532–6.

40. Aronson S, Babb L, Ames D, Gibbs RA, Venner E, Connelly JJ, et al. Empowering genomic medicine by establishing critical sequencing result data flows: the eMERGE example. J Am Med Inform Assoc. 2018;25:1375–81. https://doi.org/10.1093/jamia/ocy051.

41. Health Level Seven International. Overview—FHIR v3.0.1 [Internet]. 2018. https://www.hl7.org/fhir/overview.html.

42. Global Alliance for Genomics and Health. Work streams [Internet]. 2018. https://www.ga4gh.org/howwework/workstreams/.

43. Health Level Seven International. Genomics—FHIR v3.0.1 [Internet]. 2018. https://www.hl7.org/fhir/genomics.html.
44. Deckard J, McDonald CJ, Vreeman DJ. Supporting interoperability of genetic data with LOINC. J Am Med Inform Assoc. 2015;22:621–7. https://doi.org/10.1093/jamia/ocu012.
45. Gray KA, Yates B, Seal RL, Wright MW, Bruford EA. Genenames.org: the HGNC resources in 2015. Nucleic Acids Res. 2015;43:D1079–85.
46. Dunnen JT, Dalgleish R, Maglott DR, Hart RK, Greenblatt MS, McGowan-Jordan J, et al. HGVS recommendations for the description of sequence variants: 2016 update. Hum Mutat. 2016;37:564–9. https://onlinelibrary.wiley.com/doi/abs/10.1002/humu.22981.
47. Horaitis O, Cotton RG. The challenge of documenting mutation across the genome: the human genome variation society approach. Hum Mutat. 2004;23:447–52.
48. Stevens-Kroef M, Simons A, Rack K, Hastings RJ. Cytogenetic nomenclature and reporting. Methods Mol Biol. 2017;1541:303–9.
49. Robarge JD, Li L, Desta Z, Nguyen A, Flockhart DA. The star-allele nomenclature: retooling for translational genomics. Clin Pharmacol Ther. 2007;82:244–8.
50. Kalman LV, Agúndez JAG, Appell ML, Black JL, Bell GC, Boukouvala S, et al. Pharmacogenetic allele nomenclature: international workgroup recommendations for test result reporting. Clin Pharmacol Ther. 2016;99:172–85. https://ascpt.onlinelibrary.wiley.com/doi/abs/10.1002/cpt.280.
51. Mandel JC, Kreda DA, Mandl KD, Kohane IS, Ramoni RB. SMART on FHIR: a standards-based, interoperable apps platform for electronic health records. J Am Med Inform Assoc. 2016;23:899–908. https://doi.org/10.1093/jamia/ocv189.
52. Warner JL, Rioth MJ, Mandl KD, Mandel JC, Kreda DA, Kohane IS, et al. SMART precision cancer medicine: a FHIR-based app to provide genomic information at the point of care. J Am Med Inform Assoc. 2016;23:701–10. https://doi.org/10.1093/jamia/ocw015.
53. Alterovitz G, Warner J, Zhang P, Chen Y, Ullman-Cullere M, Kreda D, et al. SMART on FHIR genomics: facilitating standardized clinico-genomic apps. J Am Med Inform Assoc. 2015;22:1173–8.
54. Office of the National Coordinator for Health Information Technology (ONC). 2015 Edition Health Information Technology (Health IT) certification criteria, 2015 Edition Base Electronic Health Record (EHR) definition, and ONC Health IT certification program modifications [Internet]. p. 62601–759. http://www.federalregister.gov/a/2015-25597/p-307.
55. Fossey R, Kochan D, Winkler E, Pacyna JE, Olson J, Thibodeau S, et al. Ethical considerations related to return of results from genomic medicine projects: the eMERGE network (phase III) experience. J Pers Med. 2018;8:E2.
56. Wilhelmsen KC, Schmitt CP, Fecho K. Factors influencing data archival of large-scale genomic data sets. RENCI Tech. Rep. Ser. Chapel Hill, NC: University of North Carolina at Chapel Hill; 2013.
57. Tsai E, Shakbatyan R, Evans J, Rossetti P, Graham C, Sharma H, et al. Bioinformatics work-flow for clinical whole genome sequencing at partners healthcare personalized medicine. J Pers Med. 2016;6:12. http://www.mdpi.com/2075-4426/6/1/12
58. Dewey FE, Grove ME, Pan C, Goldstein BA, Bernstein JA, Chaib H, et al. Clinical interpretation and implications of whole-genome sequencing. JAMA. 2014;311:1035–45.
59. Wetterstrand K. DNA sequencing costs: data from the NHGRI Genome Sequencing Program (GSP) [Internet]. 2018. https://www.genome.gov/sequencingcostsdata.

Chapter 18
Generalizable Architectures and Principles of Informatics for Scalable Personalized and Precision Medicine (PPM) Decision Support

Steven G. Johnson, Pamala Jacobson, Susan M. Wolf, Kingshuk K. Sinha, Douglas Yee, and Constantin Aliferis

S. G. Johnson
Institute for Health Informatics, University of Minnesota,
Minneapolis, MN, USA

Division for Informatics Innovation Dissemination, University of Minnesota,
Minneapolis, MN, USA
e-mail: joh06288@umn.edu

P. Jacobson
Department of Experimental and Clinical Pharmacology, College of Pharmacy, University of Minnesota, Minneapolis, MN, USA

Division of Hematology, Oncology and Transplantation, Medical School, University of Minnesota, Minneapolis, MN, USA
e-mail: jacob117@umn.edu

S. M. Wolf
Law School, University of Minnesota, Minneapolis, MN, USA

Department of Medicine, Medical School, University of Minnesota,
Minneapolis, MN, USA

Consortium on Law and Values in Health, Environment and the Life Sciences,
University of Minnesota, Minneapolis, MN, USA
e-mail: swolf@umn.edu

K. K. Sinha
Department of Supply Chain and Operations, Carlson School of Management,
University of Minnesota, Minneapolis, MN, USA

Bioinformatics and Computational Biology, University of Minnesota, Minneapolis,
MN, USA
e-mail: ksinha@umn.edu

D. Yee
Division of Hematology, Oncology and Transplantation, Medical School, University of Minnesota, Minneapolis, MN, USA

© Springer Nature Switzerland AG 2020
T. Adam, C. Aliferis (eds.), *Personalized and Precision Medicine Informatics*,
Health Informatics, https://doi.org/10.1007/978-3-030-18626-5_18

Masonic Cancer Center, University of Minnesota, Minneapolis, MN, USA

Department of Pharmacology, Medical School, University of Minnesota,
Minneapolis, MN, USA

Microbiology, Immunology and Cancer Biology (MICaB) PhD Graduate Program,
University of Minnesota, Minneapolis, MN, USA
e-mail: yeexx006@umn.edu

C. Aliferis (✉)
Institute for Health Informatics, Department of Medicine, School of Medicine Clinical and
Translational Science Institute, Masonic Cancer Center, Program in Data Science,
University of Minnesota, Minneapolis, MN, USA
e-mail: califeri@umn.edu

Introduction

As we have seen in this book, Personalized and Precision Medicine (PPM) has huge
variability in its formats and workflows. One of the *invariants* across all PPM formats however, is the need to deliver personalized decision support at the point of
care. Related to this goal are the requirements for storing potentially massive
amounts of patient genetics and other "omics" data that go beyond traditional clinical data types, the need for protecting sensitive genetic information from abuse, the
need to ensure that decision support is based on solid and up-to-date scientific evidence, the need to translate treatment guidelines to decision rules correctly, and the
need to integrate clinical care with discovery.

In addition, PPM results and data need to be interoperable and be delivered to
patients and populations across diverse health systems, electronic health records
(EHR), and state boundaries. Furthermore, PPM delivery systems exist in an ethical, legal, and social issues (ELSI) context, including the complex and fragmented
form of the US healthcare system.

This chapter describes a general-purpose informatics architecture to enable
scalable PPM decision support, and then uses two specific customizations (pharmacogenomics for a single institution and pharmacogenomics implemented in a
state-wide network) in order to illustrate important infrastructure details. Because
the chapter is focused on general methods and not specific institutional implementations, we present methods that are institution-independent and thus have
the broadest applicability possible. We not only describe the components needed
to implement successful decision support, but also the architectures that enable
large scale PPM decision support to be deployed on a state-wide or even national
scale.

Components of a Scalable PPM Informatics Architecture

There has been significant progress over the past decade in incorporating genomic data into the process of healthcare. Results from the eMERGE Network, for example, provide important data points about what is possible and what is required to make clinical and research use of genetic information successful [1–3]. In another example, the PREDICT Project has provided a model for how to implement prospective pharmacogenomics decision support at the point of care [4].

Figure 18.1 shows high-level architectural components needed to implement scalable informatics for PPM in an application-agnostic manner [5].

The architecture consists of a Clinical Decision Support (CDS) system that computes patient-specific recommendations and enables actionable workflows, a PPM database (PPM DB) to hold individualized data about patients, a clinical knowledge repository (CKR) that describes scientific evidence connecting PPM data and recommended care actions, an EHR that creates and maintains a transactional record of

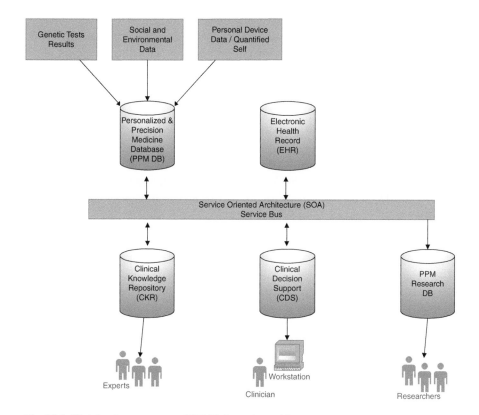

Fig. 18.1 High-level components of PPM informatics architecture

patients' clinical care data, and a research database used to conduct research to evaluate the effectiveness of the CDS and discover new knowledge related to improved patient care (also supporting Learning Health System functions). The challenge of PPM informatics is to ensure that the data and knowledge sources and the data streams that connect them, as well as the constantly changing clinical knowledge, are brought together and interpreted so that appropriate decision support can be delivered to a clinician when it is needed to have impact in the clinical workflow. Because the information is required for patient care, it must be delivered reliably, quickly, and securely.

Service Oriented Architecture (SOA)

A scalable informatics architecture must accommodate new types of data, new PPM methods, and the exponential growth of both omic data and clinical knowledge. A SOA [6] is one of the most effective ways to connect PPM components while giving flexibility for each component to evolve without interdependence on the others. A SOA is a distributed computing system that enables multiple independent components/applications (called *nodes*) to interact with each other using a communication protocol. The architecture allows any of the nodes to invoke services of any of the other nodes, subject to appropriate authentication and authorization credentials. The benefit of the architecture is that it allows additional nodes to be added and failed nodes to be removed at any time. The nodes are loosely coupled to minimize interdependency. In addition, the service-oriented architecture can facilitate *horizontal scaling*, meaning that additional nodes that perform the same function can be added in order to distribute a workload across more worker nodes.

Figure 18.2 shows a typical SOA. The architecture is split into a set of layers that are connected by a *Service Bus*. *Client* applications make requests for services. The requests can use standard protocols, such as Representational State Transfer (REST), or proprietary protocols. In either case, request messages are initially received by *Load Balancers*. The Load Balancers are the only systems that need to be exposed externally and connected to the internet. They reside in a so-called DMZ (*demilitarized zone*) to indicate that these are the only systems that hackers or malicious actors may access, while the actual servers can be more deeply protected. The Load Balancers send each incoming request message to the least busy server in the Web Layer. The Web Layer's job is to identify what type of service (API) is being requested and route the message over the service bus to the appropriate application server residing inside the Application Layer. This layer is composed of a number of application servers that communicate only via the service bus. There are different services available across the application servers. The incoming message from the client serves as a trigger to invoke a service that will then trigger additional requests on the service bus to other application servers/services. The service bus uses a *publish/subscribe design* where application servers that know how to execute a specific

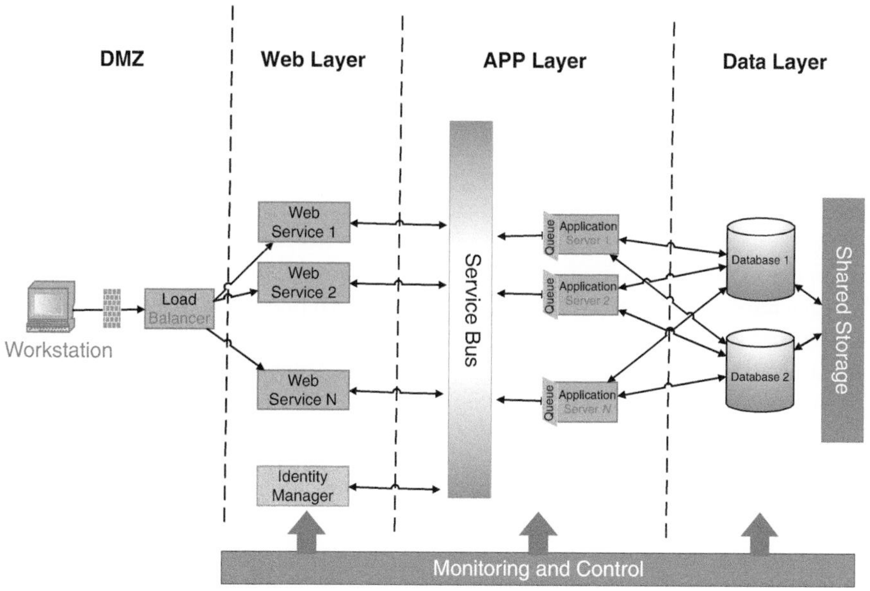

Fig. 18.2 Service-oriented architecture

type of request will subscribe to those types of events. When a message of that type comes in, the web layer will publish the event to the service bus and the next available application server will take that message and process it. The publish/subscribe paradigm also supports event-driven programming which makes it much easier and safer to keep different parts of the system loosely coupled so that changes or updates to one part of the system do not interfere with other system components [7].

The publish/subscribe architecture also allows future services to be added that respond to specific types of requests that can do additional work. For example, an incoming request to perform a CDS recommendation could be executed by a CDS application server. But that same message can also be subscribed to by a service that archives all incoming CDS requests into a research database that can be analyzed to understand the types of CDS that are being requested. Neither service needs to be aware of the other to do its job. The Web Layer may also transform and standardize the message for use by application servers. It will also hold session state and route the response message back to the client.

SOA Scalability

The advantage to the service bus approach is better application control and horizontal scaling, that is, ability to scale up the infrastructure by adding more servers performing the same tasks. Each application or service has a persistent queue where incoming requests are stored. As worker processes for that service become available, they pull the next piece of work from the queue and process it. If a queue has too much work in it, another application server/worker can be added so that work can be processed faster. This is how horizontal scaling is supported. Monitoring software can periodically check all of the queues to obtain statistics for how quickly work is being processed, types of errors and performance issues. This data can be used to dynamically add more application servers of different types to keep the overall system performant. The system is also more resilient to interruption because it can detect non-responding application servers or have some type of error condition and remove them from the service bus and add a replacement application server.

Another advantage of using the service bus architecture is improved safety when updating services. Because the services are loosely coupled, a single type of service can usually be upgraded without having to upgrade other services at the same time. This allows for safer deployments since smaller parts of the system can be changed and, if there is a problem, the change can be rolled-back to its prior version. In fact, many organizations are able to achieve continuous deployment; changes to services can be deployed into production as soon as they have been sufficiently tested. This allows the overall system to have stability, yet evolve quickly.

Security, Authentication and Encryption

Security and authentication are critical aspects of the scalable informatics architecture. In the architecture depicted in Fig. 18.3, an *Identity Manager* sits outside the system, but is callable from the system. The Identity Manager provides a service that returns a token that is unique for each individual or machine that is allowed to

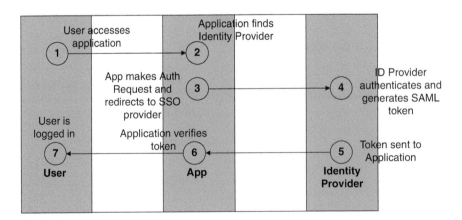

Fig. 18.3 OAuth Identity Transaction. A user (individual or application) initiates a request for a resource and is redirected to an Identity Provider where they prove their identity (via username/password and/or two-factor authentication). If authentication is successful, a token is passed back to the App indicating the user's identity

use the system. The Identity Manager can use a simple username/password authentication, or it can be more sophisticated and rely on stricter two-factor authentication or public key certificates. OAuth is a standard protocol that is used by many systems to facilitate an identity verification transaction [8].

After a user or machine's identity is verified, then the system can ask the Identity Manager what specific rights the user has for different services within the system. This information is securely available using a protocol called SAML [9]. SAML and OAuth work together to ensure incoming requests are executed only if they are appropriate. The Identity Manager can be provided as a service for just the specific application or shared by many applications across an organization (e.g., a hospital's Microsoft Active Directory).

Clinical Decision Support (CDS)

A CDS system is any software that assists in making clinical decisions [10]. Clinical decision support within an EHR evaluates data in the medical record (using CDS rules) to make recommendations. A typical CDS action is an alert that displays (1) a message explaining why the alert was triggered, (2) a substantive actionable recommendation, and (3) the evidence for the recommendation. The alert can display recommended interventions as text or simplify recommended order entries with specific attributes (such as medication doses). CDS technology can allow healthcare organizations to encode clinical best practices into rules and recommendations to inform and support clinical decisions and actions. CDS is therefore a critical mechanism for grounding PPM recommendations in a clinical knowledge repository to make information seamlessly available to the physician in the EHR within their clinical workflow [11].

Clinical Decision Support Architecture

A clinical decision support system consists of three primary components: *triggers, CDS rules, and intervention recommendations* [12]. Triggers are events that kick-off the CDS workflow. A trigger is typically an event that occurs during a clinical encounter. For example, triggers include events such as an order initiation, a patient admission, discharge or transfer, or a lab result becoming available in the EHR. PPM may require simple (e.g., medication order) or complicated (e.g., complex phenotype detection) triggers. Typically, complex trigger processing happens at a CDS external to the EHR.

When a trigger event is detected, the CDS process connected to it is launched. When the CDS process is initiated, the first thing that occurs is data that the CDS needs is retrieved from the EHR in order to compute a recommendation. The knowledge of clinical best practices is embodied within the CDS as rules stored in a Clinical Knowledge Repository (CKR). The CDS rules implement clinical guidelines and best practices to determine a recommendation. The CDS retrieves a set of rules from the CKR that ultimately produces advice and recommendations to send back to the clinician. The CDS rules need EHR-derived patient data and they may also need additional data external to the EHR such as genomic data. Once all the data are available, the CDS rules are executed one-by-one. The result of one rule can trigger another rule in a forward rule chaining cascade. At the end of the process, the CDS rules produce a set of recommendations as a response. Filtering and prioritization of CDS rules may also be applied to reduce "alert fatigue" experienced when too many rules of marginal value (for a clinician-context combination) are generated.

The recommendations can be simple messages that are displayed to the clinician or they can be complex actions that the CDS helps improve clinical performance. Some recommendations may also include assessments about the benefits and risks associated with the advice. The ultimate decision on how to use a recommendation typically rests with the clinician, but once they make that decision, the CDS can help execute it as well. For example, if the recommendation is to prescribe or administer a specific medication, the CDS may compute the appropriate dose, display the correct order for that medication, and enter it into the EHR. The clinician then has the option to agree with the recommendation to complete the order, or bypass the recommendation if in her judgment it does not apply.

Clinical decision support is implemented in two ways: *within an EHR* or as a *separate, external system* that performs the CDS functions and interfaces with the EHR.

CDS Within a Single EHR

If a healthcare system uses a single EHR throughout its entire organization, then CDS can be implemented completely within that EHR. In part due to Meaningful Use, most modern EHRs have some ability to implement CDS [13]. In such setups, the trigger events, rules and interventions are all part of the EHR. The benefit of a CDS implementation within an EHR is that the EHR vendor has ensured that the CDS works well within the defined clinical workflows and can access the necessary EHR data. But the main downside is that every EHR vendor implements CDS in different ways. Differences across different EHRs include the list of which events cause triggers, the way to specify triggers, the syntax and capabilities of the rules, and the list of possible recommendations/actions/interventions. In addition, some EHRs support powerful features such as recommendations that create orders to be signed by the clinician, while others only display informational messages. Also, some EHRs support meta-data about each alert which is saved to analyze how useful the CDS is and whether alert fatigue is a problem.

EHR vendors have in some cases created CDS content that providers can use "out of the box," such as sepsis surveillance and anti-microbial screening. However, most CDS must be implemented by each provider organization, and vendor–provided ones need to be evaluated for appropriateness for the specific population served by that provider. Currently there is no easy way to share CDS and best practices across organizations [14]. CDS Hooks is an initiative to standardize CDS across all EHRs. Its goal is to make it easier to create CDS that specifies all aspects of the triggers, rules and interventions that can be implemented in *any* EHR [15, 16]. CDS Hooks will also provide a standard way for external programs (especially SMART apps [17]) to interact with the clinician during the delivery of the CDS.

An integral dimension of a successful CDS is its evaluation. Measures of success can include improved patient outcomes, reduced complications, adverse events avoided, and reduced healthcare costs. The meta-data about how well the CDS alerts perform is held within the EHR, but it may be hard to discern from the raw EHR data what the patient outcome actually was. Organizations often have to implement various manual or automated approaches to determining patient outcomes of interest in order to analyze the effectiveness of the CDS alerts.

CDS Across Multiple EHRs

Complications occur when CDS is implemented across an organization with multiple EHRs or across multiple organizations. There are two approaches when multiple EHRs are used by an organization. The first is to implement all aspects of a CDS initiative in each EHR using that EHR's proprietary approach to CDS. When there are many organizations with many different types of EHRs, this could result in each EHR having different rule sets and different trigger events.

An attractive alternative is to implement the CDS in a centralized system outside of any of the EHRs [18]. This has the advantage of creating a single set of CDS rules, a common point for triggering the CDS, and a consistent recommendation produced by the CDS. In this approach, the CDS components of an EHR are still used to initiate a CDS process on the central CDS service. In an EHR, a trigger event will create a message to be sent to the central CDS server instead of launching the CDS process within the EHR. This message initiates a CDS service on the central server using a set of CDS rules to compute the recommendation. The central CDS still needs to see the relevant patient clinical data, which now must be sent by the EHR as part of the service request. Usually, the CDS pulls the relevant data from the EHR as a separate transaction through a protocol such as Fast Healthcare Interoperability Resources (FHIR) [19]. FHIR provides a standard way to retrieve patient data from the EHR. The central CDS computes the recommendation and then sends the result back in a response message. The EHR CDS must be able to take that message and process it into the appropriate recommendations. Most EHRs can only perform simple actions today such as displaying a message. Some can create an order to be approved by the clinician. As mentioned previously, it is the goal of CDS Hooks to make the request and response standard available on all EHR systems. The response should allow complex actions to be initiated in the EHR.

In the case of CDS across systems, it is also more efficient to have a single central repository for shared patient outcomes data to support comparative outcomes research. Data from each EHR related to the alerts and patient outcomes should be sent to the central repository on a periodic basis for reporting and analytics.

One of the major advantages of a centralized CDS is that the clinical knowledge for best practices and clinical guidelines are embodied in the rules and are in one place. If guidance needs to be updated or clinical knowledge changed, rules need to be updated only in a central repository. The rules are not scattered across multiple EHRs using different syntax and tools for maintenance. Since the same rules and data expectations are used, outcomes analysis is easier than trying to standardize across multiple systems.

The disadvantages of this approach are that since the CDS is outside the EHR, a network connection to the central CDS must always be available. In fact, the CDS should be architected with high-availability and performance in mind. The service bus architecture described earlier can be adapted to support a highly scalable, centralized CDS system (see Fig. 18.4). The design is similar to architectures already in successful use by commercial CDS vendors (such as Wolters Kluwer, Premier, and Vigilanz) that reliably support *millions of incoming transactions per day, across hundreds of diverse provider systems, with 99.9% availability, serving tens of thousands of simultaneous users and hosted in HIPAA-compliant and secure environments* [20, 21]. These results provide strong evidence in support of the premise that the presented architecture is scalable, interoperable, and overall performant.

In this architecture, the EHR must still handle the event triggers and intervention recommendations. The events of interest are set up as triggers within the EHR. When a trigger occurs, the EHR sends a request to the central CDS using the EHR's proprietary mechanisms and protocols. For example, we can use the EHR's ability to send an https request to the central CDS webservice. The EHR will send the request

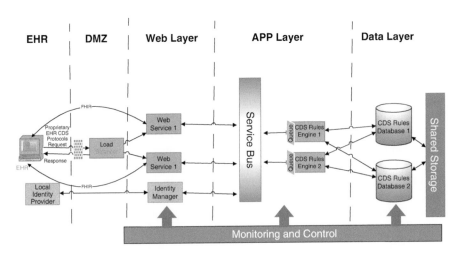

Fig. 18.4 Scalable CDS application architecture

with information such as the patient and encounter ID. Then the central CDS service can request the additional data it needs in a separate transaction using standards such as FHIR. The central CDS service initiates the request and waits for the data response. Once the data are received, the central CDS service can execute the CDS rules to generate a recommended intervention. The recommendation is sent back using the proprietary mechanisms supported by the EHR. For example, some EHRs support a *synchronous transaction model* by having the initial request wait for a response. Other EHRs work *asynchronously* and require that a separate response be sent to a queue service of the EHR. In this case, the response must contain the request transaction id so that the EHR can match-up the transactions. After the EHR receives the response, then it can display the recommended intervention. Some EHRs support returning recommended orders in the response.

PPM Database (PPM DB)

Personalized medicine data have all of the characteristics of the *three "Vs" of big data*: volume, velocity, and variety. The volume of PPM information can range from gigabytes to terabytes for a single patient. New genetic and genomic sequencing techniques make it possible to quickly and inexpensively sequence entire exomes, genomes, and microbiomes for a single individual. And this may be done more than once at different points of time, which may generate a terabyte or more of information for a single patient. New EHR technologies are needed to deal with this volume of healthcare information, which might amount to petabytes of information for an organization's patient population. EHRs are not currently equipped to handle this type and volume of information [22]. Just securely and efficiently storing this information for a typical hospital is a significant undertaking. Germline, tumor, etc., genetic and genomic PPM data are voluminous, and both assay technologies and their interpretation may evolve over time. Other types of PPM data have large data volume and change dynamically over time, including transcriptomic data, gene copy number, indels, gene fusions, germline and somatic acquired mutations, computed transcriptional assays, microbiome, data generated by patient devices, fitness and activity trackers, glucometers, and other sensors. These data need to be stored efficiently and there is not yet a standard way to represent them within the EHR. The incoming data feeds may also require monitoring and summarization layers (e.g., so that trends can be visualized and analyzed).

The variety of PPM data is quickly expanding to include whole exome and genome sequences, or restricted panel or marker genome data from retail operations (such as OneOme, Color Genetics, and 23andMe), microbiome data, and self-assessment data [23]. PPM data may also undergo computations and transformations as part of analytics, and those intermediate results may need to be stored for future use (justification of results, re-analysis or other uses).

At least as important as the big data storage considerations are privacy and security issues that must be adequately addressed [24]. PPM is by definition very specific to an individual and many of its data permanent, and contrary to a traditional data security, breach of the data cannot be rectified by a change of password. A variety of barriers against data abuse can be deployed to protect this type of information:

1. *Restricting technical access to the data only to individuals whose access the patient has approved through consent.* The data should be stored using strong encryption, such as AES-256, with keys under the control of the patient or a trusted third party authorized to act on behalf of the patient. Robust authentication and vetting of patient identities must be implemented so that linkages between the PPM data and other clinical data are correct and the risk of fraudulent access to the data is eliminated.

2. *Decoupling the genomic data not used for clinical care from the EHR.* While the part of PPM that is used for CDS will end up in the EHR as part of justification of recommendation alerts, other components (e.g., used for research or for ancestry or paternity analyses, for forensic purposes, or for pre-emptive genotyping) will remain inaccessible to entities that may have legal access to the EHR (e.g., life insurance companies authorized by the patient to access the information). The federal Genetic Information Nondiscrimination Act (GINA) protects an individual against some types of genetic discrimination by employers and health insurers, but it does not protect them against every possible type of discrimination in the event their genetic information is exposed [25].

3. *Legal protections to accompany use of a PPM database.* Informatics infrastructures for PPM should allow patients to control their PPM data that is not directly used for care, including removing (and/or destroying) the information (or portions of their information) from the PPM database at any time (except for consented research uses). The clinical recommendations and interpretations of the PPM data that are used by clinicians in care delivery should be stored in the EHR and treated the same as other parts of the medical record. PPM infrastructures must create audit logs detailing which parties (hospitals, clinicians, laboratories, etc.) accessed the data and for what reason. The PPM DB operators and data custodians should be contractually obligated to safeguard the data when it is in their possession and to abide by policies for securely destroying it after authorized use has been accomplished. As the legal frameworks designed to protect patients are evolving, there is a strong argument to be made for extending the provisions of HIPAA and GINA to define and forbid PPM data abuse.

The science and techniques for using PPM data are quickly evolving. When PPM data is used during healthcare delivery, raw genetic data should be kept separate from the genetic interpretation of that data [26]. Clinicians are most interested in using PPM data to diagnose, treat, and predict risk for a patient. Clinical interpretation can change over time as new clinical knowledge becomes available. The PPM DB must be closely coupled to the Clinical Knowledge base so that new knowledge applied to data in the PPM DB can generate new clinical interpretations. Only these interpretations should be stored in the EHR to be used by the care team for clinical decisions. But the raw and uninterpreted information of the PPM DB (for example, entire exomes) and the Clinical Knowledge base should remain separate [27]. There are also pragmatic technical reasons to maintain a separate PPM database. Genetic PPM data is very large and is not handled well in EHRs currently and in the foreseeable future [28]. Raw genomic data is considered sensitive information and best practices for which aspects of genomic data should be part of the legal medical record are still evolving [29]. Taking into account all of the above factors, keeping the PPM data outside of the EHR is an architectural model that confers a number of advantages.

Electronic Health Record (EHR)

The EHR captures and stores data related to a patient's care. Whenever the PPM DB is external to the EHR, there need to be methods to combine the important clinical data from the EHR with the PPM data. Historically, integration of external systems with the EHR has been difficult and time consuming. Most integration was accomplished using proprietary EHR protocols or with HL7 version 2.x messaging. These methods were adequate for sending and receiving routine health information to the EHR (i.e., demographics, vitals, labs, medications, etc.), but they were not designed to handle PPM data. Recently there has been significant work on the Fast Healthcare Interoperability Resources (FHIR) [19] protocol, which aims to solve this problem. FHIR holds the promise of being a single protocol that will work with all EHRs in the near future. FHIR is extensible to allow PPM data to be exchanged in a standard manner by defining a flexible record format for different types of PPM data. FHIR calls these definitions of standards "bundles". Work is currently underway to define FHIR bundles for important types of PPM data including pharmacogenomic data and patient-reported outcomes [30].

A critical issue is ensuring that a patient's EHR records are linked with the correct data in the PPM DB. The issue is getting attention from the U.S. Department of Health and Human Services' Office of the National Coordinator for Health Information Technology (ONC) [31]. It has always been important to ensure that patients are connected to the correct medical record and it is just as critical when using a patient's PPM data for care. If a patient is linked to incorrect PPM data, then CDS and predictive models may yield incorrect and possibly harmful recommendations. When the PPM DB and EHR are both contained within a single healthcare system, then a healthcare specific patient identifier assigned by the EHR (i.e., medical record number) can be used to link the data. However, if the PPM DB is external, then patient matching and linkage becomes more difficult. In the United States, patients do not have a universally unique identifier that healthcare systems can use. Instead, each healthcare system gives the patient a patient identifier that is unique only within that system. There is ongoing work to solve this issue, but until there is a solution, multiple "unique" numbers will need to be stored for each patient. Entity resolution methods may provide a solution in some cases, however a safer solution before a universal patient identifier system exists is that the EHR should store the patient's identifier from the PPM DB (and there may be multiple PPM DBs). The PPM DB, similarly, must store the patient identifier from each health system's EHR.

Clinical Knowledge Repository (CKR)

Clinical knowledge in general, and in PPM even more so, is advancing quickly. As new knowledge, evidence and clinical interpretations become available, there need to be scientifically robust policies for how and when the new information will be used in practice. Traditionally, expert panels convened by and under the auspices of clinical specialty societies or government evaluate the new information, weigh the evidence and decide when and how to turn it into practice. The recommendations are ultimately codified as practice guidelines. This review and synthesis process is often difficult and time-consuming. Most healthcare organizations currently have additional institutional review processes in place for overseeing the process of updating recommendations for medication management and order set maintenance.

The CKR contains information about the clinical interpretation of the PPM data for patient care. For example, in the case of pharmacogenomics (PGx), this knowledge is in the form of gene-drug interactions. The CKR information is comprised of text documents and guidelines that a clinician can read to understand the evidence for the clinical interpretation. The CKR should detail what is known about the interaction and the recommended action to take. There should also be information available in the CKR to help educate a patient about the clinical interpretation. In addition, the clinical knowledge must also be represented in a form that a computer can use. While there is considerable scholarly work supporting computable PGx guidelines, no universal standards are available for computationally representing clinical knowledge [32].

PPM Research Database. The research community is looking for better methods to rely on real-world evidence (RWE) in order to assess the effectiveness of treatments, medications, and interventions. The process of using PPM CDS generates data that can be potential evidence to measure effectiveness and improve outcomes [33]. A PPM research database contains data that allows researchers to study the effectiveness, safety, cost-effectiveness, and other aspects of PPM practices. It stores information about CDS use that has occurred and information about a patient's eventual clinical outcome. This database should be used to evaluate the effectiveness of the CDS and also to discover new associations in the PPM data that may lead to additional recommendations. It is outside the scope of this chapter (but covered in many other chapters of the present volume) to discuss how this data can be analyzed.

Illustrative Example: Pharmacogenomics

In order to illustrate the principles of the scalable informatics infrastructure of the section "Components of a Scalable PPM Informatics Architecture" better, we will describe general PPM infrastructure required to support PGx. PGx is a type of precision medicine with demonstrable clinical benefits, and is ready to be implemented in practice. PGx is the study of how a person's inherited genetics (i.e., germline genotype) affect their response to different drugs. There has been considerable progress in identifying gene variations associated with drug metabolism (i.e., slow metabolizers, ultrafast metabolizers), and related to those, efficacy and toxicity. Knowing whether a drug will be effective for a particular patient with a specific genetic profile guides clinicians in medication decisions. More pharmacogenes continue to be discovered and their interaction with different medications assessed. Evidence is now sufficiently strong to allow implementation of PGx in clinical settings. For example, patients who have had a heart attack are often prescribed clopidogrel (Plavix). Individuals with certain variants in the *CYP2C19* gene are poor metabolizers of the drug, increasing the risk of ineffective therapy and risk of a second heart attack or death. It is estimated that 40–50% of East Asians have one or more of these variants [34]. This suggests that most patients (and every East Asian patient) should have genetic testing for that variation before being prescribed clopidogrel. Individuals carrying these variants should be prescribed an alternative drug.

We will illustrate how to scale PPM through two use cases:

1. Implementation of PGx within a single institution.
2. A statewide implementation of PGx across a number of diverse healthcare organizations.

The architectures discussed here represent an amalgamation of architectures tested in various institutions, as well as work in progress in our institution and home state of Minnesota.

PGx Within a Single Institution

The PGx architecture for a single institution (Fig. 18.5) is very similar to the generic PPM architecture shown in Fig. 18.1.

In the case of PGx, the PPM DB holds genomic data, thus it is a Genetic Data Repository (GDR). For PGx, the CKR is a Pharmacogenomic Clinical Guideline Repository (PCGR). The PCGR holds validated PGx clinical guidelines. A number of institutions have implemented some form of PGx [4, 35]. Most of these early implementations chose a small number of gene-drug pairs as pilots to demonstrate feasibility and allow for the necessary PGx architecture development. Selection of initial drug-gene pairs for implementation varies and is highly dependent on the patient populations within the health system (e.g., pediatrics, cancer, psychiatry).

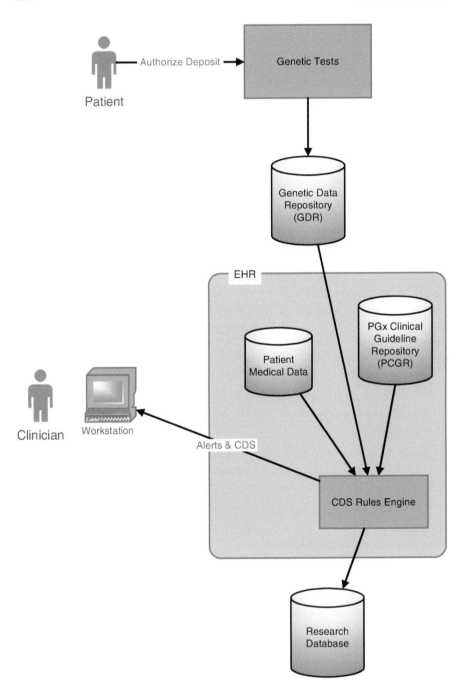

Fig. 18.5 PGx architecture at a single institution

The providers also need to ensure access to a CLIA-approved lab (internal or external) to perform clinical-grade genetic testing for the gene variations needed for clinical implementation, and a plan for how the organization will get reimbursed for the testing [36].

Pharmacogenomic Clinical Guideline Repository (PCGR)

In the case of a single institution, there is (usually) only one EHR, which simplifies the integration issues between the GDR and EHR. The PCGR should contain the actual guideline documents and allow physicians and pharmacists to easily access all of the data and evidence for their gene-drug pairs. Patient education materials, written to be understandable from a patient's viewpoint, should also be available to be printed or sent to a patient. The guidelines must be in computable form (i.e., a form that is directly useable by a computer), not just written as text that only a clinician can interpret. In the case of a single institution, the format should be written in the language that the CDS in their EHR requires. In most cases, institutions will not actually put the rules in the PCGR, but instead will just program them directly into the EHR's CDS.

Genetic Data Repository (GDR)

With PGx, there are two fundamental approaches to the timing of obtaining the genomic data needed. Patients can preemptively have their genome sequenced, or they can be tested for specific genes only when a clinician is deciding which medication to prescribe. *Preemptive genotyping* sequences an entire genome, a set of markers across the genome, or a panel of genes and saves that genetic information to be used over and over as drugs are prescribed in the future. This leads to faster PGx guidance at the point of care, and is more efficient over the lifetime of the patient since testing need only be done once for each gene of interest. *Reactive genotyping* typically tests for only one or two genes relevant to a specific medication under consideration for use or when drug therapy problems have been encountered for that medication. This may be less expensive for some patients in the short term, but adds a delay in the drug administration process that may not be acceptable in urgent situations. The PGx architecture must support both scenarios. In the case of a single institution, the results of the genetic testing can be stored in a hospital-hosted and -maintained GDR outside of the EHR. As discussed, if genotyping is performed that is not used for clinical care (especially genome-scale assays) then an alternative approach is to store the raw gene data in this separate GDR and only store the actionable variants, clinical interpretations and recommendations in the EHR.

Even in the case of a single site, the GDR must be able to accept genetic test results from both an in-house lab and external labs. Labs often send the results as text reports instead of as structured data. In that case, natural language processing

(NLP) or a direct feed to the lab's backend database may be used to extract the gene variant information from the report and put it into structured fields in the GDR in order for the CDS to use it most effectively.

PGx Clinical Decision Support

For a single institution, the CDS can exist within the organization's EHR. Most EHRs today have sufficient capability to support PGx CDS. As is typical with most clinical IT and DS systems, the organization can use a physician or pharmacist to act as champion to roll out the PGx CDS. They can be a resource to help educate the rest of the medical staff and explain why PGx is important. The medical staff needs to be trained to know when (and why) the CDS is triggered, where to look for the alerts or notes within the EHR, how to order genetic tests, how to order a PGx consult and how to read the alerts. Figure 18.6 shows an example CDS alert. It demonstrates that alerts should have a number of parts [37]:

1. The alert should *explain why the CDS was triggered*. It should state what patient condition or what medication order caused the CDS and the alert to be displayed.
2. The alert should have a short *narrative explaining the strength of evidence* for the gene-drug pair interaction and the potential adverse clinical consequence of a non-personalized administration of the drug for a patient with that gene.

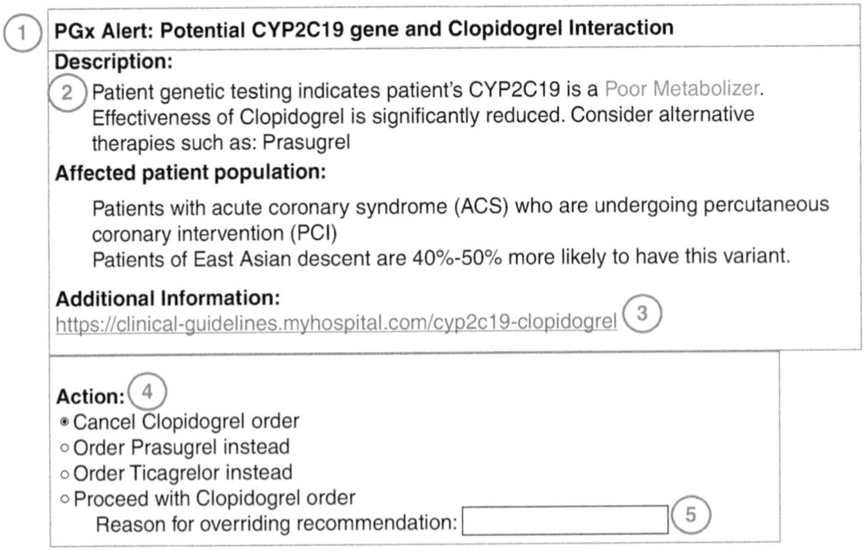

(1) **PGx Alert: Potential CYP2C19 gene and Clopidogrel Interaction**

Description:

(2) Patient genetic testing indicates patient's CYP2C19 is a Poor Metabolizer. Effectiveness of Clopidogrel is significantly reduced. Consider alternative therapies such as: Prasugrel

Affected patient population:

Patients with acute coronary syndrome (ACS) who are undergoing percutaneous coronary intervention (PCI)
Patients of East Asian descent are 40%-50% more likely to have this variant.

Additional Information:
https://clinical-guidelines.myhospital.com/cyp2c19-clopidogrel (3)

Action: (4)
◉ Cancel Clopidogrel order
○ Order Prasugrel instead
○ Order Ticagrelor instead
○ Proceed with Clopidogrel order
    Reason for overriding recommendation: [_____] (5)

Fig. 18.6 Example PGx CDS alert

3. There should be *links to additional, more in-depth information and evidence.* Usually, these will link to literature and guidelines within the PCGR.
4. The alert should display *specific recommendations for action by the clinician.* This could be dosing adjustment, a recommendation to cancel the medication order or a recommendation for an alternative medication.
5. Finally, the CDS alert should encourage the clinician to *exercise their clinical judgement* to pick a recommended action or specify a reason why they are taking a different action. This information will be valuable later in determining the effectiveness of CDS.
6. The EHR build team will also have to create an EHR display screen that shows the genomic information that the CDS used to reach its recommendation. This could include a list of the patient's gene variants related to the drug in question and the potential clinical importance of considering the drug-gene pair.

Research Database (DB)

This database stores the content of the alerts and recommendation of the CDS for secondary research use. In addition, data related to the patient's outcomes should be stored. This information may include length of stay, 30/60-day readmission, number and type of adverse drug events (ADE), and whether or not an alternative drug was used. For a single institution, these data are likely to be available in the EHR, but there are important benefits to maintaining a separate Research DB with this information. The Research DB will typically be used for assessing the PGx CDS effectiveness and for discovery of new gene-drug pair interactions.

PGx on a Statewide or National Scale

What would it take to enable deployment of PGx at the scale of a state or the nation? Previous PGx implementation pilots have typically explored deployment at single sites, typically large and cutting-edge academic medical centers. Also important initiatives (e.g., within the eMERGE, the Pharmacogenomics Research Network (PGRN) [38], and at the University of Chicago [39]) have explored the feasibility of standardizing and sharing gene variant and phenotype information to enable discovery of novel actionable gene variants in large shared databases. When considering PGx deployment at state scale and above, it is also important to consider midsize and small rural health systems that may not have the necessary expertise and technical infrastructure to implement PGx in the way that large academic medical centers can. Such entities may not have the ability to evaluate PGx clinical guidelines, implement the PGx CDS, or deal with the issues of storing and maintaining genetic

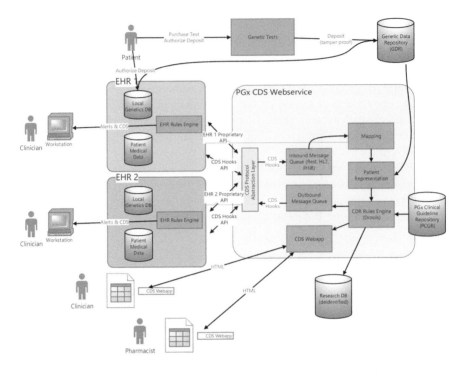

Fig. 18.7 PGx architecture on a statewide scale

data. The architecture required for PGx on a statewide or national scale needs to be highly scalable, performant, and containing securely shareable resources within the PGx Network (Fig. 18.7).

Clinical Decision Support

In a state-scale deployment, the CDS is a centralized service that all of the PGx Network participants can use. The inputs to the PGx CDS are patient demographics, patient clinical data, and the PGx Computable Guidelines. There are two ways for the CDS to be accessed:

1. *Integrated into an EHR.* Most health systems can use the CDS in this way since it will be automatic, seamless, and easy to use. The CDS process is triggered by a medication order with an actionable gene. The EHR will call the PGx CDS service and receive specific recommended actions as well as narrative explaining the recommendation. This information can be used in discussions of treatment choices with the patient. The EHR can send genetic data as part of the request (if local genetic data exists), or it can rely on the CDS service to request the patient's genetic data from the Genetic Data Repository (GDR).

2. *Providers that don't have an integrated EHR* (including retail pharmacies as part of filling a prescription) can access the CDS via a bespoke web application. In this case, the provider will manually enter the patient's identity and medication information (and possibly genetic data, if it is not already in the GDR). The identity information should include the patient's name, the number that identifies them in the GDR and information such as their data of birth as a check to protect against data entry errors. The provider will receive the same CDS recommendations as in the case of EHR integration. This mechanism is obviously more error prone and data error detection and cross-referencing mechanisms may be needed.

The PGx CDS Webservice is a horizontally scalable, transactional web application that should be hosted in the secure, HIPAA-compliant data center. Since many institutions will be depending on it for real-time CDS, it needs to be highly available (at least 99.99% availability) and high performance. Healthcare organizations that participate in such a PGx Network can connect their EHRs to the PGx CDS Webservice using secure site-to-site VPNs. Requests can be sent using the FHIR or HL7 v2.5 standards. Current work in the CDS Hooks project is one path toward the necessary standardized methods and message formats for performing CDS in an EHR [16]. In the meantime, the leading EHR vendors offer their own, proprietary, approaches to CDS integration. An abstraction layer can be built as the web layer of the webservice to translate between the appropriate EHR vendor formats and invocation methods until CDS Hooks (or similar technology) is more widely adopted. The CDS will generate the same alerts as described in the single institution scenario. But until CDS Hooks (or similar standard) is widely adopted, each organization in the PGx Network may have to do an EHR configuration to display the CDS alert messages in their EHR.

Patient Genetic Data Repository (GDR)

Health services consumers today have easy access to a number of vendors that will sequence portions of their genomes for a number of different purposes including healthcare diagnostics and ancestry. Many of these services are also moving toward clinical-grade assays. Moreover such assays are already useful to the pharmaceutical industry for conducting preliminary discovery for disease targets. It is thus reasonable to expect that the GDR will contain clinical-grade targeted panels, genome sequencing, research-grade genome-scale data, and perhaps even "recreational"/"informational" genotyping data. Patients (or their authorized healthcare or lab test providers) can choose to deposit the results of these genomic tests into the GDR. While non-CLIA compliant genetic results cannot legally and medically drive clinical decisions, they may serve as indications to the clinician that CLIA-compliant testing is warranted and needs to be ordered. Results from these genetic tests can be stored at the provider's organization or alternatively could be directed by the patient to also be deposited into the GDR. Triggering events and clinical variant related data (for CDS) and phenotypes and other genetic data (for research) will need to be harmonized for effective inter-provider use. Considerable research efforts have been devoted to such harmonization. Genome-scale assays that are executed for research or pre-emptive PGx purposes, may be deposited outside the EHR in order to overcome current technical limitations of EHR systems related to genomic data (and also conceivably protect against data privacy abuses).

Computable Guidelines

The Clinical Pharmacogenomics Implementation Consortium (CPIC) and the Dutch Pharmacogenetics Working Group (DPWG) have published clinical guidelines that are a solid starting point for the PCGR [40]. These guidelines are currently delivered only as text and require a health provider to read and interpret the evidence and recommendations. Some individual organizations have translated these guidelines into rules that can be used by the CDS within their EHR [4]. And there is work being done to develop shareable CDS rules [41], but guidelines are not currently published in a manner that can be directly put into any computer system. In general, an informatics team will need to convert these guidelines into a format that can be easily used by computers. After careful validation, the computable guidelines should be represented as versioned artifacts in the Computable Guideline Repository (CGR). The CGR should be a resource that any PGx Network participant system can use independent of whether they use the PGx CDS service. As guidelines are added or updated in the repository, subscribers to the CGR can be notified of the changes. They can then translate the changes into appropriate updates to their rules and recommendations in their internal CDS systems.

PGx Network participants that use the PGx CDS Webservice will benefit from immediately being able to use the updated guidelines, since the webservice will always use the most up-to-date version. The Computable Guideline content will typically consist of rules and decision trees. An example of the clinical decision process for the CPIC warfarin guideline is shown in Fig. 18.8 [42].

This text description of the decision process is translated into a representation that a computer can use. A good choice for software to execute CDS rules is the open source Drools Rules Engine. It is proven, performant software that can execute the Computable Guidelines. An example of a part of a Drools ruleset is shown in Fig. 18.9.

The result of executing a set of rules is a CDS action that is returned to the invoking system. The alerts and recommendations that are returned also include hyperlinks to the graded evidence for the recommendation within the context of the larger guideline paper. The recommendations should also include narratives, which are short summaries of the evidence, so that clinicians can view the evidence narrative as part of the recommendation message and don't have to click to link to the full guideline.

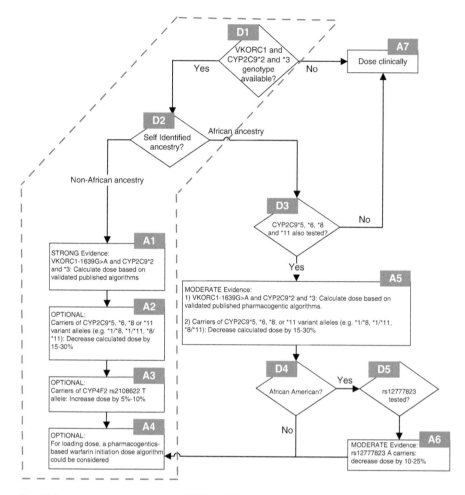

Fig. 18.8 Example decision tree for CPIC warfarin guideline (adapted from [42])

```
package CPIC_warfarin_v20180919

rule "Ancestry Dose Check - Non-African ancestry"
when
    $patient : Patient( $patient.genes.contain("VKORC1-1639G>A") && # D1
                        $patient.genes.contain("CYP2C9*2") &&       # D1
                        $patient.genes.contain("CYP2C9*3") )        # D1
                        $patient.ancestry != "African" &&           # D2
then
    new Action( "Alert", "Calculate dose based on published algorithms", evidence="strong" );   #A1
    new Action( "Info", "Carriers of CYP2C9*5, *6, *8 or *11 variant alleles (e.g. *1/*8, \     #A2
            *1/*11, *8/*11): Decrease calculated dose by 15-30%", evidence="optional" );
    new Action( "Info", "Carriers of CYP4F2 rs2108622 T allele: Increase dose by 5%-10%",\       #A3
                evidence="optional" );
    new Action( "Info", "For loading dose, a pharmacogentics-based warfarin initiation dose\      #A4
                algorithm could be considered", evidence="optional" );
end
```

Fig. 18.9 Example of a Drools Rule for a part of the CPIC warfarin guideline (the portion outlined in red in Fig. 18.8)

Computable Guideline Governance Process

In a state-wide network, there are many parties relying upon the recommendations of the clinical guidelines. There should be a centralized state-wide or nation-wide PGx Computable Guideline Advisory Board (CGAB) to oversee a robust process for examining and deploying new guidelines as new clinical and PGx evidence becomes available. Although maximum consistency across all sites/states is the ideal goal, in practice more local adaptation (to populations or more complete pharmacogene sets than national guidelines) may be occasionally warranted. In either case when new evidence is discovered, a CGAB review process can be initiated. Such a process will typically involve the following steps: First, evidence should be graded by a panel of PGx and clinical experts. Next, those experts must manually read the paper/guideline to determine if any of the rules of the associated computable guideline are impacted. If there is an impact, a new version of the guideline should be created, and the rules will be appropriately changed. The guideline must then be tested using test scenarios and simulations using previous cases. If all tests pass, the CGAB can make a decision for when to release the new guideline to the CGR. All of the subscribers to the repository should be notified of the new version accompanied by notes describing the changes and potential impacts.

Smaller institutions that may not have the expertise or larger institutions that may not have the bandwidth can rely on evidence from the CGAB. Even so, they will still need to have process governance and oversight locally.

PGx Research Database

The PGx Research Database is a repository that contains a research grade copy of all of the PGx CDS transactions. The Research DB can be used by the CGAB to assess how well the CDS is impacting outcomes. Participating healthcare organizations must also contribute patient demographics, medication, and outcome data to the Research DB. The outcome data may include key quality information such as adverse events, length of stay, readmission, and patient satisfaction. This database will also be used by researchers to discover new gene/medication interactions that may lead to new guidelines.

Conclusions

As precision medicine develops and matures, health systems will need to deliver personalized decision support to hundreds of millions and ultimately billions of patients through interoperable, reliable and performant informatics systems. This chapter introduced general concepts and methods for creating such decision support systems at large (state and national level) scales. The scalable architectures discussed in the chapter here have been proven in nation-wide deployments of CDS covering hundreds of healthcare systems, millions of patients, and thousands of providers concurrently. We discussed detailed extensions to conventional decision support requirements that are especially relevant to current and emerging forms of precision medicine. Several new informatics methods need to fully mature and be tested before end-to-end support of precision medicine is feasible.

References

1. McCarty CA, Chisholm RL, Chute CG, Kullo IJ, Jarvik GP, Larson EB, et al. The eMERGE Network: a consortium of biorepositories linked to electronic medical records data for conducting genomic studies. BMC Med Genomics. 2011;4:13.
2. Gottesman O, Kuivaniemi H, Tromp G, Faucett WA, Li R, Manolio TA, et al. The electronic medical records and genomics (eMERGE) network: past, present, and future. Genet Med. 2013;15:761–71.
3. Rasmussen-Torvik LJ, Stallings SC, Gordon AS, Almoguera B, Basford MA, Bielinski SJ, Brautbar A, Brilliant MH, Carrell DS, Connolly JJ, Crosslin DR, Doheny KF, Gallego CJ, Gottesman O, Kim DS, Leppi JC. Design and anticipated outcomes of the eMERGE-PGx project: a multi-center pilot for pre-emptive pharmacogenomics in electronic health record systems. Clin Pharmacol Ther. 2014;96:482–9.
4. Pulley JM, Denny JC, Peterson JF, Bernard GR, Vnencak-Jones CL, Ramirez AH, et al. Operational implementation of prospective genotyping for personalized medicine: the design of the Vanderbilt PREDICT project. Clin Pharmacol Ther. 2012;92:87–95.
5. Welch BM, Loya SR, Eilbeck K, Kawamoto K. A proposed clinical decision support architecture capable of supporting whole genome sequence information. J Pers Med. 2014;4:176–99.
6. Perrey R, Lycett M. Service-oriented architecture. In: Proceedings of the 2003 symposium on applications and the internet workshop. Washington, DC: IEEE; 2003. p. 116–9.
7. Taylor H, Yochem A, Phillips L, Martinez F. Event-driven architecture: how SOA enables the real-time enterprise. Boston, MA: Pearson Education; 2009.
8. The OAuth 2.0 Authorization Framework [Internet]. Internet Eng Task Force. [Cited 2018 Nov 1]. https://tools.ietf.org/html/rfc6749.
9. Oasis Security Assertion Markup Language (SAML) V2.0 Technical Overview [Internet]. [Cited 2018 Oct 18]. http://docs.oasis-open.org/security/saml/Post2.0/sstc-saml-tech-overview-2.0.html.
10. Musen MA, Middleton B, Greenes RA. Clinical decision-support systems, Biomedical informatics. London: Springer; 2014. p. 643–74.
11. Sitapati A, Kim H, Berkovich B, Marmor R, Singh S, El-Kareh R, et al. Integrated precision medicine: the role of electronic health records in delivering personalized treatment. Wiley Interdiscip Rev Syst Biol Med. 2017;9:e1378.
12. Wright A, Sittig DF, Ash JS, Sharma S, Pang JE, Middleton B. Clinical decision support capabilities of commercially-available clinical information systems. J Am Med Inform Assoc. 2009;16:637–44.
13. Mccoy AB, Wright A, Sittig DF. Cross-vendor evaluation of key user-defined clinical decision support capabilities: a scenario-based assessment of certified electronic health records with guidelines for future development. J Am Med Inform Assoc. 2015;22:1081–8.
14. Zhang M, Velasco FT, Musser RC, Kawamoto K. Enabling cross-platform clinical decision support through web-based decision support in commercial electronic health record systems: proposal and evaluation of initial prototype implementations. AMIA Annu Symp Proc. 2013;2013:1558–67.
15. Health Level Seven (HL7). CDS Hooks [Internet]. 2018 [cited 2018 Oct 15]. https://cds-hooks.org/.

16. McCallie DP, Mandel JC, Strasberg HR, Narus SP, Shekleton K, Marshall P. Beyond SMART: Remote decision support with CDS Hooks. AMIA Annu Symp Proc 2016. 2016;2121.
17. Mandl KD, Mandel JC, Murphy SN, Bernstam EV, Ramoni RL, Kreda DA, et al. The SMART platform: early experience enabling substitutable applications for electronic health records. J Am Med Inform Assoc. 2012;19:597–603.
18. Wright A, Sittig DF. SANDS: a service-oriented architecture for clinical decision support in a National Health Information Network. J Biomed Inform. 2008;41:962–81.
19. Health Level Seven (HL7). Welcome to FHIR [Internet]. 2015 [cited 2016 Feb 15]. https://www.hl7.org/fhir/.
20. PharmacyOneSource. Pharmacy OneSource/gigaspaces scalability [Internet]. [Cited 2018 Oct 10]. https://www.gigaspaces.com/sites/default/files/private/free/resource/PharmacyOneSource.pdf.
21. VigiLanz Unveils Open Enterprise Intelligence Resources (EIR) platform at HIMSS 2015 annual conference [Internet]. [Cited 2018 Oct 1]. https://www.businesswire.com/news/home/20150413005093/en/VigiLanz-Unveils-Open-Enterprise-Intelligence-Resources-EIR.
22. DuBravec D. Can EHRs handle genomics data? J AHIMA. 2015;86:28–31.
23. Whitson JR. Gaming the quantified self. Surveill Soc. 2013;11:163–76.
24. Roski J, Bo-Linn GW, Andrews TA. Creating value in health care through big data: opportunities and policy implications. Health Aff. 2014;33:1115–22.
25. Hudson KL, Holohan MK, Collins FS. Nondiscrimination act of 2008. N Engl J Med. 2008;358:2661–3.
26. Masys DR, Jarvik GP, Abernethy NF, Anderson NR, Papanicolaou GJ, Paltoo DN, et al. Technical desiderata for the integration of genomic data into Electronic Health Records. J Biomed Inform. 2012;45:419–22.
27. Starren J, Williams MS, Bottinger EP. Crossing the omic chasm: a time for omic ancillary systems. JAMA. 2013;309:1237–8.
28. Kho AN, Rasmussen LV, Connolly JJ, Peissig PL, Starren J, Hakonarson H, Hayes MG. Electronic health records. Genet Med. 2013;15:772–8.
29. Hazin R, Brothers KB, Malin BA, Koenig BA, Sanderson SC, Rothstein MA, et al. Ethical, legal, and social implications of incorporating genomic information into electronic health records. Genet Med. 2013;15:810–6.
30. Alterovitz G, Warner J, Zhang P, Chen Y, Ullman-Cullere M, Kreda D, et al. SMART on FHIR genomics: facilitating standardized clinico-genomic apps. J Am Med Inform Assoc. 2015;22:1173–8.
31. U.S. Department of Health and Human Services' Office of the National Coordinator for Health Information Technology (ONC) Patient Matching Algorithm Challenge.
32. Boxwala AA, Tu S, Peleg M, Zeng Q, Ogunyemi O, Greenes RA, et al. Toward a representation format for sharable clinical guidelines. J Biomed Inform. 2001;34:157–69.
33. Khoury MJ. Dealing with the evidence dilemma in genomics and personalized medicine. Clin Pharmacol Ther. 2010;87:635–8.
34. Bhopalwala AM, Hong RA, Khan ZR, Valentin MR, Badawi RA. Routine screening for CYP2C19 polymorphisms for patients being treated with clopidogrel is not recommended. Hawaii J Med Public Heal. 2015;74:16–20.
35. Gottesman O, Scott SA, Ellis SB, Overby CL, Ludtke A, Hulot JS, et al. The CLIPMERGE PGx program: clinical implementation of personalized medicine through electronic health records and genomics-pharmacogenomics. Clin Pharmacol Ther. 2013;94:214–7.
36. Caraballo PJ, Bielinski SJ, St. Sauver JL, Weinshilboum RM. Electronic medical record-integrated pharmacogenomics and related clinical decision support concepts. Clin Pharmacol Ther. 2017;102:254–64.
37. Sittig DF, Wright A, Osheroff JA, Middleton B, Teich JM, Ash JS, et al. Grand challenges in clinical decision support. J Biomed Inform. 2008;41:387–92.
38. Giacomini KM, Brett CM, Altman RB, Benowitz NL, Dolan ME, Flockhart DA, et al. The pharmacogenetics research network: from SNP discovery to clinical drug response. Clin Pharmacol Ther. 2007;81:328–45.

39. Danahey K, Borden BA, Furner B, Yukman P, Hussain S, Saner D, et al. Simplifying the use of pharmacogenomics in clinical practice: building the genomic prescribing system. J Biomed Inform. 2017;75:110–21.
40. Caudle K, Klein T, Hoffman J, Muller D, Whirl-Carrillo M, Gong L, et al. Incorporation of pharmacogenomics into routine clinical practice: the Clinical Pharmacogenetics Implementation Consortium (CPIC) guideline development process. Curr Drug Metab. 2014;15:209–17.
41. Linan MK, Sottara D, Freimuth RR. Creating shareable clinical decision support rules for a pharmacogenomics clinical guideline using structured knowledge representation. AMIA Annu Symp Proc. 2015;2015:1985–94.
42. Johnson JA, Caudle KE, Gong L, Whirl-Carrillo M, Stein CM, Scott SA, et al. Clinical Pharmacogenetics Implementation Consortium (CPIC) guideline for pharmacogenetics-guided warfarin dosing: 2017 update. Clin Pharmacol Ther. 2017;102:397–404.

Chapter 19
Building Comprehensive Enterprise-Scale PPM Clinical Informatics Capability and Capacity

Bruce Levy

Introduction

The terms Precision Medicine and Personalized Medicine (PPM) have significant overlap and have frequently been used interchangeably. While many equate these terms with genomics and molecular testing, they more broadly relate to the intentional design of efficient medical care focused on therapeutic benefits for patients. Precision and personalized medicine focuses on the individual patient, analyzing ever larger sets of data points from each individual to provide a specific solution tailored to that patient at a specific moment in time [1, 2].

Evidence-based medicine utilizes evidence from well-designed and well-conducted research to help optimize decision making in medicine [3]. In contrast to PPM, early evidence-based medicine efforts harkened back to the "one size fits all" approach to medical care where a patient receives diagnostic or treatment measures based on studies of average effects of treatments of populations of patients with a given disease or condition. Given the innumerable differences between individual patients and the growing quantity of health data from every patient, it is highly unlikely there is any such evidence in the literature that is specific for a given patient at a given point in time. Thus, early evidence-based medicine was population based.

However, as shall be shown, in attempting to move patient-centered activities from small pilots to institutional, enterprise-wide or multi-enterprise/state levels, principles of both evidence-based medicine and PPM need to both be applied together in combination, and evidence based medicine and PPM need be reconciled and re-inforce one another. Geisinger, in its multi-year efforts in developing an enterprise level portfolio of initiatives commonly referred to as ProvenCare®,

B. Levy (✉)
Geisinger Commonwealth School of Medicine, Geisinger Health, Danville, PA, USA
e-mail: blevy2@geisinger.edu

© Springer Nature Switzerland AG 2020
T. Adam, C. Aliferis (eds.), *Personalized and Precision Medicine Informatics*,
Health Informatics, https://doi.org/10.1007/978-3-030-18626-5_19

has utilized both concepts of evidence-based medicine and PPM to provide better care at a lower cost. The key lessons learned through these experiences will be presented and described.

Clinical Microsystems: The Concept Underlying ProvenCare®

"Clinical Microsystems is shorthand for a comprehensive approach to providing value for individuals and families by analyzing, managing, improving and innovating in health care systems" [4]. Traditionally, patients receive their care in a variety of settings involving different healthcare providers. Examples of these settings include the patient's primary care provider's office, a specialists' office, an urgent care center, a hospital, or an outpatient surgical center. Each of these locations represent a clinical microsystem. The patient enters each clinical microsystem with a given health status at a specific time and exits after a series of activities (registration, assessment, treatment) with some change to their health status [5].

Traditionally, most health systems have had limited coordination and collaboration between and across different clinical microsystems, whether within the same health system or across multiple health systems. It has been shown that the performance of a clinical microsystem is linked to the microsystem's intelligent use of data, detailed knowledge of its individual patients and populations of patients, quality of its connections to related microsystems, and the engagement of its employees in both performing their work and striving to improve their work. Excellent clinical microsystems are a prerequisite for high performing health care organizations [4].

Many health systems may already have high performing clinical microsystems that take excellent care of patients while within their microsystem. Yet the quality of care delivered by a single microsystem within a health system may vary greatly from patient to patient or even between different encounters for the same patient. The microsystem might not even know of this variation in care if no quality data is being shared with them. One common challenge for these microsystems lies in their ability to effectively and efficiently handoff patients to another clinical microsystem, which is all too often ineffective. Also, individual employees within microsystems are typically not empowered by leadership to innovate and improve their operations.

Advancing clinical microsystems to the next level requires that the health system develop a patient-centric perspective to its operations. This reorientation leads to the linking of each patient's microsystems into a larger *mesosystem* that is designed specifically to that patient and their health needs. For example, the microsystems for a patient with advanced coronary artery disease (CAD) might include their PCP, a cardiologist, an interventional cardiologist, a cardiac surgeon, and a nutritionist. The patient may also interact with other clinical microsystems, such as a gastroenterologist for a routine colonoscopy screening. Patients with similar conditions, such as CAD, will tend to require similar medical services and visit the same microsystems for care [4]. These disease-based mesosystems represent common pathways that patients with similar conditions may follow [6].

Ultimately, the quality of care and its value will be determined not just by how well care is delivered within each microsystem, but by how well the different microsystems can coordinate care, communicate efficiently during handoffs and exchanges, and innovate. A health system is comprised of various mesosystems and microsystems all working together with the patient at its center. The *macrosystem* provides the leadership, resources and accountability to enable the clinical microsystems and mesosystems to operate, and it provides patients with high quality, efficient and satisfying health care [7, 8].

One key feature for the success of clinical microsystems, mesosystems and macrosystems is the effective use of data and information technology. The systems need to be supported by a rich source of data and analytics that are focused on the needs of each microsystem to deliver care. This is not limited to just direct patient care, but also includes feedback and measures of performance for each microsystem. The data and analytics needs to be relevant and provide real-time meaningful intelligence. Having providers within a clinical microsystem sufficiently expert at informatics can help facilitate the value of the data environment [4–8].

ProvenCare®: More Than a Decade of Experience Building PPM to an Enterprise Level

In the early 2000s, Geisinger, a rural health system in central Pennsylvania, began to re-examine how it was providing medical services to its patients. There was growing recognition that there was significant waste in the delivery of healthcare in the United States and that there was an inverse relationship between cost and quality. Geisinger's leadership realized that if they could identify and reduce suboptimal care, they could both improve the quality of the healthcare delivered and lower the total cost of providing that care.

This transformation did not happen overnight. The first step was to create a compelling shared vision for the entire enterprise, from the lowest paid worker to the chairman of the board, with the benefit of the patient being the key goal. Shared governance was employed with the formation of leadership dyads and triads for each implementation [9]. There was recognition that the front-line employees needed to be empowered to make their own contributions to the vision, and that this was as much a bottom up as a top down effort. All employees would share in the successes of the program and learn from the failures along the route. Rapid innovative cycles would be required to quickly identify effective solutions and stop work on ideas that were not bearing fruit [10]. Finally, the need for large quantities of data and advanced analytics around meaningful metrics that were focused on patient outcomes was identified as critical to evaluate this process [11].

ProvenCare CABG®

The first area that Geisinger focused on was coronary artery bypass graft (CABG) surgery. While the cardiac surgery program already showed excellent outcomes and the surgeons were a cohesive and collegial group, there were several identified issues. Each surgeon individually decided whether to include evidence-based medicine (EBM) into their own practice, leading to multiple different care pathways for patients. While the various microsystems around CABG patients had implemented improvements, there was no meaningful communication or coordination between the microsystems [11–13].

The phases that were developed as part of the ProvenCare® process included [6, 11]:

1. Identification of best practice evidence.
2. Process redesign.
3. Data analytics.
4. Implementation.

Phase 1: Evidence

The relevant literature was reviewed, including the American College of Cardiology (ACC)/American Heart Association (AHA) guidelines for CABG. The focus was on the Class I and Class IIa ACC/AHA recommendations. The cardiac surgeons from all Geisinger facilities discussed the evidence, agreed by consensus which of the guidelines to follow, and identified the steps needed to meet the guidelines. Gaining 100% consensus among the clinicians is critical to mitigate criticism of "cookbook medicine," and to achieve acceptance of the process. This effort resulted in 19 clinically applicable recommendations that had 40 measurable process elements.

Phase 2: Process Redesign

Multidisciplinary teams consisting of a physician, surgery physician assistant, critical care registered nurse, operating theatre registered nurse, cardiac rehabilitation technician, electronic health record programmer and clinical process improvement specialists were formed at each facility and met weekly by videoconferencing. Each surgeon's process flows were observed and documented. The surgeons were surprised by the variations identified in their practices. Patients were also engaged to provide input into the process redesign. Non-value-added work was eliminated, and the system was "idealized" to incorporate the process elements identified in Phase 1. New workflows were designed that emphasized the use of technology solutions and delegating specific elements to the appropriate members of the care team. Clinical decision support, care flow maps and specially-designed history and physical templates were built. The new process and all the developed tools were extensively tested.

Phase 3: Data Analytics

Data regarding the metrics needed to be collected and analyzed to provide feedback to the care team regarding adherence to the implemented best practice guidelines. The metrics not only monitored compliance with the guidelines themselves, but also collected financial data that allowed comparison of costs before and after implementation. It was initially decided that compliance with the measures would be all or none, and that the feedback be provided as close as possible to real time. Providers were allowed to deviate from the default best practices; however, the reason(s) for the deviation had to be documented in the EHR and justified to the provider's colleagues. These deviations were tracked and evaluated.

Phase 4: Implementation and Results

ProvenCare CABG® went live approximately 18 months after initiation of the process. Due to the extensive involvement of the entire care team throughout the development process everyone knew the goals, process elements and compliance monitoring that were being deployed. In the first month following go-live, 59% of the CABG patients had all the ProvenCare® elements met, which increased to 100% by the fourth month [13].

Studying the data comparing the elective CABG patients in 2005 (prior to implementation) and 2006 (post-implementation) showed a 78% reduction in deep sternal wound infection, 67% decrease in in-hospital mortality, 50% reduction in intra-op blood products, and a 37% reduction in reoperation due to bleeding. While postoperative mean length of stay did not significantly decrease, a significantly higher number of patients were discharged to home [11, 13].

Expansion of ProvenCare®

In the decade since the initial CABG process improvement, Geisinger has deployed numerous additional ProvenCare® products throughout its health system. ProvenCare® now covers not only multiple additional surgical procedures, but also processes for treating a variety of acute and chronic diseases.

One example, ProvenCare Diabetes®, includes [11]:

- All-or-none set of 14 evidence-based guidelines for managing diabetes patients.
- Clinical process redesign to eliminate, automate, delegate, incorporate and activate.
- Clinical decision support in the form of evidence-based alerts and health management reminders for providers and clinic nurses.

After a few years, data that demonstrated a real impact on patient outcomes began to be generated. In the first 3 years of ProvenCare Diabetes® the process improvement measures resulted in 306 prevented heart attacks, 141 prevented strokes, and 166 prevented cases of retinopathy compared to what would have been expected from that population prior to implementation [11]. This is in addition to the thousands of patients that now had documented 100% compliance with all the evidence-based processes defined for their condition(s).

ProvenCare® also enabled Geisinger to offer competitive bundled pricing for their ProvenCare® portfolio, resulting in both improved quality and lower costs. ProvenCare has expanded to many additional offerings, each of which has contributed to higher healthcare quality and safety, greater consistency and efficiency in delivering care, lower costs to provide that care, and increased patient satisfaction [14–19]. Geisinger has also demonstrated that their ProvenCare® products can be implemented at other health care institutions utilizing different vendor's electronic health records [11, 15]. Finally, while documenting that patients consistently receive the best evidence-based care processes is an important first step, it is necessary to recognize that the ultimate goal is to have a positive impact on patient outcomes, and that requires metrics that focus on outcomes in addition to the process steps.

Data and Analytics Foundation for PPM at Enterprise Level

One significant challenge at the current time that inhibits the evolution of PPM to the enterprise level in many health care institutions is the relative lack of appropriate data warehouse and analytics capabilities within many health systems. The engine on which process care improvement depends is the capability to measure performance and results visually and in as close to real-time as is practical. For example, Yale-New Haven Hospital was able to improve its 11:00 AM discharge rate from 10.4% to 21.2% in 4 years through the application of a simple visual (red-yellow-green) tool to identify patients likely to be discharged the next day [20].

One of the key requirements of a successful PPM initiative is access to data in as close to real time as possible. For example, once a clinician enters a new diagnosis on a patient the decision support system immediately looks to identify the next best practice steps, evaluate which of those steps may have already been performed, and recommends what should occur next, all while the patient is still in the office. Unfortunately, many data warehouse systems currently rely on relatively infrequent data imports that occur on a daily or other periodic basis. This impairs the ability of the care team to react in a timely manner.

Even if the data is made quickly available, the analytics that need to be performed typically requires data from multiple sources. As part of ProvenCare® Geisinger not only looked at patient data in the EHR, but also focused on other sources of data such as data in other clinical systems and claims data present within Geisinger's health insurance electronic system. It is not difficult to envision a time when additional outside sources of data, such as social determinants of health, may be important to incorporate into the data warehouse for integration with clinical data and analysis. With these combined sources of data, health systems can begin to ask questions such as: Do patients miss necessary appointments because of difficulties in travel? Do patients not fill all their prescriptions due to financial issues? and Do these issues have an impact on patient outcomes? Most data warehouses are proprietary and when common data models or other interoperability measures have not been implemented, they make it difficult to import data from sources beyond the EHR. A robust data warehouse that enables importing and integration of data from multiple disparate sources is necessary.

Finally, the analytics that are required can be quite complex, especially when multiple sources of data need to be analyzed in combination. This typically requires significant on-site expertise. However, the development of PPM tools and analytics that are EHR vendor neutral and can be easily implemented by multiple health systems, such as ProvenCare®, will help to reduce this dependence. The developed intelligence needs to be easily visualized so that individuals can understand the data at a high level with a single glance (e.g., the percentage of patients where the metrics were met along with a color code to easily identify problems). At the same time, the visualized data need to have drill down capabilities, so that individuals more deeply studying the data can easily review it without having to go to another source. Finally, it is critical to have data transparency where all involved parties can have access to and review the data and analytics.

Developing the Informatics Capacity to Achieve PPM at Enterprise Level

The data and analytics requirements of an enterprise level PPM necessitates an informatics trained and experienced workforce. This cannot be limited to the technical side of Health Information Technology (HIT), but must include healthcare providers, operations managers and support staff at multiple levels. Currently, most health systems are challenged to identify, employ and organize a sufficient number of professionals that have adequate training in informatics.

Physicians

Currently, most medical schools provide little or no education in clinical informatics [21, 22]. In many cases, the "informatics" education provided to medical students does not go beyond some combination of education in evidence-based medicine or the standard vendor-specific EHR training that all providers receive. Similarly, there is little informatics education being provided to residents. One notable exception is within the pathology residency community, who have included informatics into the ACGME Program Requirements for Pathology, Pathology Milestones, as well as the American Board of Pathology certification examination, and have created a pathology informatics curriculum called Pathology Informatics Essentials for Residents

[23–25]. The recent approval of a new medical subspecialty in Clinical Informatics and the creation of ACGME-accredited Clinical Informatics Fellowships represents a significant step forward in physician informatics education necessary for PPM [26, 27].

As it becomes more broadly recognized that clinical informatics is an integral part of the daily practice of medicine, educational opportunities in the field of clinical informatics will continue to expand. Some medical schools and residency programs have begun to incorporate informatics education into their curricula, and institutions are starting to utilize an educational version of the electronic health record as an important educational tool for medical students and residents [28–30]. The Medical University of South Carolina modified its curriculum to engage second year medical students in the development of a clinical decision support (CDS) tool [31]. This not only provides the student with a practical exercise involving evidence-based medicine and CDS tool development, but also prepares them for a future utilizing informatics to support their practice of medicine.

Nurses, Physician Extenders, Pharmacists and Health Care Technicians

Nurses, physician extenders, pharmacists and many other health care workers have also started to incorporate informatics into their practice of medicine [32, 33]. Informatics education has been variably incorporated into the primary degree programs for many health professionals [34–36]. Additional opportunities are typically available for more advanced degree programs for these health professionals [37]. In addition, many health professionals, including physicians, will participate in graduate certificate or master's degree programs in clinical informatics offered both live and online through a variety of institutions of higher learning. However, like medical education for physicians, informatics needs to be better incorporated into the educational program for these health professionals.

Health Informatics Technology (HIT) and Computer Science Professionals

It is incorrect to assume that individuals educated in computer science or HIT will necessarily have expertise in clinical informatics. There is a distinct difference between the areas of HIT and informatics. HIT's primary focus is the technology that enables the acquisition, entry, editing, retrieving and simple analysis of health data. The exact nature and content of the data and its use is secondary to the systems that HIT needs to maintain. In contrast, informatics' primary focus is on the data and how it can be used to generate intelligence that supports patient care and the efficient operation of the health system. From an informatics perspective, information technology is a tool that is used to accomplish the primary goals of informatics.

As a result, most computer scientists and IT professionals, while experts regarding the hardware and IT software used in healthcare, may have little knowledge regarding clinical workflows and informatics needs of a health system. These professionals typically require additional informatics training to become maximally effective in these positions.

Given the multidisciplinary nature of PPM initiatives and the informatics educational requirements of the various members of the team, the concept of multidisciplinary education in informatics is attractive. Having health and technical professionals learn and train in informatics together can provide not only a broader informatics educational base but also encourage multidisciplinary team activities starting during education [38–40].

Informatics Teams

The presence of appropriately trained individuals, while required, is only the first step in developing the needed informatics expertise to support PPM. It is also necessary to form multidisciplinary teams of informaticists to work together and with their non-informatics healthcare colleagues to fully develop the informatics capabilities that support PPM at the enterprise or state level. The formation and organization of these teams is critical to the success of these efforts. One such model of organization is presented below.

A team of physician informaticists (PI) should be organized under a Chief Medical Informatics Officer (CMIO). The CMIO should be a physician board certified in clinical informatics and be provided with the resources and administrative support to organize and lead the PI team. While it is acceptable to start small and build the PI team, the eventual goal is for the team to represent a broad spectrum of the clinical specialties. These physicians should be spending a significant amount of their time practicing medicine in their clinical specialty. This provides the team direct insight into the clinical workflows and provides the clinical departments a known and hopefully respected colleague representing the specialty's interests. For systems that have multiple physical locations, it is also important to consider representation from each of the platforms in the system. The majority of physician informaticists should aspire towards board certification in clinical informatics. Some institutions, such as Geisinger, have expanded physician informaticists to include physician extenders, creating teams of provider informaticists.

Similarly, a team of nurse informaticists should be organized under a Chief Nursing Informatics Officer (CNIO). Typically nurse informaticists are more intimately involved in the analyst role and may spend significant time building within the EHR, in contrast to their physician colleagues. As nurses they have insight into and access to different aspects of the health system. As greater numbers of other health professionals become more directly involved with informatics, teams representing other groups such as pharmacists may form independently. In the interim, inclusion of these informatics colleagues into the provider or nurse informaticist teams is acceptable.

While having these independent teams of informaticist is a necessary first step, the collaboration and ultimate integration of these teams is the required next step. One of the reasons behind the success of ProvenCare® has been ascribed to the creation of multidisciplinary informatics teams. Triad informatics teams consisting of a nurse informaticist, a provider informaticist and an EHR analyst that are responsible for a certain aspect of informatics or a clinical service has been shown to be extremely effective. Expanding that team to include key clinical and operational leaders in a given service area for the development of PPM in a shared governance structure is a key aspect to help maximize success [9].

Conclusions

While the creation of large scale Personalized Precision Medicine (PPM) capabilities may appear to be a daunting task, in reality most health systems already have the necessary components to initiate and sustain their own journeys to enterprise level PPM. The success of ProvenCare® is actually based on the application of relatively simple, yet currently disconnected processes.

1. **Create the appropriate vision and leadership structures:** While it may be tempting to focus the vision on cost savings, experience has shown that clinicians respond best to visions that surround the patient rather than the financial picture of the institution. This effort needs to empower front-line staff as well as leadership to create real and sustained change.
2. **Identify the existing evidence-based best practice**: There are numerous examples of good medical and scientific evidence to support best practice available in the literature or through professional societies. What is currently lacking is the blueprint that takes you from a guideline to specific action steps and their implementation. The challenge is to get your clinicians together to review and achieve consensus on best practices.
3. **Hardwire the identified best practices**: Once the best practices are identified, the processes need to be hard wired into both the clinical workflows and the electronic health record. Involvement of information technology in the entire process helps ensure that appropriate electronic tools are built and tested.
4. **Develop appropriate metrics**: While it is important to monitor and report on metrics involving the individual process steps, don't forget the ultimate goal of improving patient outcomes. This is one area where health systems may need to develop or acquire resources to collect and report on appropriate metrics in real time.

5. **Innovate, innovate, innovate**: Rapid cycle innovation enables a health system to quickly identify useful projects, allows the system to quickly abandon projects that are not providing value, and permits continual improvement of the measures and metrics as knowledge is gained.

6. **Maintain and update**: The work is not completed once go-live is over. Medical evidence is continually changing, so it is necessary to establish a schedule to review and update best practice and the tools necessary to achieve improved patient outcomes.

References

1. United States National Library of Medicine. What is the difference between precision medicine and personalized medicine? What about pharmacogenomics? Bethesda, MD: National Institutes of Health; 2019. https://ghr.nlm.nih.gov/primer/precisionmedicine/precisionvspersonalized. Reviewed Apr 2015, accessed Aug 2018.
2. Bresnick J. What are precision medicine and personalized medicine? Health IT Analytics. https://healthitanalytics.com/features/what-are-precision-medicine-and-personalized-medicine. Copyright 2012–2018, accessed Aug 2018.
3. Masic I, Miokovic M, Muhamedagic B. Evidence based medicine—new approaches and challenges. Acta Inform Med. 2008;16:219–25.
4. Nelson EC, Godfrey M, Batalden PB, et al. Clinical microsystems, part 1: the building blocks of health systems. Jt Comm J Qual Patient Saf. 2008;34:367–78.
5. Nelson EC, Batalden PB, Godfrey MN. Quality by design: a microsystems approach. San Francisco, CA: Jossey-Bass; 2007.
6. McKinley KE, Berry SA, Laam LA, et al. Clinical microsystems, part 4: building innovative population-specific mesosystems. Jt Comm J Qual Patient Saf. 2008;34:655–63.
7. Wasson JH, Anders SG, Moore LG, et al. Clinical microsystems, part 2: learning from micro practices about providing patients the care they want and need. Jt Comm J Qual Patient Saf. 2008;34:445–52.
8. Godfrey MM, Melin CN, Muething SE, et al. Clinical microsystems, part 3: transformation of two hospitals using microsystem, mesosystem and macrosystem strategies. Jt Comm J Qual Patient Saf. 2008;34:591–603.
9. Nolan R, Wary A, King M, et al. Geisinger's ProvenCare methodology. JONA. 2011;41:226–30.
10. Steele GD, Haynes JA, Davis DE, et al. How Geisinger's advanced medical home model argues the case for rapid-cycle innovation. Health Aff. 2010;29:2047–53.
11. Steele GD, Feinberg DT. ProvenCare: how to deliver value-based healthcare the Geisinger way. New York: McGraw-Hill; 2018.
12. Berry SA, Doll MC, McKinley KE, et al. ProvenCare: quality improvement model for designing highly reliable care in cardiac surgery. Qual Saf Health Care. 2009;18:360–8.
13. Casale AS, Paulus RA, Selna MJ, et al. ProvenCare^SM a provider-driven pay-for-performance program for acute episode cardiac surgical care. Ann Surg. 2007;246:613–23.
14. Borade A, Kempegowda H, Tawari A, et al. Improvement in osteoporosis detection in a fracture liaison service with integration of a geriatric hip fracture care program. Int J Care Injured. 2016;47:2755–9.
15. Katlic MR, Facktor MA, Berry SA, et al. ProvenCare lung cancer: a multi-institutional improvement collaborative. CA Cancer J Clin. 2011;61:382–96.
16. Berry SA, Laam LA, Wary AA, et al. ProvenCare perinatal: a model for delivering evidence/guideline-based care for perinatal populations. Jt Comm J Qual Patient Saf. 2011;37:229–39.

17. Gionfriddo MR, Pulk RA, Sahni DR, et al. ProvenCare psoriasis: a disease management model to optimize care. Derm Online J. 2018;24:1–5.

18. Khurana S, Gaines S, Lee TH. Enhanced cure rates for HCV: Geisinger's approach. NEJM Catalyst. https://catalyst.nejm.org/geisinger-provencare-hcv-cure/. Published 11 Jul 2018, accessed Aug 2018.

19. Geisinger and Medacta International. Geisinger announces it will stand behind cost of hip surgery for a lifetime. https://www.geisinger.org/about-geisinger/news-and-media/news-releases/2018/03/08/21/51/geisinger-announces-it-will-stand-behind-cost-of-hip-surgery-for-a-lifetime. Published 8 Mar 2018, accessed Aug 2018.

20. Mathews KS, Corso P, Bacon S, et al. Using the red/yellow/green discharge tool to improve the timeliness of hospital discharges. Jt Comm J Qual Patient Saf. 2014;40:243–52.

21. Richardson JE, Bouquin DR, Tmanova LL, et al. Information and informatics literacies of first-year medical students. J Med Lib Assoc. 2015;103:198–202.

22. Badgett RG, Paukert JL, Levy LS. Teaching clinical informatics to third-year medical students: negative results from two controlled trials. BMC Med Educ. 2001;1:3.

23. Accreditation Council for Graduate Medical Education. ACGME program requirements for Graduate Medical Education in Anatomic Pathology and Clinical Pathology. 2018; approved 4 Feb 2018; effective 1 Jul 2018. https://acgme.org/Portals/0/PFAssets/ProgramRequirements/300PathologyCore2018.pdf?ver=2018-02-19-085552-553. Accessed Sept 2018.

24. American Board of Pathology. Clinical pathology exam blueprint. 2018. http://abpath.org/index.php/taking-an-examination/primary-certificate-requirements. Accessed Sept 2018.

25. Henricks WH, Karcher DS, Harrison JH Jr, et al. Pathology informatics essentials for residents: a flexible informatics curriculum linked to Accreditation Council for Graduate Medical Education milestones. J Pathol Inform. 2016;7:27.

26. Gardner RM, Overhage JM, Steen EB, et al. Core content for the subspecialty of clinical informatics. J Am Med Inform Assoc. 2009;16:153–7.

27. Longhurst CA, Pageler NM, Palma JP, et al. Early experiences of accredited clinical informatics fellowships. J Am Med Inform Assoc. 2016;23:829–34.

28. Wald HS, George P, Reis SP, et al. Electronic heath record training in undergraduate medical education: bridging theory to practice with curricula for empowering patient-a and relationship-centered care in the computerized setting. Acad Med. 2014;89:380–6.

29. Biagioli FE, Elliot DL, Palmer RT, et al. The electronic health record objective structured clinical examination: assessing student competency in patient interactions while using the electronic health record. Acad Med. 2017;92:87–91.

30. Hersch W, Biagioli F, Scholl G, et al. From competencies to competence: model, approach, and lessons learned from implementing a clinical informatics curriculum for medical students. In: Shachak A, Borycki EM, Reis SP, editors. Health professionals' education in the age of clinical information systems, mobile computing and social networks. London: Elsevier; 2017. p. 269–87.

31. Crabtree EA, Brennan E, Davis A, et al. Connecting education to quality: engaging medical students in the development of evidence-based clinical decision support tools. Acad Med. 2017;92:83–6.

32. Yang L, Cul D, Zhu X, et al. Perspectives from nurse managers on informatics competencies. ScientificWorldJournal. 2014;2014:391714.

33. Chonsilapawit T, Rungpragayphan S. Skills and knowledge of informatics, and training needs of hospital pharmacists in Thailand: a self-assessment survey. Int J Med Inform. 2016;94:255–62.

34. Breeden EA, Clauson KA. Development and implementation of a multitiered health informatics curriculum in a college of pharmacy. J Am Med Inform Assn. 2016;23:844–7.

35. Spenser JA. Integrating informatics in undergraduate nursing curricula: using the QSEN framework as a guide. J Nurs Educ. 2012;51:697–701.

36. Cummings E, Shin EH, Mather C, et al. Embedding nursing informatics education into an Australian undergraduate nursing degree. Nursing Inform. 2016;3:329–33.
37. Flynn A, Fox BI, Clauson KA, et al. An approach for some in advanced pharmacy informatics education. Am J Pharm Educ. 2017;81:6241.
38. Breil B, Fritz F, Thiemann V, et al. Multidisciplinary education in medical informatics—a course for medical and informatics students. Stud Health Technol Inform. 2010;160:581–4.
39. Myers MK, Jansson-Knodell CL, Schroeder DR, et al. Using knowledge translation for quality improvement: an interprofessional education intervention to improve thromboprophylaxis among medical inpatients. J Multidiscip Healthc. 2018;11:467–72.
40. Williams MS, Ritchie MD, Payne PRO. Interdisciplinary training to build an informatics workforce for precision medicine. Appl Transl Genom. 2015;6:28–30.

Chapter 20
Personalized and Precision Medicine Informatics Education

Terrence Adam

Introduction

Education in PPM informatics is a novel informatics training area aiming to develop a broad knowledge base in precision medicine as well as to provide sufficient depth of training in several core informatics areas in order to produce successful PPM informatics practitioners. Because of the aimed breadth and depth of knowledge and skills, PPM informatics training is generally best delivered via graduate-level education and it benefits from a substantial amount of hands on work.

Other education modalities are also important as the field of PPM and the informatics that supports it continue to expand and diffuse into clinical practice. The availability of high quality online, mixed online and traditional classroom learning approaches can address students' needs, as they seek educational opportunities while being part of the workforce or, in some cases, while being geographically separated from educational settings. In addition, PPM informatics education addresses important workforce needs and helps address the known gaps in PPM knowledge among practitioners [1–3].

In addition to the setting, there are other content management issues to address. Several unique challenges complicate precision medicine informatics education, including problems surrounding data access, data privacy management and other issues that impose restrictions on work in the PPM space. As this

T. Adam (✉)
Department of Pharmaceutical Care and Health Systems, College of Pharmacy, University of Minnesota, Minneapolis, MN, USA

Institute for Health Informatics, University of Minnesota, Minneapolis, MN, USA

PhD Program in Precision Medicine Informatics, University of Minnesota, Minneapolis, MN, USA

Minneapolis Veterans Administration, Minneapolis, MN, USA
e-mail: adamx004@umn.edu

© Springer Nature Switzerland AG 2020
T. Adam, C. Aliferis (eds.), *Personalized and Precision Medicine Informatics*, Health Informatics, https://doi.org/10.1007/978-3-030-18626-5_20

area is rapidly expanding, it is expected that there will be ongoing innovations in data sharing and management to help facilitate data and application access for students.

Background

Standard core content areas for PPM informatics education have not yet been fully developed to date, but prior reviews have identified several focus areas. One such review defined seven areas of importance for the support and delivery of precision medicine [4]. This work reflected stakeholder input including researchers, providers, payers and patients. The key areas of importance included (1) electronic consent and specimen for tracking of biospecimens for research, (2) data standards for data privacy, security and integrity for data integration and exchange, (3) advanced methods for biomarker discovery and translation, (4) implementation and enforcement of protocols and provenance, (5) precision medicine knowledge base construction, (6) enhancement of electronic health records to promote precision medicine and (7) consumer engagement [4]. Other recommendations of what should be included in precision medicine informatics training curricula have been offered by Frey et al. [5]. Four roles were defined for informatics including "(1) managing big data, (2) creating learning systems for knowledge generation, (3) providing access for individual involvement, and (4) ultimately supporting optimal delivery of precision treatments derived from translational research" [5]. Each of these roles requires knowledge not only of the informatics methods and technology but also of the context in which such methods and technology are developed, implemented and maintained.

It is also reasonable to see big data as a common requirement across most approaches to PPM informatics education given its role in helping to define disease as well as tailor treatments for patients. Definitions of big data have changed over the years based on the evolving capacity of information systems to both acquire and use data, but the scale of potential data currently available even at the individual level would certainly fit most definitions of big data. Volume of data along with the variability/complexity of the data, the ability to verify and standardize the data as well to analyze it, are important determinants of the use of data and the ability to extract scientific and health care value from it. Big data skills are important for PPM informatics learners to acquire and develop throughout their careers.

Other published reviews of informatics education have identified a number of additional focus areas supporting an interdisciplinary approach to education. These include the need to address the changes in electronic medical records systems, integration of medical devices and consumer devices and changes in the reimbursement models for health care [6]. Each of these elements of the health system require data in order for the innovations to be measured and have impacts on care delivery.

Having available data that is of high quality and is well integrated can help drive innovation in clinical decision making and the underlying clinical and basic sciences to facilitate novel approaches to health care.

Prerequisites to PMI Education

Core field prerequisites establish the minimal background requirements that PMI students will need to have previously acquired in order to successfully complete the PMI learning objectives. The prerequisites include (a) a mix of biological and clinical context knowledge, and (b) foundational computational and quantitative training.

Biological training prerequisites ensure that students have an understanding of the fundamentals of the biological and health sciences with needed coverage of several common context areas. Ideally, they will have a working knowledge of genetics, both to understand the context for the work, but also to appreciate the historical evolution of genetics and the ways in which new methods can be applied to understand clinical disorders with a genetic basis. The understanding that much of genetics has been historically driven by the identification of clinical patterns is useful to put current work into perspective.

Quantitative and computational skills are essential to support data analytic and computational work in the field. There are a number of approaches which may allow students to acquire this knowledge, including mathematical prerequisites such as linear algebra, probability, calculus, discrete math as well as statistical training (including common statistical methods and research designs). In addition, PPM informatics students will need a foundation of computer programming skills and an introduction to data structures and algorithms in order to effectively engage in graduate level computational courses and PPM methodological research.

Clinical knowledge (including pharmacology) provides PPM informatics students with a level of understanding of the potential implications of research findings on patients and on health systems in the precision medicine space. This includes skills for acquiring, developing or converting data; creating data interpretations; identification of actionable results; and management of corresponding actions. As scientific knowledge advances, the clinical signature of PPM tests evolves, and students should be able to first understand and then manage this evolution. The need to re-evaluate prior work on a regular basis is not typically part of clinical training which tends to focus on immediate and binary decision-making, but the nuance in the setting of PPM is important. Other clinical fields such as genetic counseling have incorporated result reinterpretation into their workflows to address variants of uncertain significance providing an approach to study for use in PPM.

Overall, the number of prerequisites will vary by the educational program, but with graduate training at the master's degree level, it is expected that most identified prerequisites would be completed prior to starting the degree training and any deficiencies can be addressed by a small number of remedial courses and/or directed study.

Core Educational Competencies

Biological Sciences, including Genetics and Molecular Biology training will typically be part of PPM informatics training to provide a contextual background. An understanding of genetics will also be needed to help students appreciate the basis for heritability and its historical development (Table 20.1).

Genetic and Genomic Data Analysis training courses can take a number of forms but will invariably teach at least basic sequence alignment and genome assembly working with a variety of data sources. Students should work with a number of different platforms and gain knowledge of how to work with DNA and RNA sequences and other molecular data. They should also gain an understanding of how to analyze genomic data sets to link inheritable genetic and somatic variation with clinical phenotypes. These topics can be part of a graduate-level bioinformatics course.

Principles of Clinical Practice and Healthcare Systems can be taught via specialized courses tailored to the needs of non-clinicians. Alternatively, advanced undergraduate or graduate courses in physiology, pharmacology and nosology can provide the necessary knowledge.

Foundational Concepts and Methods in Clinical Informatics and Bioinformatics are standard survey courses that introduce fundamental informatics concepts, methods, systems, tools, and standards required to immerse PPM students in the field of informatics.

Knowledge Representation and Data Standards address basic competencies related to the fundamentals of knowledge representation and the coding of knowledge elements into data standards [7]. For PPM informatics, this covers typical clinical knowledge representation including core terminologies and ontologies used

Table 20.1 Precision medicine informatics core competencies

• Biological Sciences (including Genetics and Molecular Biology)
• Genetic and Genomic Data Analysis
• Principles of Clinical Practice and Healthcare Systems
• Foundational Concepts and Methods in Clinical Informatics and Bioinformatics
• Knowledge Representation and Data Standards
• Data Governance, Quality, Security, and Integration
• Principles of Software Engineering of Clinical Information Systems and Clinical Decision Support Systems
• Machine Learning and Statistical Methods
• Legal and Ethical Topics

to describe and manage the basic components of clinical care for disease diagnostics and treatment. Most of these components would typically overlap with the foundational concepts and methods in clinical informatics and bioinformatics offerings. However, for PPM informatics training, it is important to add the capability to link to other knowledge representation resources such as Gene Ontology or Online Mendelian Inheritance in Man to facilitate better disease subtyping and data integration work [8, 9]. Ontological analysis and data integration methods [10] as well as basic familiarity with NLP methods are also important components of PPM informatics training.

Data Governance, Quality, Security, and Integration. Data Governance principles are needed for PPM informatics students to understand, implement and create data governance agreements related to data which is generated and/or shared. This is needed to ensure compliance but also to help with resource management. In addition, PPM informatics professionals will also need to work with other professionals such as legal and regulatory experts for data governance. **Data Quality** assessment methods cover methods and practices needed to identify and manage missing data elements, difficult to reconcile data, data standard and terminology deficiencies, conversion problems and other common issues in complex information systems. This part of the training program teaches mapping, tracking, and general data quality benchmarking principles. This type of training aims to ensure that institutional data will be a viable and valuable resource for both operational and research work.

Data Integration can be taught as part of a clinical informatics survey course or program project work, but the program may also incorporate more advanced data integration in order to teach how to track and cross-reference patients across systems including electronic health records, biobanks, OMICs servers, research databases, consumer applications and other resources and how to create multi-modal datasets for analysis or decision support. Data integration topics may also include methods to support the capacity to re-interpret prior results in the context of new scientific understanding, and to determine which raw and processed data elements need to be made available for diagnostics and result reinterpretation. Students will also be trained in OMICs data management that resides outside the (clinical) electronic health record.

Principles of Software Engineering of Clinical Information Systems and Clinical Decision Support Systems cover the architectures, data structures, functionalities and methods used in the creation, deployment and evaluation of Clinical Information Systems such as EHRs, Provider Order Entry, and Clinical Decision Support Systems. Human Computer Interaction topics are also included for their role in the creation of highly functional and widely adopted systems for professionals but also for consumer applications to facilitate information acquisition and provision to consumers.

Machine Learning and Statistical Methods. This part of the program requires students to have a minimum quantitative background. Coverage of specific learning algorithms in both the predictive and causal modeling realms, feature selection, clustering/subtyping, model selection methods, loss functions, error estimators, theory of generalization and overfitting, with application to genome annotations and comparisons are key educational focus areas. The methods can also be applied to structural prediction, gene expression analysis and integrated functional genomics work. **Statistical Methods** and research designs are another core methods area for PPM informatics students to support work in designing studies, hypothesis testing and evaluation of pertinent outcomes. Statistical methods which work well with PPM informatics data may differ in emphasis from a traditional statistical training sequence and specialized electives may be needed.

Legal and Ethical Issues are another core training component which needs to be addressed in a PPM informatics training curriculum to ensure that students have awareness, sensitivity and training covering the management of data security as well as other clinical and research risks to patients and family members, and enforcing institutional compliance [11].

Graduate Training

Current offerings for graduate education specializing in PPM informatics are very limited. The lack of availability is mainly due to the recent development of PPM informatics as an identifiable area of professional activity. At present, most students can pursue training with a more general informatics degree and then add targeted, elective PPM-specific training in areas which address students' career goals. Limited electives in graduate training programs may make it difficult for students to acquire PPM informatics training via formal didactics due to limited support for their studies, timing related issues or the cost burden of adding courses to a traditional core informatics program.

Case Study: University of Minnesota Precision and Personalized Medicine Informatics PhD Specialty Track. The recognition of market and student needs for tailored training opportunities in PPM informatics, combined with a strategic focus in PPM informatics research starting in 2015, led the University of Minnesota to develop a specialized PPM informatics educational offering. The initial effort led to the creation of a doctoral degree specialty track with eventual plans to add terminal PPM informatics master's degree-level training for students in future offerings.

The University of Minnesota is in a large metropolitan community of over two million people and is home to one of the largest core hubs of biomedical device and healthcare companies including a large local presence from companies such as Medtronic, Boston Scientific, United Health Group and others. It is also a location for a number of startup companies which have emerged due to the large concentration of biomedical talent and large pools of early-stage investment capital. These companies have employed graduates of the long standing University of Minnesota Health Informatics program, but they have also become a source of students in the program as employees decide to acquire additional informatics skills to supplement their prior technical and healthcare backgrounds.

Our experience in working with these adult students is that they have had a variety of reasons to pursue graduate training in PPM informatics. Some were seeking additional educational credentials either to open up new job opportunities in growth areas in their companies or they were looking to make a transition to different work roles and viewed informatics training as a means to facilitate their personal career development. Many of them had strong technical backgrounds and were seeking additional health science knowledge to complement their technical capabilities. Traditional health informatics offerings provided useful educational content to this group of both trainees and traditional graduate students, but did not address a growing community and institutional training need for PPM informatics education. In an effort to better position the program for future workforce needs, the Health Informatics graduate program underwent a substantial review of its educational capacity and designed a number of new curricular components based on the skills of available faculty as well as the expected needs of the community.

After a review of work force needs, institutional needs, faculty capacity and related course offerings, the Precision and Personalized Medicine Informatics track evolved and was approved by faculty and the University as a specialty track for the PhD program and provides a formal degree mechanism for PPM informatics training.

The *Precision and Personalized Medicine Informatics track* provides a didactic program for students to develop specialized knowledge in PPM informatics methods applied to personal and population health-focused problems. They develop skills in quantitative methods and biomedical sciences for their application to precision medicine. In addition, they gain an understanding of the medical and biological sciences to provide needed context on which to apply informatics methods.

Students pursuing a PhD in the Precision and Personalized Medicine track are expected to earn a Health Informatics MS degree as part of their PhD training. In this training pathway, they consult with their program advisor to identify pertinent didactic and experiential work for their personalized training program which is tailored to their background. Since students may come from clinical, basic science, technology or other backgrounds, it is important that they can address any areas of limited proficiency to allow them to fill those needs with elective courses to obtain sufficient training to meet program expectations as well as their career goals.

The training in the program follows a similar path as in other specialty training tracks at the informatics doctoral level reflecting both common core informatics methods offerings and similar training requirements as the University of Minnesota Master of Science and Master of Health Informatics degrees. The common core methods training include general foundational courses in Health Informatics, Applied Health Care Databases, and Informatics Methods for Health Care Quality Outcomes and Patient Safety. The program adds some distinctive elements including a Foundations of Translational Bioinformatics and Foundations of Precision Medicine Informatics with supplemental hands-on labs. Other core training includes pharmacogenomics, health data analytics and clinical data mining courses. Finally, students are expected to complete an advanced statistical sequence, electives and thesis credits to complete their training as well as a seminar series.

Additional suggested electives which are recommended include advanced statistical offerings, correlated data analysis, mathematical analysis for biological networks, Bayesian decision theory, advanced machine learning topics (causal modeling, latent variable modeling, etc.) and advanced statistical genetics and genomics. The didactic work is supplemented with an internship to allow students to get supplemental hands-on experience to build on their work in formal didactics.

The University of Minnesota program conducts regular curricular reviews to ensure that PPM informatics-related content is meeting the needs of students and potential employers in the community. Engagement with a professional external advisory committee and formal and informal alumni networks provide important quality improvement guidance to make sure that the program is meeting student needs.

Mentored Research Training

For advanced graduate training at the doctoral and post-doctoral levels, students gravitate to centers of excellence and well-regarded labs to maximize their training opportunities with mentors at PPM informatics sites who support their work of interest. Support for such efforts in the form of sustained pre-doctoral and post-doctoral funding streams will generally support those working at the most advanced levels of PPM informatics. For those working in more operational capacities such as building enterprise scale systems, it is less clear how to support such training in clinical and research settings.

Practical Training Requirements

Hands-on training enables students to translate abstract knowledge into practical solutions across the spectrum of PPM informatics. Most will begin this process in laboratory work and structured course projects and assignments followed by practice opportunities provided via partnerships with other organizations or health systems to provide real world exposure through internships. Such work provides invaluable exposures to clinical and bio-molecular data along with payer data to provide a full view of patient data and health systems [12].

In educational program development for all types of PPM informatics offerings, it is useful to identify and make available de-identified data sources which can be used in a protected environment or made available as de-identified synthetic data sets. Fortunately, there are a growing number of available public use data files for use in educational settings and these resources provide a means for students to work directly with data and understand good data documentation practices.

Students spend time doing their own data exploration after getting an initial introduction to the data. This can either be done as individual-focused tasks or alternatively can be done in a group setting where they work with others from different backgrounds if the setting allows for it. Having the ability to partner the more clinically-oriented with the more technically-oriented allows both parties to learn from each other. Formal informatics training programs often have such diverse students; however, in more targeted settings, such as a research or skill-based training conference, participants may be more homogenous and this may not allow as much cross-discipline learning within groups. Even in these cases, where student backgrounds are similar, variations in their clinical, technical and scientific knowledge may be addressed with pre-conference survey work to maximize group learning.

Professional Continuing Education

Continuing Education provides learning for practitioners who are looking to acquire targeted skills pertinent to their professional practices and needs. Such education in PPM may focus on targeted methods such as the interpretation of a specific test, or may be more broad-based such as a focus on the type of testing which a practitioner may consider in their daily work. It may also entail a very broad-based or in-depth review of method(s) which may be part of an extended conference or training series. In developing such content, it is important to have an understanding of the skills and background knowledge of the audience in order to tailor the content appropriately. Such content can be delivered through a variety of delivery mechanisms; however, it will generally require a review process for formal continuing education credits based on the professional organization for which the professional educational content is delivered. For content delivery, there may be opportunities to develop and re-use content across a variety of professions where backgrounds may be similar, but will require multiple content accreditation reviews. For instance, in a study of 10 pharmacogenomics continuing education programs within the eMERGE network, sites employed face-to-face content delivery, point-of-care education using alerts and messaging, and online education resources as part of their training [13].

Continuing education also provides an opportunity to pursue a more prolonged educational effort. Using a multi-modal approach addresses educational needs in a coordinated manner and translates evidence into practice [14]; however, the ability to affect change in clinical practice and improve practice guideline adherence has been variable [15, 16]. For example, some continuing education offerings include the use of self-directed, planned, pre-course offerings to ensure that participants will have a base level of knowledge prior to undertaking more advanced educational offerings. These continuing education programs may include content which takes place over a longer period of time, and trainees typically will need to meet objectives at each phase before moving on in order to ensure that they are able to manage more advanced education. Another continuing education approach is to use massively open online course (MOOC) offerings. Prior MOOC offerings demonstrated the importance of having actual clinical scenarios which were tailored to the health-care provider point of view when providing PPM educational content [17]. Such offerings could be a means to provide students with a base of knowledge on which to build toward more advanced work.

The development and management of a prolonged educational series can also take the form of a live course offering which may be used as part of a formal semi-nar series to facilitate active learning. Such offerings have the advantage of an interactive experience which allow trainees to direct targeted questions to experts and facilitate greater format flexibility. Such seminar series are frequently used in other areas of clinical practice, especially for medicine, nursing, and pharmacy, which have specific clinical continuing education requirements. These offerings are typically only available in large academically-oriented centers for specialized content offerings such as PPM informatics. The seminar series approach also has the advantage of reaching a large audience in a manner that provides flexibility for both presenters and participants and can allow the hosting site to make data and software available, which may otherwise be impossible to replicate in a remote setting.

Advanced educational offerings for health professionals with board certification may become another option for training in the field. The development of accredited clinical informatics fellowships for physicians have provided a pathway to informatics training, but have generally not been heavily focused on PPM. The early experiences with these fellowships has been previously described, including a number of issues regarding program funding, didactic training, experiential rotations, scholarship, and health system alignment [18], which may also prove to be obstacles in having such physician training for PPM informatics.

PPM Certificates provide another training opportunity. Certificates are generally more flexible than traditional degree offerings and can be developed and implemented faster than a traditional degree offering. Given the advanced knowledge bases required for many areas of PPM informatics and rapid scientific evolution, educational content focused on emerging PPM informatics specialties are good fits for certificate training. Certificate programs do have downsides such as variable workplace value; however, these concerns can be mitigated with careful content development work and rigorous program design. Strong prerequisite requirements can also help ensure program quality and facilitate continuity between certificate programs and formal degree programs for PPM informatics training.

Conclusion

PPM informatics education is a new and evolving area of informatics which incorporates new types of information into the clinical and research space to translate data into PPM knowledge and PPM knowledge and information into clinical action.

Though many of the same methods which have served informatics trainees are still as relevant and needed now as in the past, the growth in the types of information and quantities of information will require the involvement of specialist informaticists to identify and manage these data resources to ensure that these investments create value to patients, researchers, and health systems. PPM informatics education will continue evolving to meet these challenges well into the future.

References

1. McCullough KB, Formea CM, Berg KD, Burzynski JA, Cunningham JL, Ou NN, et al. Assessment of the pharmacogenomics educational needs of pharmacists. Am J Pharm Educ. 2011;75:51. http://www.ncbi.nlm.nih.gov/pubmed/21655405.
2. Shields A, Lerman C. Anticipating clinical integration of pharmacogenetic treatment strategies for addiction: are primary care physicians ready? Clin Pharmacol Ther. 2008;83:635–9. http://doi.wiley.com/10.1038/clpt.2008.4.
3. Stanek EJ, Sanders CL, Taber KAJ, Khalid M, Patel A, Verbrugge RR, et al. Adoption of pharmacogenomic testing by US physicians: results of a nationwide survey. Clin Pharmacol Ther. 2012;91:450–8. http://doi.wiley.com/10.1038/clpt.2011.306.
4. Tenenbaum JD, Avillach P, Benham-Hutchins M, Breitenstein MK, Crowgey EL, Hoffman MA, et al. An informatics research agenda to support precision medicine: seven key areas. J Am Med Inform Assoc. 2016;23:791–5. http://www.ncbi.nlm.nih.gov/pubmed/27107452.
5. Frey LJ, Bernstam EV, Denny JC. Precision medicine informatics. J Am Med Informatics Assoc. 2016;23:668–70. https://academic.oup.com/jamia/article-lookup/doi/10.1093/jamia/ocw053.
6. Fenton SH, Tremblay MC, Lehmann HP. Focusing on informatics education. J Am Med Inform Assoc. 2016;23:812. https://academic.oup.com/jamia/article-lookup/doi/10.1093/jamia/ocw094.
7. Valenta AL, Meagher EA, Tachinardi U, Starren J. Core informatics competencies for clinical and translational scientists: what do our customers and collaborators need to know? J Am Med Inform Assoc. 2016;23:835–9. http://www.ncbi.nlm.nih.gov/pubmed/27121608.
8. Amberger JS, Bocchini CA, Schiettecatte F, Scott AF, Hamosh A. OMIM.org: Online Mendelian Inheritance in Man (OMIM®), an online catalog of human genes and genetic disorders. Nucleic Acids Res. 2015;43:D789–98. http://academic.oup.com/nar/article/43/D1/D789/2439148/OMIMorg-Online-Mendelian-Inheritance-in-Man-OMIM.
9. The Gene Ontology Consortium. Expansion of the Gene Ontology knowledgebase and resources. Nucleic Acids Res. 2017;45:D331–8. https://academic.oup.com/nar/article-lookup/doi/10.1093/nar/gkw1108.
10. Manzoni C, Kia DA, Vandrovcova J, Hardy J, Wood NW, Lewis PA, et al. Genome, transcriptome and proteome: the rise of omics data and their integration in biomedical sciences. Brief Bioinform. 2018;19:286–302. https://academic.oup.com/bib/article/19/2/286/2562648.
11. Korngiebel DM, Thummel KE, Burke W. Implementing precision medicine: the ethical challenges. Trends Pharmacol Sci. 2017;38:8–14. https://www.sciencedirect.com/science/article/pii/S0165614716301651?via%3Dihub.
12. Williams MS, Ritchie MD, Payne PRO. Interdisciplinary training to build an informatics workforce for precision medicine. Appl Transl Genomics. 2015;6:28–30. http://www.ncbi.nlm.nih.gov/pubmed/27054076.
13. Rohrer Vitek CR, Abul-Husn NS, Connolly JJ, Hartzler AL, Kitchner T, Peterson JF, et al. Healthcare provider education to support integration of pharmacogenomics in practice: the eMERGE Network experience. Pharmacogenomics. 2017;18:1013–25. https://www.future-medicine.com/doi/10.2217/pgs-2017-0038.

14. Davis D, Evans M, Jadad A, Perrier L, Rath D, Ryan D, et al. The case for knowledge translation: shortening the journey from evidence to effect. BMJ. 2003;327:33–5. http://www.ncbi.nlm.nih.gov/pubmed/12842955.

15. Cabana MD, Rand CS, Powe NR, Wu AW, Wilson MH, Abboud PA, et al. Why don't physicians follow clinical practice guidelines? A framework for improvement. JAMA. 1999;282:1458–65. http://www.ncbi.nlm.nih.gov/pubmed/10535437.

16. Davis DA, Thomson MA, Oxman AD, Haynes RB. Changing physician performance. A systematic review of the effect of continuing medical education strategies. JAMA. 1995;274:700–5. http://www.ncbi.nlm.nih.gov/pubmed/7650822.

17. McCarthy JJ. Driving personalized medicine forward: the who, what, when, and how of educating the health-care workforce. Mol Genet Genomic Med. 2014;2:455–7. http://doi.wiley.com/10.1002/mgg3.113.

18. Longhurst CA, Pageler NM, Palma JP, Finnell JT, Levy BP, Yackel TR, et al. Early experiences of accredited clinical informatics fellowships. J Am Med Informatics Assoc. 2016;23:829–34. https://academic.oup.com/jamia/article-lookup/doi/10.1093/jamia/ocv209.

Part V
Conclusion

Chapter 21
The Landscape of PPM Informatics and the Future of Medicine

Constantin Aliferis and Terrence Adam

The Current State of PPM and the Role of Informatics

The previous 20 chapters of the present volume describe a rich tapestry of diverse PPM formats across the spectrum of health sciences and healthcare. The different forms of PPM exhibit varying degrees of maturity and proximity to clinical deployment at health system scale. Informatics methodologies for knowledge discovery, support of care delivery, and patient engagement are critical for the eventual success of the PPM paradigm. The concept of a learning health system is intrinsically linked with PPM and as such it is also dependent on and facilitated by informatics.

Classic and Emerging PPM workflows have been and are widely used in the forms of **genetic counseling, clinical risk assessment, outcome risk stratification and (on a limited basis) pharmacogenomics**. Well established mechanisms, including informatics systems and methods, are already in place for the

C. Aliferis
Institute for Health Informatics, Department of Medicine, School of Medicine Clinical and Translational Science Institute, Masonic Cancer Center, Program in Data Science, University of Minnesota, Minneapolis, MN, USA
e-mail: califeri@umn.edu

T. Adam (✉)
Institute for Health Informatics, University of Minnesota, Minneapolis, MN, USA

Department of Pharmaceutical Care and Health Systems, College of Pharmacy, University of Minnesota, Minneapolis, MN, USA

PhD Program in Precision Medicine Informatics, University of Minnesota, Minneapolis, MN, USA

Minneapolis Veterans Administration, Minneapolis, MN, USA
e-mail: adamx004@umn.edu

© Springer Nature Switzerland AG 2020
T. Adam, C. Aliferis (eds.), *Personalized and Precision Medicine Informatics*, Health Informatics, https://doi.org/10.1007/978-3-030-18626-5_21

support of clinical care delivery. PPM informatics methods and existing systems support these areas at the present scales and timelines of development and deployment.

In the realm of **genomic PPM oncology,** major strides have been accomplished in tumor sequencing, molecular tumor subtyping and molecular profiling and biomarker discovery, as well as highly targeted treatments that work only for parts of the population. Moreover a new paradigm of **genomic clinical trials** is being explored in oncology, and massive discovery datasets incorporating clinical and genomic information are being assembled and mined. PPM informatics is an essential backbone of the discovery process (e.g., by providing support for precision and pragmatic trials and the analysis and modeling of genomic data), is helping to provide access to growing pools of standardized data resources, and is moving toward genomic medical records built on generalized architectures.

As the capture and storage of practice data and genomic information has grown, the ability to create a **precision learning health system** increasingly becomes a reality both at the individual level and to the practice, facility, regional and national health system levels.

Emerging PPM Areas Mature Enough for Broad Adoption: The Challenges of Implementation at Scale

PGx is accepted scientifically for a small number of actionable genetic variants, and has been adopted by a small number of providers for a small fraction of patients. Broad adoption of PGx across all patients and providers is far from being a reality, however. Similarly, whereas **clinical risk modeling** has a long history of success and adoption, the vast majority of risk models are yet to be discovered and implemented in practice. Along the same lines, **genomic and adaptive trials** represent a very small percentage of all clinical trials.

In addition, **molecular profile tests** in clinical practice represent a small fraction of all disease-drug combinations. Finally, **clinico-genomic cohorts and datasets** are only now emerging and much work needs be done until large, representative datasets exist for PPM clinico-genomic exploration are ready and available.

The above observations are not surprising and are a reflection of two fundamental factors determining successful implementation of new medical technologies and discoveries: (1) the fundamental operational adaptations to how medicine is conducted that needs to occur for disruptive science and technology to be adopted. (2) Issues of scaling, e.g., developing and validating a single molecular profile, PGx variant decision rule, or clinical risk model is distinctly easier and faster than establishing scalable "assembly line" processes for the rapid development, validation, and deployment of such modalities.

The phenomenon is neither new nor is it PPM-specific. Prior studies have shown that the translation of health research takes on average 17 years [1]. There is strong evidence to support, but it remains to be seen whether newer informatics methodologies such as the new capability to analyze comprehensive datasets automatically or semi-automatically, can expedite the R&D cycles while concurrently increasing the number of PPM modalities delivered in practice.

Among the barriers to broad implementation of mature PPM forms we emphasize three main areas: economics of PPM; knowledges barriers; and ethical, legal, and social implications.

The Economics of PPM. A recent health economics review of precision medicine, argues that three areas are likely to have the most impact in the next decade including complex algorithms, health apps and omics based biomarkers [2]. There are a number of difficulties with completing economic and outcome evaluations for these and other areas of PPM including problems with multiple results, different utility measures, secondary findings, downstream impacts and interactive effects [3]. These difficulties affect the ability to make policy decisions about insurance coverage, economic value and other preference assessments such as care guidelines that determine which technology is to be adopted and supported. A highly instructive example is in the pre-emptive application of PGx which exhibits small costs over the lifetime of an individual; however, because of provider fragmentation, population movement, and limited decision time-frames by payors does not always a have a favorable cost-effectiveness profile in the short term. PGx cost and reimbursement were cited as reasons for failure for pre-emptive adoption [4]. Another instructive example of a positive flavor is provided in Chap. 8 where it is shown that adoption of a molecular profile can reduce health system costs without adversely affecting outcomes. Even in this case though, the fragmentation of the market share of the corresponding drug and the highly variant pricing policies by pharmaceutical companies may work against widespread adoption of such useful forms of PPM.

Knowledge Barriers. Clinicians in practice typically lack the necessary background in PPM directly preventing their support of implementation [2–22]. The same is true for a variety of clinical support staff, informaticists supporting current electronic health record systems, omics data managers, researchers, and others. Ultimately, PPM informatics will need to come as close to seamless as possible and just be another component of day-to-day health care delivery. From a workforce standpoint, those in direct clinical care delivery will need to be able to efficiently access needed information for clinical decision making and have a trust in the data they access to make good decisions. The work will also need to be readily completed by generalist clinicians in care delivery and by generalist information technology support personnel since it is not feasible to have all such work done by genetic specialists and creative approaches may be needed to address knowledge gaps in the current workforce [5].

Ethical Legal Social Implications (ELSI) related factors. A third major barrier to broad adoption and implementation of mature PPM forms and workflows is ELSI factors. For example, concerns about patient data privacy, especially as it relates to misuse by third parties (life insurers, employers, law enforcement, etc.) are considered important impediments to genetic data collection and sharing for care and scientific discovery [23]. Similar adverse effects may occur, for example, by linking known genetic factors determining clinically relevant medication responses to other phenotypes in the EHR such as propensity to addiction, dangerous behaviors, etc. A case of a family with an early death in a family member and subsequent testing of family members and a diagnosis of long QT syndrome focused on the genotypic results without strong phenotypic correlations provides an important reminder of the potential unintended consequences of genetic testing [6].

PPM Areas of Significant Scientific Research Opportunity

Contrary to the mature PPM areas discussed previously where adoption and implementation are the main concerns, several forms of PPM are not yet fully mature to the point where they can be deployed. Significant work needs be completed before clinical adoption is warranted. These areas represent the biggest opportunities for research exploration.

Based on the discussion in the section "Emerging PPM Areas Mature Enough for Broad Adoption: The Challenges of Implementation at Scale" the research potential in the following areas is readily apparent (details omitted since they have been covered previously):

- Development of molecular profiling to cover the full spectrum of disease-drug combinations.
- Exploration of new assaying technologies and related informatics methods that can increase the accuracy of PPM tests. Currently developing assays which may enhance testing capacity include: single cell assays, extracellular vesicles (EVs) assays, and micro RNAs [24, 25].
- Development of enhanced ELSI frameworks, including policy for data privacy and consenting, for preventing the misuse of PPM data in both research and clinical settings.
- Developing methods and supporting data management and analytics for adaptive and genomic precision trials.
- Studying and establishing the health economic cost-effectiveness of various PPM forms and workflows as a necessary step toward adoption.
- Creating highly functional and interoperable genomic and PPM EHRs.
- Creating scalable and interoperable PPM decision support methodologies and systems.

- Educating the clinical as well as informatics workforce, using PPM-rich curricula and learning-on-demand.

In addition to the above the following PPM areas have great potential:

Learning Health System Research (LHSR) Extensions to "Personome" and Exosome". As evidenced throughout this volume, the goals of PPM are in complete alignment with the objectives of LHSR for facilitating the collection of rich standardized care data which are amenable to analysis, re-use and sharing and can provide the foundation on which a learning health system can operate. Disease outcome risk modeling as covered in this volume is one of the many types of determinations that can lead to better decisions on an individual basis, thus enabling the whole system to achieve better outcomes and reduced costs [7–10, 15]. A PPM lens can provide tangible improvements to traditional methods used by the science of health services improvement. For example, PPM makes possible the critical distinction between unwanted/negative versus desirable/positive variation (the former to large extent has driven early literature on cost and outcome improvements). The care data can furthermore be enhanced with personal characteristics, life circumstances, behaviors, personality, support networks, social networks, environmental factors, and resilience to improve overall health, however. This data can exist in "personal data clouds" [11] as part of the currently unmeasured "*personome*" [12] as well as shared "*global environment*" measurements with health significance, the mining of which can confer individualized and system-level preventative and long-term care advantages that go beyond simply improving the care system by narrowly focusing on medical encounter data.

Participatory Medicine. Outside of medicine, widespread availability of computing, internet access and mobile phones has made it possible for individuals to participate in large-scale scientific endeavors [26]. Because of the complexity of the health data and its analysis, it is reasonable to expect that in the foreseeable future, the main contribution of citizen scientists for PPM will be in advocating for capturing and sharing data with the professional scientific community, however. Large-scale programs such as All of Us are expected to create large research databases to identify genotype/phenotype relationships for use in clinical care and as part of a learning health system. It is hard to overstate the potential of this type of project for advancing PPM and overall health.

Health Care Delivery Evolution: Personalized e-visits. E-visits allow patients to engage in a more flexible manner with providers and may also yield additional information on the patient environment, especially if real-time audio-video is used. Technical limitations (e.g., bandwidth) currently create some barriers to synchronous communication, but other alternatives such as patient portals or asynchronous messaging and mobile apps [16, 19] can also be used in supporting the approach. The use of online telemedicine counseling may also be a viable alternative or complement to training genetic counseling, and return of results [13, 14].

Table 21.1 summarizes the successes and opportunities of PPM research across all major forms of PPM.

Table 21.1 Summary of successes and opportunities of PPM informatics across all major forms of PPM

PPM informatics successes		
Main forms of PPM/ components of PPM workflows	**Successes to date and significant Informatics contributions to implementation**	**Successes to date and significant Informatics contributions to scientific discovery**
Classic PPM: • Genetic counseling • Clinical risk assessment • Outcome risk stratification • Pharmacogenomics	• Databases with literature and genetic variants role in disease predisposition and response to Rx • Delivery of guidelines and computerized decision support for risk assessment	
Emerging PPM: • Genomic PPM oncology • Tumor sequencing • Molecular tumor subtyping, molecular profiling and biomarker discovery • Targeted molecular treatments • Genomic clinical trials • Massive discovery datasets incorporating clinical and genomic information • Health system-wide PGx • Precision learning health system	• Limited support for genomic EHR via Omic Ancillary Systems • PGx guideline repositories • Small-scale EHR-enabled Delivery of PGx clinical decision alerting and support • Data standardization	• Data standardization • Methods for data privacy and security • Informatics for biospecimen management • (Limited) Clinico-genomic cohorts and datasets • Bioinformatics databases • Bioinformatics discovery methods and tools • Bioinformatics in support of high-throughput omics assay technologies
PPM informatics opportunities		
Main forms of PPM/ components of PPM workflows	**Future opportunity for significant Informatics contributions to implementation**	**Future opportunity for significant informatics contributions to scientific discovery**
• Development of molecular profiling to cover the full spectrum of disease-drug combinations • Using PPM to enhance drug research and development	• "Closed loop" seamlessly integrated delivery of molecular profiling tests at the bedside	• Analysis and modeling of omic and multi-modal data to discover, validate and de-risk biomarkers and clinical-grade signatures • Exploration of new assaying technologies and related informatics methods that can increase the accuracy of PPM tests. E.g.: single cell assays, extracellular vesicles (EVs) assays, and micro RNAs

(continued)

Table 21.1 (continued)

• Development of enhanced ELSI frameworks, including data privacy and consenting, for preventing the misuse of PPM data in both research and clinical settings	• Enhanced reporting systems to identify ELSI concerns	• Enhanced methods for data privacy and security that protect individuals/patients while allowing for effective research
• Developing methods and supporting data management and analytics for adaptive and genomic precision trials • Pragmatic trials and practice based evidence		• Next-generation CTMSs that natively support adaptive and genomic trials • Data capture and analysis of practice data and practice-based-evidence discovery
• Studying and establishing the health economic cost-effectiveness of various PPM forms and workflows as a necessary step toward adoption	• Development and validation of widely and computable accepted standards for PPM valuation of cost and benefits	• Simulation and other methods for estimating health economic costs and value • Methods to incorporate patient preferences into PPM policy and clinical decisions
• Creating effective and widely accessible genomic and PPM-capable EHRs • Data Integration for Diagnosis and Treatment	• Omic Ancillary Systems and other genomic EHR extension technologies • Enhanced patient data linkage and universal identifiers • Scalable and interoperable PPM decision support methodologies and systems	
Overcoming knowledge barriers: • Educating the workforce: clinical as well as informatics • Educating citizens and patients • Educating administrators and policy makers	• Targeted and learning-on-demand educational tools for broader societal adoption of PPM	• New PPM-rich curricula for clinicians, informaticists and administrators and just-in-time • Personalized learning approaches to both students and established clinical practitioners
• Improving Cost (Inefficiencies) and Outcomes/ Quality in the Health system. Learning Health System research (LHSR).	• Rapid, closed loop data measurement/capture analysis and delivery systems	• New automated predictive, causal, trajectory, sub-population and outlier analytics with forecasting, explanatory, and intervention outcome estimation capabilities with low risk and high transparency
• High-granularity Individualization of Health Care		• Personome informatics
• Health Care Delivery Evolution	• Systems to facilitate high quality integrated, continuous e-health care delivery	

Known and Unknown Determinants of PPM Success; Intended and Unintended Consequences

Efforts to predict the direction of whole fields, industries and complex systems are routinely hampered by the inherent unpredictability of such systems. We therefore acknowledge that at least some of our projections to the future of PPM may fail to materialize either in forms or timeframes that current evidence suggests. In this section we discuss, briefly, several factors and "known unknowns" that may accelerate or decelerate the rate and degree of success of the "PPM programme". We also present plausible developments that may tip the scales of PPM in various directions. In order to emphasize that this section is the single most speculative part of the present volume it is presented as a set of numbered conjectures and predictions which can also be viewed as testable hypotheses (Table 21.2).

Table 21.2 Conjectures (and testable hypotheses) about the future of PPM and the role of informatics

• *Hypothesis 1*: Certain forms of health system (e.g. single payer versus market-driven, vs. hybrids) are more amenable to large-scale PPM development, validation and adoption. The rate and extent of development and adoption of PPM will be greatly affected by the evolution of the health system's structure and policies
• *Hypothesis 2* (corollary to 1): If hypothesis 1 is true, then because different countries have different forms of health systems, global leadership in PPM science will be closely linked to countries with health systems highly enabling PPM
• *Hypothesis 3*: PPM-enabled fragmentation of drug markets may be catalyzed by national health policy requiring or enabling such fragmentation when medically and societally beneficial
• *Hypothesis 4*: The genomic EHR of the future will shift data access control to patients and thus with it also shift effective ownership of medical data
• *Hypothesis 5*: High profile cases of PPM data misuse may decelerate the progression toward PPM (or force expansion of current legal protections)
• *Hypothesis 6*: The principle of variation reduction as a means for improving costs and outcomes will become less relevant in light of the benefits of personalization by PPM. Alternatively the concept of variation will be redefined to focus on departures from the PPM-optimal care
• *Hypothesis 7*: Diminishing returns will start being observed in PPM disease subtyping and other PPM studies beyond which further personalization will be ineffective or inefficient. Finding the point of diminishing returns will become an important principle in future PPM research
• Hypothesis 8: The clinician of tomorrow will be deeply versed in the principles of PPM, irrespective of specialty or profession. Alternatively, certain existing specialties may become the "heavy lifters" of PPM. Alternatively, a sub-specialty in PPM will be made available for every specialty
• *Hypothesis 9* (corollary to 8): Every clinician will be versed in the informatics methods, and tools needed to support PPM. Every informaticist will be deeply versed in PPM informatics
• *Hypothesis 10*: In order to achieve broad societal support of PPM, every citizen and especially decision makers (legislators, judges, managers) as well as educators, journalists and other opinion makers and "influencers" will be well-versed in the main tenets of PPM

(continued)

- *Hypothesis 11:* The PPM scientific body of knowledge may develop so quickly and may be so compelling that traditional provider systems cannot adapt quickly enough. This may spur alternative or supplementary PPM health care systems that will co-exist in parallel with traditional ones

- *Hypothesis 12*: The Pharma industry of tomorrow may become entirely PPM in nature

- *Hypothesis 13*: Traditional EHRs may be entirely replaced by genomic and PPM ones, or alternatively, traditional EHRs will be permanently supplemented by omic ancillary systems (OAS)

- *Hypothesis 14*: The use of postmortem testing with molecular autopsies can provide important data on the causes of sudden death in the young and contribute to our understanding of the correlations between genotypes and phenotypes [17, 18]. Continued reduction in testing cost may expand testing to older populations

- *Hypothesis 15*: Gene therapy methods by in vivo modification of the genome will be coupled with PPM diagnostics to create a new class of PPM with unprecedented power

Conclusion: The Future of PPM

We posit that this volume, and the underlying body of literature that supports it, make it clear that PPM is an inevitable part of the future of medicine, one that promises to radically improve the length and quality of human life by preventing and optimally treating disease and by enhancing well-being and longevity. PPM comes in many forms, variants and workflows that this book catalogues and describes in considerable detail. Critical to the nature and importance of PPM are its close relationships with efficient healthcare delivery, clinical genomics, learning healthcare systems, and legal/ethical/societal frameworks and factors. PPM is therefore a true "systems" and collaborative interdisciplinary endeavor in one of the largest scale imaginable in the health sciences.

Because PPM relies on deep measurement and analysis of numerous interacting factors (e.g., clinical, omic, social, legal, environmental), and because it requires discovery and delivery mechanisms that are highly data and information-processing oriented, informatics is an indispensable and intrinsically linked foundation of PPM. PPM informatics spans the spectrum from PPM discovery to PPM delivery adding fundamental value all along.

The future of PPM has great promise, but also many challenges that need to be overcome. One set of challenges discussed in the present chapter relates to implementation and another to scientific development and evolution of the health system to enable and accommodate PPM.

The informatics research opportunities are many, diverse and identifiable, yet they still can unfold in unpredictable trajectories. Regardless of many remaining unknowns, PPM informatics research is certain to produce major improvements to health sciences and healthcare, making this a most worthy and exciting area of scientific exploration.

References

1. Morris ZS, Wooding S, Grant J. The answer is 17 years, what is the question: understanding time lags in translational research. J R Soc Med. 2011;104(12):510–20. https://doi.org/10.1258/jrsm.2011.110180.
2. Love-Koh J, Peel A, Rejon-Parrilla JC, Ennis K, Lovett R, Manca A, et al. The future of precision medicine: potential impacts for health technology assessment. Pharmacoeconomics. 2018;36(12):1439–51. https://doi.org/10.1007/s40273-018-0686-6.
3. Phillips KA, Douglas MP, Trosman JR, Marshall DA. "What Goes Around Comes Around": lessons learned from economic evaluations of personalized medicine applied to digital medicine. Value Health. 2017;20(1):47–53. https://doi.org/10.1016/j.jval.2016.08.736.
4. Dunnenberger HM, Crews KR, Hoffman JM, Caudle KE, Broeckel U, Howard SC, et al. Preemptive clinical pharmacogenetics implementation: current programs in five US medical centers. Annu Rev Pharmacol Toxicol. 2015;55:89–106.
5. McCarthy JJ. Driving personalized medicine forward: the who, what, when, and how of educating the health-care workforce. Mol Genet Genomic Med. 2014;2(6):455–7. https://doi.org/10.1002/mgg3.113.
6. Ackerman JP, Bartos DC, Kapplinger JD, Tester DJ, Delisle BP, Ackerman MJ. The promise and peril of precision medicine: phenotyping still matters most. Mayo Clin Proc. 2016. https://doi.org/10.1016/j.mayocp.2016.08.008.
7. Krumholz HM. Big data and new knowledge in medicine: the thinking, training, and tools needed for a learning health system. Health Aff (Millwood). 2014;33(7):1163–70. https://doi.org/10.1377/hlthaff.2014.0053.
8. Wennberg J, Gittelsohn. Small area variations in health care delivery. Science. 1973;182(4117):1102–8.
9. NHS-Confederation. Variation in healthcare: does it matter and can anything be done. London: NHS Confederation; 2004.
10. Fisher ES, Wennberg DE, Stukel TA, Gottlieb DJ, Lucas FL, Pinder EL. The implications of regional variations in Medicare spending. Part 1: the content, quality, and accessibility of care. Ann Intern Med. 2003;138(4):273–87.
11. Flores M, Glusman G, Brogaard K, Price ND, Hood L. P4 medicine: how systems medicine will transform the healthcare sector and society. Pers Med. 2013;10(6):565–76. https://doi.org/10.2217/pme.13.57.
12. Ziegelstein RC. Personomics. JAMA Intern Med. 2015;175(6):888–9. https://doi.org/10.1001/jamainternmed.2015.0861.
13. Olson JE, Ryu E, Lyke KJ, Bielinski SJ, Winkler EM, Hathcock MA, et al. Acceptability of electronic visits for return of research results in the Mayo Clinic biobank. Mayo Clin Proc Innov Qual Outcomes. 2018;2(4):352–8. https://doi.org/10.1016/j.mayocpiqo.2018.07.004.
14. Otten E, Birnie E, Ranchor AV, van Langen IM. Online genetic counseling from the providers' perspective: counselors' evaluations and a time and cost analysis. Eur J Hum Genet. 2016;24(9):1255–61. https://doi.org/10.1038/ejhg.2015.283.
15. Aronson SJ, Rehm HL. Building the foundation for genomics in precision medicine. Nature. 2015;526(7573):336–42. https://doi.org/10.1038/nature15816.
16. Orsama AL, Lahteenmaki J, Harno K, Kulju M, Wintergerst E, Schachner H, et al. Active assistance technology reduces glycosylated hemoglobin and weight in individuals with type 2 diabetes: results of a theory-based randomized trial. Diabetes Technol Ther. 2013;15(8):662–9. https://doi.org/10.1089/dia.2013.0056.
17. Rueda M, Wagner JL, Phillips TC, Topol SE, Muse ED, Lucas JR, et al. Molecular autopsy for sudden death in the young: is data aggregation the key? Front Cardiovasc Med. 2017;4:72. https://doi.org/10.3389/fcvm.2017.00072.
18. Torkamani A, Muse ED, Spencer EG, Rueda M, Wagner GN, Lucas JR, Topol EJ. Molecular autopsy for sudden unexpected death. JAMA. 2016;316(14):1492–4. https://doi.org/10.1001/jama.2016.11445.

19. Turner-McGrievy GM, Beets MW, Moore JB, Kaczynski AT, Barr-Anderson DJ, Tate DF. Comparison of traditional versus mobile app self-monitoring of physical activity and dietary intake among overweight adults participating in an mHealth weight loss program. J Am Med Inform Assoc. 2013;20(3):513–8. https://doi.org/10.1136/amiajnl-2012-001510.
20. McCullough KB, Formea CM, Berg KD, Burzynski JA, Cunningham JL, Ou NN, et al. Assessment of the pharmacogenomics educational needs of pharmacists. Am J Pharm Educ. 2011;75(3):51.
21. Shields AE, Lerman C. Anticipating clinical integration of pharmacogenetic treatment strategies for addiction: are primary care physicians ready? Clin Pharmacol Ther. 2008;83(4):635–9.
22. Stanek EJ, Sanders CL, Taber KA, Khalid M, Patel A, Verbrugge RR, et al. Adoption of pharmacogenomic testing by US physicians: results of a nationwide survey. Clin Pharmacol Ther. 2012;91(3):450–8.
23. McGuire AL, Fisher R, Cusenza P, Hudson K, Rothstein MA, McGraw D, et al. Confidentiality, privacy, and security of genetic and genomic test information in electronic health records: points to consider. Genet Med. 2008;10(7):495–9.
24. Kuipers J, Jahn K, Beerenwinkel N. Advances in understanding tumour evolution through single-cell sequencing. Biochim Biophys Acta Rev Cancer. 2017;1867(2):127–38.
25. Witwer KW, Buzas EI, Bemis LT, Bora A, Lasser C, Lotvall J, et al. Standardization of sample collection, isolation and analysis methods in extracellular vesicle research. J Extracell Vesicles. 2013;2 https://doi.org/10.3402/jev.v2i0.20360.
26. Gura T. Citizen science: amateur experts. Nature. 2013;496(7444):259–61.

Index

© Springer Nature Switzerland AG 2020
T. Adam, C. Aliferis (eds.), *Personalized and Precision Medicine Informatics*,
Health Informatics, https://doi.org/10.1007/978-3-030-18626-5